NEUROLOGY - LABORATORY AND CLINICAL RESEARCH DEVELOPMENTS

HANDBOOK OF STROKE AND NEUROCRITICAL CARE

NEUROLOGY - LABORATORY AND CLINICAL RESEARCH DEVELOPMENTS

Additional books in this series can be found on Nova's website
under the Series tab.

Additional E-books in this series can be found on Nova's website
under the E-book tab.

CEREBROVASCULAR RESEARCH AND DISORDERS

Additional books in this series can be found on Nova's website
under the Series tab.

Additional E-books in this series can be found on Nova's website
under the E-book tab.

NEUROLOGY - LABORATORY AND CLINICAL RESEARCH
DEVELOPMENTS

HANDBOOK OF STROKE AND NEUROCRITICAL CARE

VIVIEN H. LEE
EDITOR

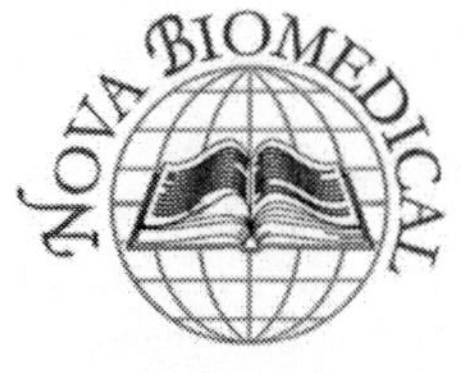

Nova Science Publishers, Inc.
New York

For permission to use material from this book please contact us:
Telephone 631-231-7269; Fax 631-231-8175
Web Site: http://www.novapublishers.com

NOTICE TO THE READER

The Publisher has taken reasonable care in the preparation of this book, but makes no expressed or implied warranty of any kind and assumes no responsibility for any errors or omissions. No liability is assumed for incidental or consequential damages in connection with or arising out of information contained in this book. The Publisher shall not be liable for any special, consequential, or exemplary damages resulting, in whole or in part, from the readers' use of, or reliance upon, this material. Any parts of this book based on government reports are so indicated and copyright is claimed for those parts to the extent applicable to compilations of such works.

Independent verification should be sought for any data, advice or recommendations contained in this book. In addition, no responsibility is assumed by the publisher for any injury and/or damage to persons or property arising from any methods, products, instructions, ideas or otherwise contained in this publication.

This publication is designed to provide accurate and authoritative information with regard to the subject matter covered herein. It is sold with the clear understanding that the Publisher is not engaged in rendering legal or any other professional services. If legal or any other expert assistance is required, the services of a competent person should be sought. FROM A DECLARATION OF PARTICIPANTS JOINTLY ADOPTED BY A COMMITTEE OF THE AMERICAN BAR ASSOCIATION AND A COMMITTEE OF PUBLISHERS.

Additional color graphics may be available in the e-book version of this book.

Library of Congress Cataloging-in-Publication Data

Handbook of stroke and neurocritical care / editor, Vivien H. Lee.
      p. ; cm.
   Includes bibliographical references and index.
   ISBN 978-1-61324-786-0 (hardcover : alk. paper)   1.   Cerebrovascular disease--Treatment. 2. Neurological intensive care. I. Lee, Vivien H.
   [DNLM: 1. Stroke--therapy. 2. Critical Care--methods. WL 355]
   RC388.5.H363 2011
   616.8'1062--dc23
                                 2011016755

Published by Nova Science Publishers, Inc. †New York

Contents

Preface

'Handbook of Stroke and Neurocritical Care' is a thorough-source of referenced material in handbook format that provides useful material on the topic of stroke and neurocritical care for the trainee level. This handbook was written for the fellow, resident or medical student and is meant to be a quick source of detailed information on the topic of stroke and neurocritical care. The concise organization and relianaceon abundant figures and images are useful to the trainee. Although detailed, the size of the handbook allows it to be easily carried with the trainee, making it practical and useful. (Imprint: Nova Biomedical)

In: Handbook of Stroke and Neurocritical Care   ISBN: 978-61324-786-0
Editor: V. H. Lee   © 2012 Nova Science Publishers, Inc.

Chapter I

Normal Anatomy

Vivien H. Lee
Department of Neurological Sciences, Section of Stroke and
Neurocritical care,
Rush University Medical Center, Chicago, IL, USA

Arterial Anatomy

Great Vessels

1) Aortic Arch (Figure 1)
    a) Brachoicephalic trunk (innominate artery)
        (i) First vessel that arises from the aortic arch.
        (ii) Bifurcates into the Right Subclavian Artery (SCV)
            and Right Common Carotid Artery (CCA)
            1) Major branches that arise from the right SCV are
                the right VA, internal thoracic arteries, and the
                thyrocervical and costocervical trunks
            2) Right CCA divides into the right ECA and right
                ICA
    b) Left Common Carotid Artery
        (i) Usually the 2nd major vessel that arises from the aortic
            arch

           (ii) Arises from aortic arch apex just distal to the brachiocephalic artery origin

           (iii) At upper border of thyroid cartilage, the left CCA bifurcates into the left ICA and ECA

    c) Left Subclavian Artery

           (i) Arises from the aortic arch a few millimeters distal to the left CCA origin

           (ii) gives off the left VA and internal thoracic arteries and the left thyrocervical and costocervical trunks

    d) Normal variant- Bovine arch- shared origin of the brachiocephalic trunk and left CCA is the most frequently encountered normal variant in aortic arch, occurs in 27% of cases

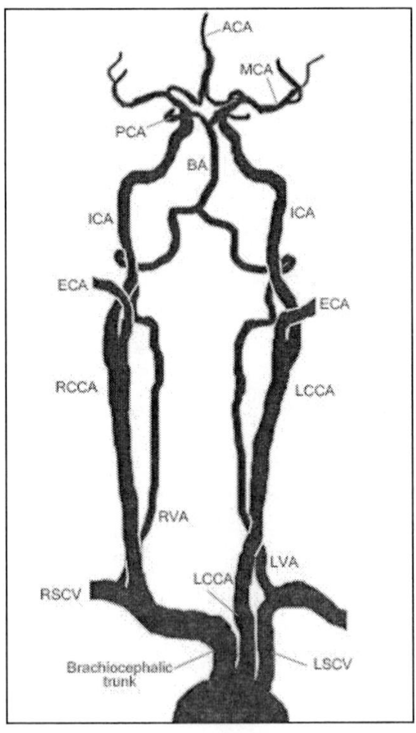

Figure 1. Aortic arch, great vessels, and their major branches (AP view).

   2) Vertebral artery (VA)

     a) VA is divided into 4 segments (Figure 2)

b) V1 (extraosseous) segment
    (i) Arises from SCV, courses posterosuperiorly to enter the transverse foramen of C6 vertebrae
c) V2 (foraminal) segment
    (i) Ascends vertically, passing through the foramina of the C3-6 transverse processes, then course through C2, then runs through C1 transverse foramina
    (ii) Exits from C to curve backward and course above the posterior arch of the atlas
d) V3 (extraspinal) segment
    (i) Begins as the VA exit from C1 and end where VA penetrates the dura
    (ii) Enter the skull visa the foramen magnum
e) V4 (intradural) segment
    (i) intracranial portion ends at the medullopontine junction where the 2 VAs join to form the midline basilar artery
f) VA has cervical, meningeal, and intracranial branches
    (i) Cervical- 2 types of branches
        1) muscular branches –V2 segment gives off multiple small unnamed muscular branches that supply the deep cervical musculature
        2) spinal branches- supply the spinal cord and its coverings, anastomosing with spinal arteries from other vessels (such as the ascending pharyngeal artery & thyrocervical trunk)
            (i) Meningeal branches- anterior an posterior meningeal branches arise from the distal extracranial VA to supply part of the posterior fossa dura.
            (ii) Intracranial branches   (see circle of willis)

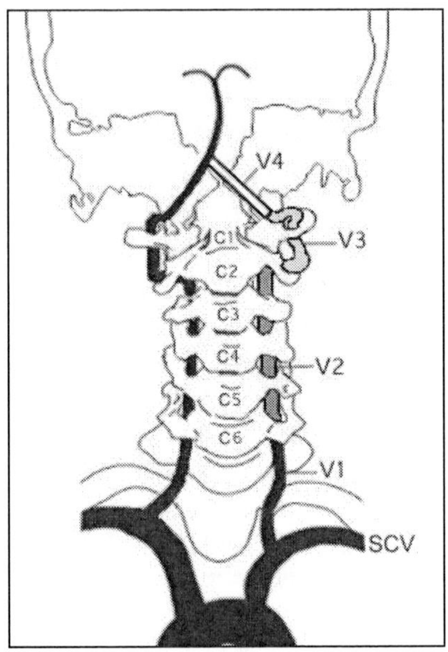

Figure 2. Vertebral artery segments (AP view). VA enters the transverse foramens of the C6 (or C5 veretebrae) and runs within the intervertebral foramina, exiting to course behind the atlas, then piercing the dura mater to enter the foarmen magnum. he 2 VAs then unite to form the BA.

Carotid Arteries

1) Common Carotid Artery (CCA)
   a) Normal CCA bifurcation is at midcervical level ~ C4, typically around C3-5 (may occur as high as C1 or as low as T2)
   b) Bifurcates into ECA and ICA
2) External Carotid artery (ECA) (Figure 3)
   a) Supplies most extracranial structures of the head and neck
   b) ECA trunk rapidly decreases in size as it gives off branches to the tongue, deep face, and neck. It terminates medial to the parotid gland by diving into it 2 main distal branches (Superficial temporal artery and Maxillary artery)
   c) ECA has 8 major branches
      (i) Superior thyroid artery – 1st ECA branch, supplies the larynx & most of the upper thyroid gland

(ii) Ascending pharyngeal artery- supplies the pharynx and eustasian tube, tympanic cavity, and prevertebral muscles, dura & lower cranial nerves

(iii) Lingual artery – supplies tongue & oral cavity

(iv) Facial artery – supplies most of face, palate, lip & cheek

    1) FA terminates near the medial canthus of the eye by becoming the angular artery, and anastomoses with branches of the ophthalmic artery, a branch of the ICA

    2) The anastomosis between orbital branches of the ICA and the ECA is an important potential pathway for collateral blood flow in the event of ICA occlusion

(v) Occipital artery – supplies musculocutaneous structures of the posterior neck & scalp

(vi) Posterior auricular artery – supplies the scalp, pinna & external auditory canal

(vii) Superficial temporal artery (STA)– cutaneous artery that supplies the anterior $2/3^{rd}$ of scalp, part of ear & parotid gland

    1) Transverse facial artery- branch of the STA

(viii) Internal maxillary deep face & artery – supplies nose

3) Internal Carotid Artery (ICA)- (Figure 3)

  a) originates from CCA at C3-4 or C4-5 level

  b) ICA is divided into 7 segments

  c) C1 Ascending cervical ICA segment

    (i) Carotid bulb- The carotid bulb is the most proximal aspect of the cervical ICA. It forms a significant focal dilatation where the ICA originates from the CCA at a slight angle

    (ii) From the bulb, the cervical ICA courses cephalad within the carotid space (CS), a fascially defined tubular shaped sheath that contains all 2 layers of the deep cervical fascia

      1) CS contents include the ICA, Internal Jugular vein (IJ), lymph nodes, postganglionic sympathetic nerves, and several of the lower cranial nerves.

(iii) C1 initially lies posterolateral to ECA but then courses medial to ECA as it ascends towards skull base

(iv) C1 Lies in front of Internal Jugular (IJ) vein and slightly medial to it

(v) C1 terminates as the ICA enters the carotid canal in the petrous temporal bone

(vi) No branches in neck

d) C2 Petrous ICA segment (Figure 4)

(i) C2 enters the skull through the carotid canal within the petrous temporal bone and forms an S shaped curve

(ii) C2 has 2 subsegments- Vertical (ascending) segment & Horizontal segment

(iii) 2 Branches- Caroticotympanic artery & Vidian artery (inconstant)

e) C3 Lacerum ICA segment (Figure 4)

(i) Begins where the petrous carotid canal ends

(ii) Ends at the petrolingual ligament (a small refelction of periosteum that runs between the lingual of the sphenoid bone anteriorly & the petrous apex posteriorly)

(iii) Usually no branches

f) C4 Cavernous ICA segment

(i) Begins at the superior margin of the petrolingual ligament

(ii) C4 has 3 subsegments- a ascending vertical portion, a horizontal segment, & a short vertical portion (2 bends called the posterior genu and the anterior genu)

(iii) Courses within the cavernous sinus, surrounded by venous channels

(iv) Exits the cavernous sinus through a dural ring

(v) Branches

1) Posterior trunk (meningohypophyseal artery) supplies branches to the pituitary gland, tentorium, and clivus

2) Lateral trunk (inferolateral trunk)- supply the 3rd, 4th, and 6th cranial nerves, as well as the gasserian ganglion and cavernous sinus dura

3) Medial braches- small inconsistent branches (capsular arteries of McConnell) found in only

28% of anatomic specimens, supply the pituitary gland

(vi) Cavernous sinus (Figure 5)
1) CN III, IV & VI course lateral to cavernous ICA. Only CN VI courses within the cavernous sinus proper
2) Carotid artery is the most medial structure within the cavenous sinus, surrounded by endothelial lined sinusoids and thin walled venules. The sphenoid sinus is medial to the cavernous sinus

g) C5 Clinoid ICA segment
(i) C5 is the shortest of all the ICA segments, comprises only a small wedge-shaped areas along the superior aspect of the anterior genu
(ii) Begins at the proximal dural ring
(iii) Ends at the distal dural ring where the ICA enters the subarachnoid space
(iv) C5 segment is an interdural structure, located in a collar of dura
(v) No discernible branches

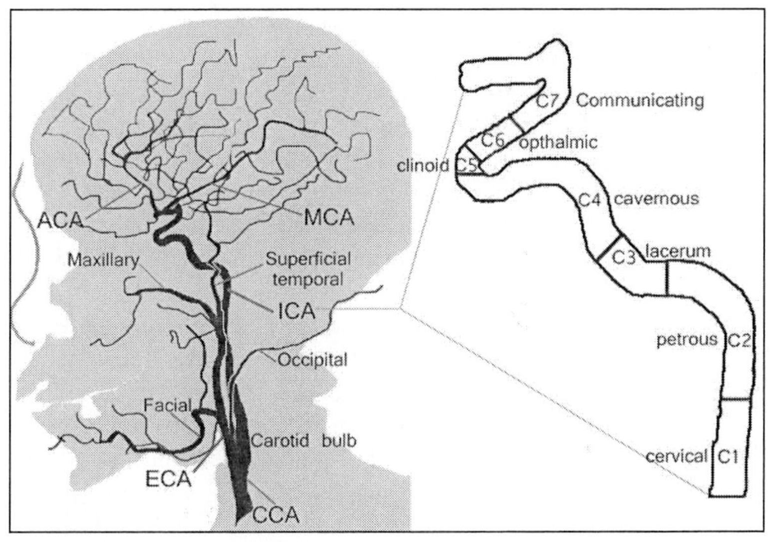

Figure 3. Lateral view of the CCA including ECA and ICA segments. ECA divides into 2 main distal branches (STA and maxillary artery). The 7 anatomically distinct ICA segments are shown.

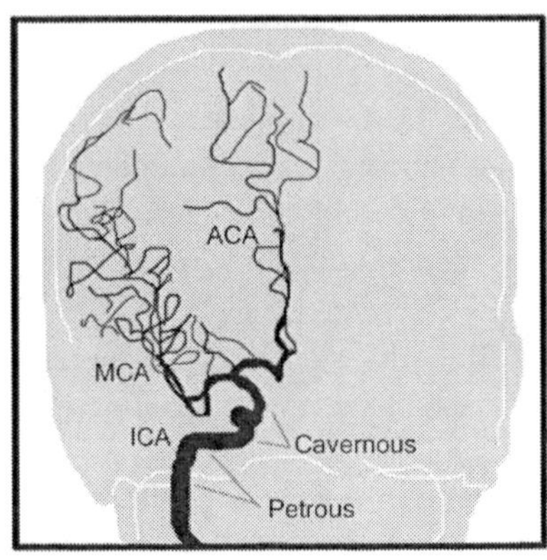

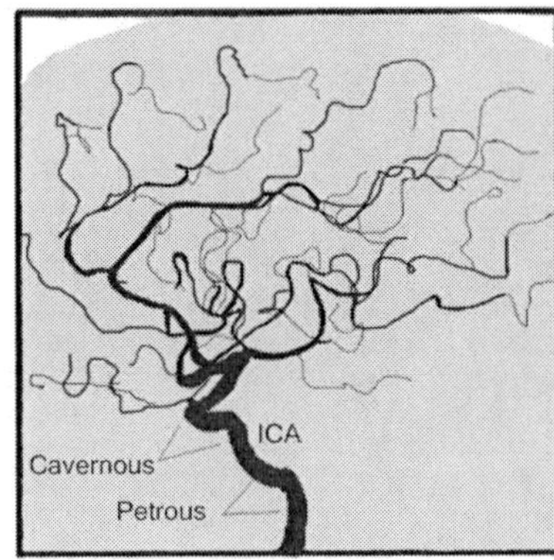

Figure 4. AP and lateral views of petrous and cavernous segments of ICA.

    h)   C6 Ophthalmic ICA segment
- (i) Intradural ICA (supraclinoid)
- (ii) Begins at the distal dural ring and terminates proximal to the PCOM origin
- (iii) Terminates just proximal to the PCOM origin
- (iv) Represents the most proximal intradural portion of the supraclinoid ICA
- (v) 2 important Branches from C6
  - 1) Ophthalmic artery- 1st major intracranial ICA branch, originates from C6 segment, courses through the optic canal into the orbit, intradural in 90% of anatomic dissections. OA has 3 major branches:
    - a) Ocular branches (supply retina and choroid of the eye)- includes the central retinal artery and ciliary arteries
    - b) Orbital branches – lacrimal artery & group of unnamed muscular branches (supply extraocular muscles & oribital periosteum)
    - (i) Recurrent meningeal artery (branch of lacrimal artery) passes backward through the

> superior orbital fissure & anastomoses with branches of the middle meningeal artery
>
> c) Extraorbital branches – have extensive anastomoses with ethmoidal and facial branches of the ECA
>
> 2) Superior hypophyseal arteries – supply anterior pituitary lobe, pituitary stalk, optic nerve & chiasm
>
> (vi) Angiographic carotid siphon- an S shaped curve that is formed by the cavernous & supraclinoid ICA segments, best visualized on lateral cerebral angiograms.

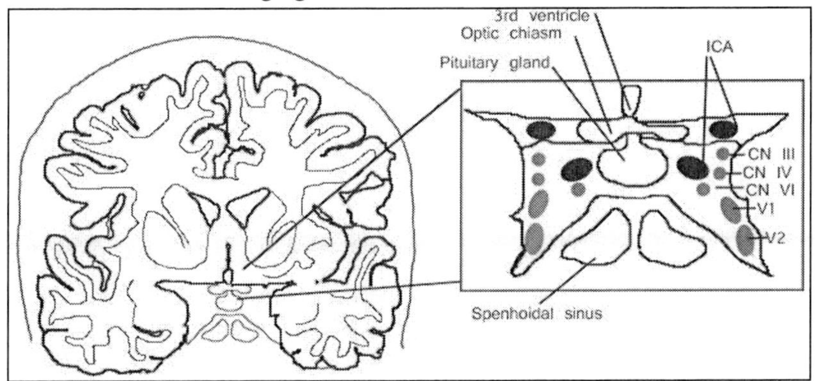

Figure 5. Cavernous sinus (AP view). C4 ICA segment is surrounded by the endothelial lined venous sinusoids that comprise the caverbous sinus. The abducens nerve is the only cranial nerve that lies within the cavernous sinus properl the other carnial nerves (III, IV, V1, V2) are contained within the lateral dural wall.

> i) C7 Communicating ICA segment
>
> (i) C7 begins proximal to the origin of the PCOM & ends as the ICA bifurcates into its 2 terminal branches (ACA & MCA)
>
> (ii) 2 Branches
>
> 1) PCOM
>
> a) PCOM arises from the posterior aspect of the intradural ICA and anastomoses with the PCA, connects the anterior and posterior circulation

        b)   Gives rise to several small branches (anterior thalamoperforating arteries) that supply the medial thalamus and walls of the 3rd ventricle

    2)   Anterior choroidal Artery

        a)   Arises from the posteromedial aspect of the supraclinoid ICA a short distance above the PCOM origin

        b)   Supplies the optic tract, cerebral peduncle, uncal & parahippocampal gyri of temporal lobe, part of thalamus & posterior limb of internal capsule

Circle of Willis (Figure 6)

    1)   Interconnecting arterial "polygon"

    2)   Complete circle of willis is seen in only 20-25%, anomalies are common including hypoplasia

    3)   Anomolies

        a)   Persistent trigeminal artery (PTA)- most common carotid-basilar anastromosis, usually associated with small PCOMS and vertebral arteries and hypoplastic basilar artery

        b)   Fetal origin PCA from ICA with hypoplastic/absent P1 segment

            i.   Most common anomaly, seen in 15-20% of cases

    4)   Anterior Cerebral Artery (ACA)

        a)   A1 segment (horizontal) – segment from ACA origin to its junction with the ACOM

            (i)   Medial lenticulostriate arteries arise from A1 and supply head of caudate nucleus and anterior limb o internal capsule

        b)   A2 segment – includes segment from junction of ACOM to its bifurcation into pericallosal and callosomarginal arteries

            (i)   Recurrent artery of Heubner- the largest and longest ACA penetrating branch

                1)   Is a lenticulostriate branch that typically arises from proximal A2 segment (50% of cases) or the A1 segment

    c) Perforating branches- medial lenticulostriate arteries and the recurrent artery of Heubner, supply caudate head, anterior limb of internal capsule, & part of basal ganglia

    d) Anterior communicating artery (ACOM)- connects the two horizontal ACA segments

    e) Azygous ACA is a solitary unpaired vessel that arises as a single trunk from the A1 segment of the right or left ACA (occurs in up to 4%)

5) Middle Cerebral Artery (MCA)

    a) MCA courses laterally giving off lenticulostriate artery branches to basal ganglia and internal capsule, then MCA trifurcates (near sylvian fissure) into small anterior temporal branches and larger superior and inferior trunks (M2)

    b) MCA bifurcates (50% of cases) or trifurcates (25% of cases) near the insula

    c) M1 segment (horizontal)

        (i) Deep perforatoring branches lateral lenticulostriate arteries arise from M1, supply the lentiform nucleus, part of internal capsule, & caudate nucleus

        (ii) Anterior temporal artery- arises from M1 segment before bifurcation at ~ same level as the lenticulostriate arteries, passes directly anteriorly and inferiorly over the temporal tip and usually does not enter the sylvian fissure

    d) M2 segment (insular branches)

        (i) Superior trunk – supplies lateral portions of the cerebral hemispheres above the sylvian fissure

        (ii) Inferior trunk- supplies the temporal and inferior parietal lobes below the sylvian fissure

6) Intracranial Vertebral artery (VA)

    a) Intracranial VA branches include a number of small meningeal arteries, the posterior and anterior spinal arteries, perforating arteries, and the posterior inferior cerebellar artery (PICA)

    b) Posterior spinal artery arises from distal VA or PICA.

    c) Anterior spinal artery arises from the distal VA, gives off small perforating branches that supply the anterior surface of the medulla (pyramids). In half of cases, the ASA unites with the ASA from the opposite VA then runs caudal in the anteromedian sulcus of the spinal cord.

   d) Posterior inferior cerebellar artery (PICA) arises from the VA at the anterolateral aspect of the brainstem

      (i) supplies the posterior and inferior surfaces of the cerebellum and inferior vermis

7) Basilar Artery (BA)

   a) Normallly terminates near pontmesencephalic junction by dividing into its 2 terminal branches (right and left PCAs)

   b) BA gives off numerous pontine perforating arteries- 2 sets of pontine branches

      (i) median and paramedian pontine perforating arteries

      (ii) lateral pontine arteries

   c) BA gives rise to 2 important cerebellar arteries

      (i) Anterior inferior cerebellar arteries (AICA)- supplies the smallest area of the cerebellum, the petrosal surface

      (ii) Superior cerebellar arteries (SCA)- supplies the superior surface of the cerebellum and upper vermis

   d) Perforating branches- Distal BA and proximal PCAs give risk to posterior thalamoperforating arteries and thalamogeniculate arteries, which supply midbrain and thalamus

8) Posterior Cerebral Artery (PCA)

   a) P1- segment extends from origin at basilar bifurcation to its junction with PCOM

      (i) Lies within the interpeduncular cistern, represents the most proximal aspect of the PCA

      (ii) Posterior thalamoperforating arteries arise from basilar bifurcation & P1 segments, supply the thalamus and midbrain

      (iii) Medial posterior choroidal artery originates either from P1 or proximal P2 segment, supply the tectal plate, part of midbrain, posterior thalalmus, pineal gland, & tela choroidea of 3rd ventricle

   b) P2 segment – extends from the junction between PCOM and PCA to the posterior aspect of the midbrain

      (i) 80% of thalamogeniculate arteries originate from P2 segment

   c) PCOM

(i)   Perforating branches- Anterior thalamoperforating arteries arise from PCOM, supply part of thalamus, infralenticular limb of internal capsule, & optic tracts

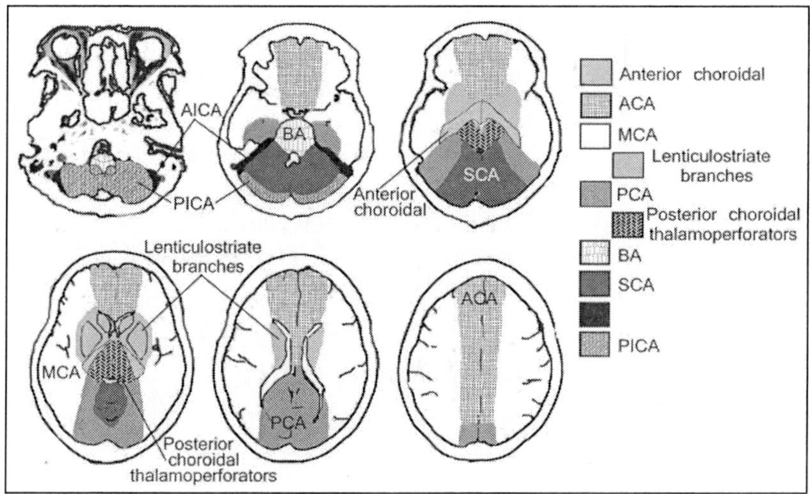

Figure 6. Vascular territories on axial CT brain.

Venous Anatomy

1) Dural sinuses (Figure 7)
    a) Dural venous sinuses are tracbeculated, endothelial-lined channels whose fibrous walls are formed by the inner and outer layers of the dura matter
    b) Situated at the junctions and edges of the falx ceebri and the tentorium cerebelli
    c) Superior sagittal sinus (SSS)
        (i)   Courses in an arc in the superior margin of the falx cerebri and ends at the internal occipital protuberance by draining into the confluence of the sinuses (torcula herophili)
        (ii) SSS drains most of the blood from the cerebral hemispheres
    d) Inferior sagittal sinus (ISS)
        (i)   Runs in the inferior margin of the falx

    (ii) Joins with the great cerebral vein of Galen to form the straight sinus

e)   Straight sinus (SS)

f)   Transverse Sinus (TS)

    (i) The paired transverse sinuses originate at the torcula and course anteriolaterally along the skull between the attachments of the tentorium cerebellu, empties into the sigmoid sinuses

    (ii) One of the TS (most often the left) is hypoplastic or absent

g)   Sigmoid sinuses (SS)- drain into the jugular veins

h)   Cavernous sinuses (Figure 4)- Ophthalmic and facial veins drain into the cavernous sinuses

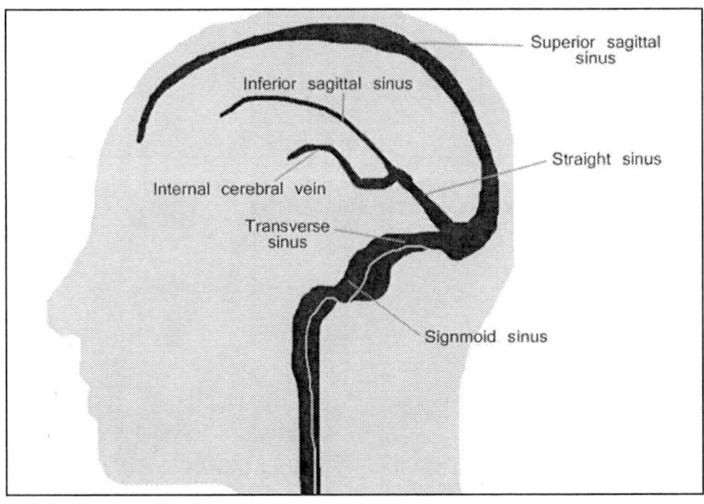

Figure 7. Dural sinuses (lateral view).

2)   Cerebral Veins

a)   Superficial (cortical veins)- most unnamed, although the following 3 are often identified

    (i) Superficial middle cerebral vein – runs along sylvian fissure

    (ii) Vein of Trolard- large anastomotic cerebral vein that courses cephalad from sylvian fissure to the SSS)

    (iii) Vein of Labbe- courses posterolaterally from sylvian fissure to the transverse sinus

   b) Deep cerebral veins
       (i)   Medullary veins
       (ii) Subependymal veins
       (iii) Basal veins
       (iv) Vein of Galen
   c) Posterior fossa veins

References

[1]   Osborn AG. *Diagnostic Neuroradiology*. CV Mosby, 1944.

[2]   Osborn AG. *Diagnostic Cerebral Angiography*. Lippincott Williams & Wilkins, Philadelphia, PA: 1999.

[3]   Caplan, LR. *Caplan's stroke, a clinical approach*, 3rd ed, Butterworth-Heinemann, Boston 2000.

In: Handbook of Stroke and Neurocritical Care   ISBN: 978-61324-786-0
Editor: V. H. Lee   © 2012 Nova Science Publishers, Inc.

Chapter II

Ischemic Stroke - Epidemiology

Vivien H. Lee
Department of Neurological Sciences, Section of Stroke and
Neurocritical care,
Rush University Medical Center, Chicago, IL, USA

Ischemic stroke is a heterogenous group of disorders. Stroke prognosis, risk of recurrence and management are influenced by Ischemic stroke subtype.

1) TOAST study (Trial of Org 10172 in Acute stroke treatment)[1]
    a) a randomized blinded placebo controlled trial of IV infusion of a low molecular weight heparinoid (danaparoid, ORG 101732) versus placebo
    b) Although the study was negative, it provided a useful classification of ischemic stroke with high Inter-rater agreement.
2) TOAST Subtypes (Figure 1)
    a) Large-artery atherosclerosis (LAA)
    b) Cardioembolism
    c) Small-vessel occlusion
    d) Stroke of undetermined etiology (Cryptogenic)
    e) Stroke of other determined etiology (rare causes)
3) Epidemiological Studies

a) Rochester, MN stroke epidemiology study (Table 1) provides Stroke recurrence, functional outcome, and mortality.[4]
  (i) Among the stroke subtypes, LAA had the highest stroke recurrence rate (early and late), but paradoxically had the best long-term survival rates
    1) Stroke recurrence rate for the LAA stroke subtype was 18.5% at 1-month and 40.2% at 5 years, which was higher compared to the other subtypes. [4]
    2) Northern Manhattan Stroke Study (NOMASS) was a large epidemiological study reporting subtypes of ischemic stroke, recorded a recurrence rate for LAA 14.4%. [5]
  (ii) Good functional outcome (defined as modified Rankin score of 1-2) at 1-year was seen in 53% of patients with LAA subtype compared to 82% of patients with lacunar subtype and only 27% in the cardioembolic subtype. [4]

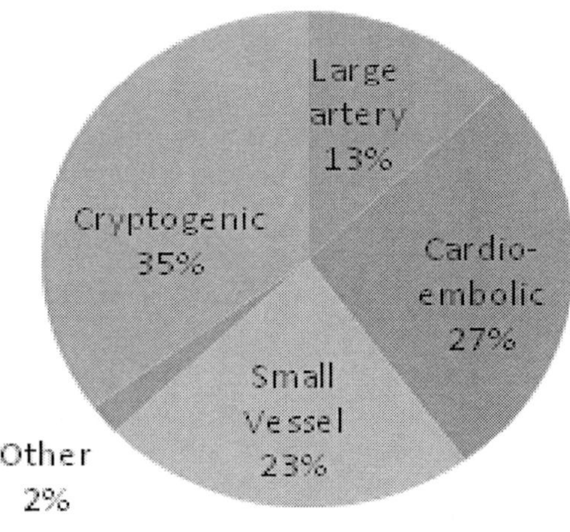

Figure 1. 5 TOAST subtypes [2,3].

Table 1. Cerebral infarction subtype specific recurrence risks, death, and functional outcome [4]

	Large-artery atherosclerosis	Cardioembolic	Lacunar	Uncertain cause
Stroke recurrence				
30-days	18.5%	5.3%	1.4%	3.3%
1-year	24.4%	13.7%	7.1%	13.2%
5-years	40.2%	31.7%	24.8%	33.2%
Good Functional Outcome (defined as mRS of 1 or 2)				
1-year	53.4%	26.7%	81.9%	50.3%
Death rates				
30-days	8.1%	30.3%	1.4%	14%
1-year	10.8%	53%	6.9%	25.6%
5-years	32.2%	80.4%	35.1%	48.6%

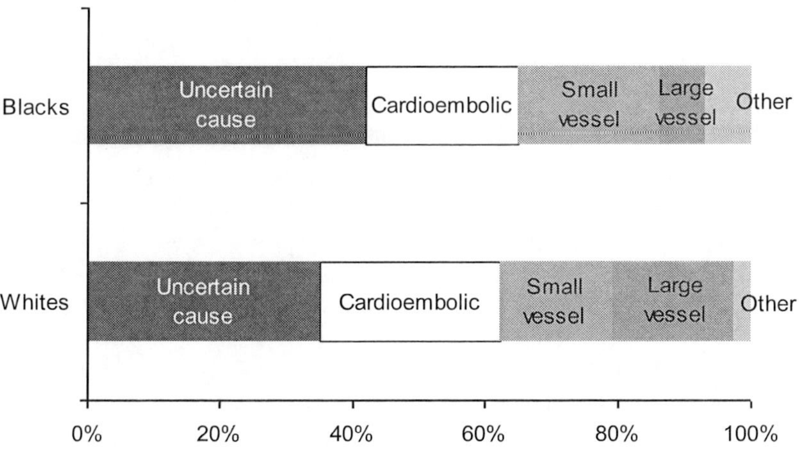

Figure 2. Age- and sex-adjusted annual incidence rates (per 100 000 population) for first-ever ischemic stroke (Rochester, MN versus Cincinnati, OH, respectively) were as follows: large-artery (27 vs.17); cardioembolic (40 vs. 56); small-vessel (25 vs. 52), uncertain cause (52 vs. 103), other cause (4 vs.17) [6,7].

      b)   Germany Study showed that 2 years after onset, patients in the small-vessel occlusion subgroup were 3 times more likely to be alive than those with cardioembolism. [2]

      c)   Overall, small vessel occlusion group has best functional outcome, survival and lowest recurrence rate

4)   Racial and gender differences

a) Men have a 4 times greater age-adjusted incidence rate of ischemic stroke due to LAA subtype than women (47 vs 12 per 100,000) [6]

b) LAA stroke subtype is more common in whites compared with blacks(Figure 2).[6,7]

(i) annual incidence rate of first ischemic stroke due to large-vessel atherosclerosis was 27 per 100,000 in Rochester, MN, a population that was 96% white (Figure 2) versus only 17 per 100,000 in the black population of the greater Cincinnati/northern Kentucky stroke incidence study.[6,7]

References

[1] The Publications Committee for the Trial of ORG 10172 in Acute Stroke Treatment (TOAST) Investigators. Low molecular weight heparinoid, ORG 10172 (danaparoid), and outcome after acute ischemic stroke: a randomized controlled trial. *JAMA.* 1998;*279:1265-*1272.

[2] Peter L. Kolominsky-Rabas, MD; Margarete Weber, MD; Olaf Gefeller, MSc, PhD; Bernhard Neundoerfer, MD, PhD; Peter U. Heuschmann, MD, MPH Epidemiology of Ischemic Stroke Subtypes According to TOAST Criteria. Incidence, Recurrence, and Long-Term Survival in Ischemic Stroke Subtypes: A Population-Based Study. *Stroke.* 2001;32:2735-2740.

[3] Adams, Jr, HP, Bendixen BH, Kappelle LJ, Biller J, Love BB, Gordon DL, and Marsh EE. Classification of subtype of acute ischemic stroke. Definitions for use in a multicenter clinical trial TOAST.

[4] Petty GW, Brown RD Jr, Whisnant JP, Sicks JD, O'Fallon WM, *Wiebers DO. Ischemic stroke subtypes: a population-based study of functional outcome, survival, and recurrence. Stroke.* 2003;31:1062-8.

[5] Sacco RL, Shi T, Zamanillo MC, Kargman DE. Predictors of mortality and recurrence after hospitalized cerebral infarction in an urban community: the Northern Manhattan Stroke Study. *Neurology.* 1994;44:626–634.

[6] Petty GW, Brown RD Jr, Whisnant JP, Sicks JD, O'Fallon WM, Wiebers DO. Ischemic stroke subtypes: a population-based study of incidence and risk factors. *Stroke. 1999;30:2513-6.*

[7]   Woo D, Gebel J, Miller R, Kothari R, Brott T, Khoury J, Salisbury S, Shukla R, Pancioli A, Jauch E, Broderick J. Incidence rates of first-ever ischemic stroke subtypes among blacks: a population-based study. *Stroke.*1999;30:2517-2522.

In: Handbook of Stroke and Neurocritical Care   ISBN: 978-61324-786-0
Editor: V. H. Lee   © 2012 Nova Science Publishers, Inc.

Chapter III

Ischemic Stroke-Large-Artery Atherosclerosis

Vivien H. Lee

Department of Neurological Sciences, Section of Stroke and
Neurocritical care,
Rush University Medical Center, Chicago, IL, USA

Large Artery Atherosclerosis (LAA)

1) Background/Demographics
   a) Large artery atherosclerosis (LAA) includes
      (i) intracranial atherosclerosis (ICAS)
      (ii) extracranial artery disease (i.e. carotid disease).
   b) In autopsy studies, atherosclerosis develops earlier than in
      the extracranial carotid compared to intracranial arteries,
      and its progression parallels that of atherosclerosis in the
      aorta (Figure 1).[1]
   c) In Northern Manhattan Stroke Study (NOMASS) of 438
      mixed-ethnicity stroke patients, 9% of acute strokes were
      due to extracranial atherosclerosis and 8% were due to
      intracranial atherosclerosis.[2]

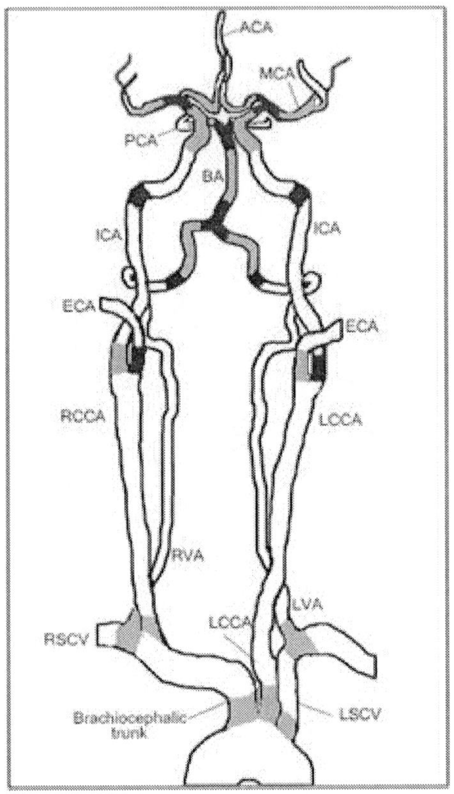

Figure 1. Sites of atherosclerosis (Severity indicated by coloring, black>grey).

Table 1. Racial distribution of carotid disease

Study/Author	Population	Results
Angiogram studies		
International Study of Extracranial to Intracranial Bypass[11]	STA-MCA bypass	MCA occlusive disease more common indication in Japan than in North America
Gorelick[5]	106 patients with symptomatic unilateral carotid occlusive disease	In asymptomatic vessels, Black patients had more lesions of supraclinoid ICA, ACA stem, and MCA; White patients had more extracranial carotid disease

Study/Author	Population	Results
Gorelick6	26 Whites, 45 Blacks mixed racial population in Chicago	Whites had more severe ICA origin disease; Blacks had more severe MCA and supraclinoid ICA disease
Feldmann[8]	24 Whites, 24 Chinese symptomatic cerebrovascular disease	In symptomatic vascular territories, Whites had more severe extracranial lesions, Chinese had more severe intracranial lesions
Northern Manhattan Stroke Study[2]	438 Residents of Manhattan > age 39 years hospitalized for acute stroke	The proportion of intracranial atherosclerosis by race: 1% of whites, 6% of blacks, and 11% of Hispanics. Rate of extracranial atherosclerosis by race: 11% of whites, 8% of blacks, and 9% of Hispanics.
Autopsy studies		
International Atherosclerosis Project [1,7]	2166 autopsies performed on Blacks and Whites (from New Orleans, Jamaica, Norway)	In the 65-69 year old age group, intracranial lesions (stenosis) occurred in 43% of Blacks compared to 8.5% of Whites

ICA =internal carotid artery, ACA = anterior cerebral artery MCA = middle cerebral artery.

    d)   Among the stroke subtypes, LAA had the highest stroke recurrence rate (early and late).[3]

  2) Ethnic differences have been demonstrated in many angiographic and autopsy studies

    a)   Data consistently demonstrates that Blacks, Asians, and Hispanics have more intracranial atherosclerotic disease in contrast to whites who may be prone to extracranial carotid disease. [1,4,5,6,7,8,9,10]

(Table 1).

Intracranial Atherosclerotic Stenosis (ICAS)

Intracranial atherosclerotic stenosis (ICAS) can be divided into asymptomatic status and symptomatic status.

  1) Asymptomatic ICAS Natural history

   a)   Asymptomatic ICAS has a lower risk of stroke compared with symptomatic ICAS.
- (i) prospective study of 102 patients with MCA stenosis or occlusion
    1) symptomatic MCA disease had an overall stroke risk of 12.5% per year (ipsilateral 9.1%)
    2) risk for asymptomatic MCA disease was only 2.8%/year (ipsilateral 1.4%). [12]

   b)   Most series confirm a relatively low risk of stroke, with an annual ipsilateral stroke risk ranging from 0 to 3.5% (Table 2).

Table 2. Annual stroke rate in asymptomatic and mixed asymptomatic/symptomatic ICAS

Author	1 year Stroke rate	1 year ipsilateral Stroke rate	Summary
Asymptomatic ICAS			
Nahab [13]*	--	3.5%[+] MRA 0%[+] CA	65 pts with symptomatic ICAS and coexistant ICAS by MRA (14 by CA) from WASID,
Kern [12]	2.8%	1.4%	56 pts with MCA stenosis by TCD
Kremer [14]	0%	0%	50 pts MCA stenosis by TCD (>50% stenosis in 12)
Mixed Asymptomatic and Symptomatic ICAS			
Craig [15]**	19	7.6[+]	58 pts with ICA stenosis by CA (81% symptomatic)
Marzewski [16]*	4%	3%[+]	66 patients* ICA stenosis by CA (41% symptomatic)
Moufarrij [17]*	3%	2%[+]	45 distal VA or BA stenosis by CA (73% symptomatic)

pts= patients, MRA= MR angiogram head, CA= cerebral angiogram, MCA= middle cerebral artery, ICA= internal carotid artery, VA= vertebral artery, BA= basilar artery, TCD= Transcranial Doppler, in territory of stenosis[+], 50-99% stenosis*, >1/3 stenosis **

   c)   Asymptomatic ICAS often coexists with symptomatic ICAs, and in the Warfarin versus Aspirin for Symptomatic

Intracranial Disease (WASID) study, coexisting asymptomatic ICAS was detected in up to 27.3% (n=65/238) of patients with symptomatic ICAS undergoing MR angiogram (MRA).[13]

2) Symptomatic ICAS Natural History

    a) Studies suggest that symptomatic ICAS is estimated to have an annual ipsilateral stroke rate of 7% to 12% (Table 3)

Table 3. Annual stroke rate in symptomatic ICAS

Author	1 year Stroke rate	1 year ipsilateral Stroke rate	Summary
Symptomatic ICAS			
Retrospective WASID Study [18]*	15% BA 13.7% VA	10.7%[+] BA 7.8%[+] VA	68 pts with ICAS posterior circulation
Prospective WASID, Chimowitz [19]*	14% Warfarin 15% Aspirin	11%+++	569 pts with ICAS
Kern [12]	12.5%	9.1%	46 pts with MCA disease by TCD
Bogousslavsky [20]	9.5%	7.8%	164 medically treated pts from EC-IC bypass (53% MCA stenosis)
Corston [21]	3.5%	-	21 pts with MCA (33-66% stenosis by CA)
Mazighi [22]*	6.8%	-	122 pts with ICAS
Thijs [23]*	14%	-	52 pts with ICAS
Kwon [24]	0%	0%	135 pts with MCA or BA stenosis (by MRA)

pt = patients, MRA= MR angiogram head, CA= cerebral angiogram, MCA= middle cerebral artery, BA= basilar artery, TCD= Transcranial Doppler, in territory of stenosis[+], 50-99% stenosis*, >1/3 stenosis **, stroke in the territory of the symptomatic artery+++.

    b) Extracranial to Intracranial Bypass Trial [11]

        (i) 1377 patients with symptomatic carotid atherosclerotic disease randomized to medical versus bypass surgery followed for an average of 56 months

(ii) In the medical group of 714 patients, 59% were internal carotid artery occlusions, 24% with MCA occlusive disease (stenosis and occlusion) and 17% with intracranial ICA stenosis (above the C-2 vertebral body), of which 13.8% of the medical arm suffered stroke or death at the end of one year.

(iii) In patients with MCA stenosis, annual stroke rate was 9.5% and ipsilateral stroke rate was 7.8%

c) The retrospective WASID study [10]

(i) Non-randomized Retrospective review of 68 patients with 50- 99% ICAS treated with warfarin (n542) or aspirin (n526), with a median follow-up of 13.8 months

(ii) 15 patients (22%) had an ischemic stroke .

d) The prospective Warfarin and Aspirin for Symptomatic Intracranial atheromatous Disease (WASID) trial [19]

(i) Prospective, multicenter, randomized trial comparing warfarin and aspirin in patients with symptomatic ICAS (>50% on cerebral angiogram) [19]

(ii) 106 (19%) developed subsequent ischemic stroke, of which 77 (14%) were in the territory of the stenotic artery.[25]

(iii) rate of ischemic stroke in the territory of the stenotic artery overall was 11% at 1 year and 14% at 2 years.[25]

(iv) factors associated with a higher subsequent stroke risk in symptomatic ICAS, included degree of stenosis and recent symptoms.[26]

e) Degree of stenosis

(i) factor associated with higher subsequent ischemic stroke risk in the territory of the stenotic artery included degree of stenosis.[26]

(ii) Patients with symptomatic stenosis >70% has a higher 2 year risk of stroke (19% vs 10%)

(iii) In the high-grade stenosis subgroup (>70% stenosis) with a qualifying event as stroke, the 2 year risk of stroke is in the territory of the artery was 25%.[26]

(iv) data is comparable with symptomatic extracranial carotid artery stenosis, where the degree of stenosis significantly impacts the rate of recurrent ipsilateral stroke, with higher risk corresponding to higher degrees of stenosis.

f) Timing

   (i)   majority (78%) of recurrent strokes occurred within the first year [26]

   (ii) In the >70% stenosis subgroup, 23% of the stroke risk was in the 1st year, with only an additional 2% risk in the second year

   (iii) Patients with recent symptoms ($\leq$ 17 days) had a higher risk of 2-year stroke (17% vs 10%) [26]

   (iv) patients are at highest risk soon after their qualifying event

   (v)   the recurrent stroke risk drops dramatically thereafter for patients who are 1 year out from their event

g) Qualfying event

   (i)   Type of qualifying event (TIA versus stroke) was not associated with recurrent risk of stroke in the territory of the stenosis [26]

h) Sex

   (i)   Men have 4 times higher incidence rate of first ischemic stroke due to large-vessel atherosclerosis than women [27] However, in ICAS women may have greater recurrent stroke risk than men.

   (ii) Subgroup analysis of WASID showed that women with symptomatic ICAS were at significantly higher risk for recurrent ischemic stroke and for the combined end point of stroke or vascular death compared with men (2-year rates 28.4% versus 16.6%, p = 0.017).[28]

      1) increased risk persists even after adjusting for sociodemographic features, lifestyle, vascular risk factors, angiographic findings, and features of the qualifying event.[28]

   (iii) Female gender was also a significant risk factor associated with subsequent ischemic stroke in the territory of the stenotic intracranial artery.[26]

i) Other factors - not significantly associated with risk of subsequent ischemic stroke in the territory of the stenotic artery included length of stenosis, use of antithrombotic medication at the time of the qualifying event, and medication treatment (aspirin versus coumadin).[19,26]

j) Radiographic progression of stenosis- Progression of symptomatic ICAS has been suggested to predict patients who are at increased risk of recurrent clinical events.

   (i) Among 21 patients (48% presented with stroke) with 45 intracranial stenoses, repeat angiography done at a mean of 26.7 months demonstrated an increase in the mean stenosis of intracranial lesions from 43.9% to 51.8% (p 0.03).[29] Based upon a 10% change, 40% of the intracranial stenoses progressed, 40% were stable, and 20% regressed. There were 4 TIAs and no strokes in the follow-up period [29]

   (ii) Among 40 patients with angiogram confirmed symptomatic MCA stenosis followed by TCD for a median of 26 months, one-third progressed radiographically and 60% remained stable. Progression of MCA stenosis detected by TCD was independently associated with recurrent ischemic events in the territory of the MCA stenosis and occurred in 8 patients (20%).

   (iii) Findings should be interpreted with caution, given the relatively small numbers [30]

k) Location of stenosis

   (i) some studies have suggested that the early stroke risk may be higher in patients with vertebrobasilar (VB) stenosis. The "higher" early stroke risk may be due to a higher prevalence of large artery stenosis in patients with posterior circulation events compared with carotid territory events. [31,32]

   (ii) In a population based study, 37/141(26.2%) symptomatic patients with VB events were found to have >50% vertebral or basilar stenosis compared with only 41/357(11.5%) of anterior circulation event patients found to have carotid stenosis.[Y] Furthermore, 17/37 (46%) patients who had symptomatic VB stenosis had a recurrent TIA or ischemic stroke in the posterior circulation within 90 days compared with 22/104 (21%) patients without VB stenosis. [32]

  (iii) subgroup analysis of patients with symptomatic intracranial VB stenosis in the retrospective WASID study suggested VB stenosis as a subgroup with a high risk of recurrent stroke (22%). [33] However, in the prospective WASID study, the location of stenosis (anterior versus posterior) was not a significant factor in the risk of recurrent stroke in the territory of the stenotic artery.[26]

3) Secondary stroke prevention
 a) The prospective WASID study [19]
  (i) patients with symptomatic ICAS (>50% on cerebral angiogram).
  (ii) Aspirin 1300mg per day vs warfarin dose adjusted to a target INR between 2 -3
  (iii) primary end point was ischemic stroke, brain hemorrhage, or death from vascular causes
  (iv) stopped early after enrolling 569 patients due to concerns about safety in the warfarin group
  (v) Warfarin was associated with significantly higher rates of adverse events and provided no benefit over aspirin
  (vi) primary end point occurred in 22.1% of aspirin group and 21.8% of warfarin group
  (vii) Conclusion: Aspirin should be used in preference to warfarin for patients with ICAS.
  (viii) Criticisms of the study
   a) unusual dosing of aspirin (1300mg per day)
   b) patients randomized to warfarin reached target INR only 63% of the time.
  (ix) Subgroups analysis [34]
   1) subset of basilar artery stenosis was the only group that showed decreased rate of primary outcome in the warfarin arm compared to the aspirin arm (18% vs 9%, p 0.04).
   2) However, many variables were tested without adjusting for multiple comparisons, and the wide confidence intervals and small sample size are problematic for definitive conclusions. Furthermore, there was no significant difference between aspirin and warfarin in the rates of

ischemic stroke in the territory of the symptomatic basilar artery. The lower rate of primary endpoint in the warfarin arm for the basilar stenosis subgroup is likely a result of chance.

3) Warfarin likely has no benefit in stroke reduction in patients with basilar artery stenosis.

b) Vascular risk factor modification

(i) reduces progression of disease, as well as for the added benefit of reducing overall cardiovascular risk.

(ii) In WASID Specific risk factors were associated with an increased risk of vascular events among patients with ICAS.[35]

1) Hyperlipidemia- cholesterol levels ($\geq$ 200 mg/dL) were associated with an increased risk of major vascular event (stroke, myocardial infarction, vascular death) in symptomatic ICAS [35]

2) Hypertension

a) elevated systolic blood pressure (SBP) ($\geq$ 140 mm Hg) were associated with an increased risk of major vascular event (stroke, myocardial infarction, vascular death) in symptomatic ICAS

b) clinical practice of maintaining high blood pressure in patients with intracranial stenosis to maintain perfusion is not recommended given the WASID subgroup analysis which found higher blood pressure is associated with increased risk of recurrent ischemic stroke[36]

(i) this increased stroke risk in the territory of the stenotic artery with elevated blood pressure persists even after adjustment for risk factors.

c) increased risk of stroke with higher blood pressure was driven mostly by patients in the highest SBP group (> 160 mmHg).[36]

d) optimal timing of the blood pressure lowering, remains uncertain and a subset of patients may benefit from permissive hypertension in the acute and early subacute periods following the event.

3) Other risk factors

   a) In WASID, hemoglobin A1c > 7% was associated with higher risk of major vascular event (31% vs 20%), although this difference was not significant, likely due to low statistical power.[35]

c) Future studies

   a) Despite medical therapy, symptomatic ICAS is associated with a high recurrent stroke risk. Interventional treatments are currently being studied as potential options to improve outcomes.

   b) SAMMPRIS is an ongoing randomized trial evaluating stenting versus medical management in symptomatic ICAS

Carotid Atherosclerosis

1) Prevalence- Over the age of 65 years, the prevalence of significant carotid stenosis is likely between 5-7% in women and 7-9% in men.

2) Non-modifiable predictors- The most notable non-modifiable predictors of carotid atherosclerosis include advancing age, male sex, family history, and race.

   a) Advancing age is perhaps the most influential non-modifiable risk factor for cerebral and cervical atherosclerosis.[1,4,37,38]

   b) Gender. Male sex is a significant independent predictor associated with increased rates of extracranial carotid atherosclerosis.[38]

   c) Family history. In the Framingham Offspring Study, 1662 adult children (mean age 57 years) of the original parental cohort were studied, and a family history of premature coronary heart disease in a parent was significantly associated with higher offspring carotid IMT on carotid ultrasound, even after adjustment for cardiovascular risk factors.[39]

3) Modifiable predictors
    a) Hypertension, cigarette smoking, and diabetes are established risk factors for carotid atherosclerosis and have been demonstrated in many studies.[40, 41,42,43,44,45]
    b) Hyperlipidemia
       (i) meta-analysis reported that each 10% reduction in low-density lipoprotein cholesterol reduced the risk of stroke by 15.6% and carotid intima–media thickness by 0.73% per year, supporting the suggestion that statin use may reduce progression of carotid atherosclerosis [46,47]
    c) Socioeconomic status (SES)
       (i) Studies demonstrate a strong association between SES and carotid atherosclerosis that is evident at early and advanced stages [48,49,50]
       (ii) Socioeconomic status not only affects the prevalence of symptomatic carotid atherosclerosis, but also the treatment, as the higher rate of symptomatic carotid disease in lower socioeconomic groups does not correspond with an increased rate of carotid endarterectomy [51]

4) Stroke Mechanism in carotid disease
    a) 2 distinct patterns of infarct in carotid disease include cortical (micro-embolism) and watershed/hemodynamic (low-flow) distribution. Evidence from clinical cerebral perfusion studies, ultrasound studies, and neuropathology studies support both mechanisms, suggesting an additive effect.[LLL]
       (i) Hemodynamic mechanism - positron emission tomography (PET) studies demonstrating increased oxygen extraction suggestive of decreased perfusion.[52]
       (ii) Micro-embolism mechanism- Clinically silent microemboli have also been demonstrated on transcranial Doppler in symptomatic carotid disease.[53, 54]
    b) Both explanations may be involved, with microemboli may be more likely to cause small cortical infarcts in the

setting of hypoperfusion due to decreased clearance of microemboli.[52]

Asymptomatic Carotid Stenosis

1) Prevalence- Extracranial asymptomatic carotid stenosis prevalence ranges from 3% to 15%, depending upon population studied (Table 4).
2) Carotid Bruit
   a) In the Framingham cohort, carotid bruit was observed in 3.5% of those age 44 - 54 years and in 7% age 65 - 79 years [58]
   b) Studies suggest that cervical bruits are not specific for the presence of extracranial carotid stenosis
      a) Presence of carotid bruit correlated positively with ultrasound in only 61%. False positive results (a bruit was audible) occurred in 23% in patients with normal Doppler exams, and false negative results (no bruit was heard) occurred in 16% with abnormal Doppler studies. Only 28% of asymptomatic patients would be correctly diagnosed if the presence of cervical bruit is used as the only sign of associated extracranial artery disease [59]
      b) Carotid bruits were correlated with the carotid arteriograms on 1004 patients.[vv] Positive predictive values of carotid bruit for ipsilateral extracranial carotid atherosclerosis were 64-77%, and for intracranial carotid atherosclerosis were 16-18%. A carotid bruit was audible in 30% of patients with 50-89% stenosis, and in 43% of those with 90-99% stenosis.[60] Confounding the issue is the fact that bruits can be audible in over 21% of occluded arteries [60]
   c) Screening for carotid occlusive disease
      (i) Some studies suggest that ultrasound screening for asymptomatic carotid stenosis (>60%) may be cost-effective when performed in high-prevalence populations (20% prevalence).[61,62,63] The benefit of screening low-prevalence asymptomatic

populations ($\leq$5%) is lost with angiographic or surgical complications [63]

(ii) Mass screening for asymptomatic carotid stenosis in the general population is not recommended as cost-effective

3) Natural history- Asymptomatic significant carotid stenosis is well-recognized to have significantly lower risk of future cerebral ischemia compared to symptomatic carotid disease.

a) Asymptomatic Carotid Atherosclerosis Study (ACAS) [64]

(i) Medical cohort on daily aspirin had an aggregate risk for ipsilateral stroke of 11% over 5 years, which yields an annual stroke rate of approximately 2%.

b) Asymptomatic Carotid Surgery Trial (ACST) [65]

(i) 5-year stroke risk in the arm assigned to deferred surgery was approximately 12%.

c) North American Symptomatic Carotid Endarterectomy Trial (NASCET) [66]

(i) 5-year risk of first stroke in co-existing asymptomatic contralateral stenosis was 8% in those with stenosis < 60% and 16.2% in those with a stenosis of 60-99%.

(ii) Highest 5-year stroke rate at 18.5% was seen in the patients with a stenosis of 75-94%

d) Annual rate of ipsilateral stroke in extracranial carotid stenosis is approximately 2-4%, based upon these observational studies (Table 5)

Table 4. Summary of carotid atherosclerotic disease prevalence studies

Author/Study	Population studied	Prevalence
Fine-Edelstein [42] Framingham Study	general population, almost exclusively white aged 66 to 93 years in the Framingham Study	$\geq$50% stenosis in 7% women, 9% men
O'Leary [55] Cardiovascular Health Study	5,201 patients >65 years in the Cardiovascular Health Study	$\geq$50% stenosis in 7% men, 5% women
Jungquist [56]	478 Men from Malmo Sweden, aged > 69 years	60-99% stenosis in 3% 1.5% occlusion
Roederer [43] University of Washington	patients referred to the vascular laboratory	$\geq$50% stenosis in 8% mild cervical bruits 14%

Hillen [57] Berlin Aging Study	225 healthy volunteers, aged 70-100, Population-based cross-sectional survey Berlin Aging Study	$\geq$ 50% stenosis in 15% $\geq$ 75% stenosis in 4%

4) Asymptomatic carotid stenosis and Carotid endarterectomy (CEA)

   a) Benefit of carotid endarterectomy in reducing the incidence of cerebral infarction for asymptomatic carotid stenosis >60% has been established by ACAS and ACST

   b) 3 Class I studies available (ACAS, ACST, VAS), and 2 other studies (MACE, CASANOVA) were stopped prematurely or poorly designed

      (i) ACAS and ACST had different primary endpoints. ACAS and the previous symptomatic trials utilized ipsilateral stroke as the primary endpoint whereas ACST included all strokes, including contralateral events and vertebrobasilar strokes. If the ACST analysis was limited to ipsilateral stroke only, the absolute benefit would be reduced.

   c) Asymptomatic Carotid Atherosclerosis Study (ACAS) [64]

      (i) 1,662 patients with 60 - 99% stenosis defined angiographically for the surgical group and primarily with ultrasound for the medical group.

      (ii) Study was halted by the Data Safety and Monitoring Board after 2.7 years median follow-up because of a projected 5.9% ARR at 5 years favoring CE (NNT = 17).

      (iii) 5-year projected rate of ipsilateral stroke was 11.0% for the medical group and 5.1% for surgical group (p = 0.004).

      (iv) NNH of 43

      (v) Very low perioperative stroke/death rate of 2.3%

      (vi) No benefit for CEA in women

   d) Veterans Affairs Study [67]

      (i) 444 men with angiographically proven 50 - 99% asymptomatic stenosis.

      (ii) There was a nonsignificant trend favoring CEA for prevention of ipsilateral stroke (9.4% vs 4.7% at 4 years). However, this was a secondary endpoint.

           (iii) The primary endpoint included TIA, which most clinicians consider as an inappropriate endpoint.

           (iv) The 30-day perioperative stroke and death rate was 4.7%, NNH of 21

e) Asymptomatic Carotid Surgery Trial (ACST) [65]

           (i) 3,120 patients randomized, 1,560 each group (immediate CEA vs indefinite deferral of CEA) with 5-year follow-up

           (ii) Determination of stenosis made by carotid ultrasound and expressed as percent diameter reduction. Eligibility included carotid artery diameter reduction of at least 60% on ultrasound and no symptoms within the past 6 months.

           (iii) Combining the perioperative events (stroke and death within 30 days) and the nonperioperative strokes, the 5-year risks were 6.4% (immediate CEA) vs 11.8% (deferred CEA) for all strokes (ARR 5.4% p , 0.0001)

           (iv) 2,044 men and 1,076 women. Men and women both benefited but there were only a total of 40 nonperioperative strokes in women

           (v) 5-year benefit of CE appeared to be as great for those with <80% diameter reduction (mean 69% stenosis) as for those with 80 to 99% (mean 87%) reduction.

f) Mayo Asymptomatic Carotid Endarterectomy (MACE) [69]

           (i) stopped prematurely after only 71 patients due to a high rate (22%) of myocardial infarction in surgical group (due to trial policy of withholding aspirin from the surgical group)

g) Carotid Artery Stenosis with Asymptomatic Narrowing: Operation Vs Aspirin (CASANOVA) [68]

           (i) suboptimal study design and conduct.

           (ii) 410 patients with 50 - 90% stenosis

           (iii) High rate of crossovers: 7% of surgical patients never received a CEA and 20% of the medical patients were given a unilateral or bilateral CEA. This deprived the study of the high risk patients who were of greatest interest and confused the overall interpretation of the data.

Table 5. Summary of Studies indicating the natural history of asymptomatic carotid stenosis

Study/Trial	Population	Risk
ACAS [64] 1662 patients	stenosis ≥ 60% Medical Surgical	Aggregate risk** over 5 years 11.0% (2% per year) 5.1% (1% per year)
NASCET [66] 1820 patients	stenosis < 50% 50-59% 60-74% 75-94% 95-99% occlusion	First Ipsilateral stroke over 5 years 7.8% (1.5% per year) 12.9% (2.5% per year) 14.8% (2.9% per year) 18.5% (3.7% per year) 14.7% (2.9% per year) 9.4% (1.8% per year)
Veterans Affairs study [67] 444 Men	stenosis ≥ 50% Medical Surgical	Ipsilateral stroke over 4 years 9.4% (2.4% per year) 4.7% (1.2 % per year)
ACST [65] 3120 patients	stenosis ≥ 60% Deferred (Medical) Surgical	5-year risk of any stroke 11.8% (2.3% per year) 6.4% (1.2% per year)
CASANOVA [68] 410 patients	stenosis ≥ 50%, complex design, over half of the non-surgical patients underwent CEA, inconclusive	
MACE [69] 71 patients	[†]trial policy of withholding ASA from surgical group lead to high rate of MI (26%)	

[†]Stopped prematurely,**stroke or death.

Symptomatic Carotid Stenosis

1) Natural history
   a) NASCET study for 70-99% carotid stenosis demonstrated a recurrent ipsilateral stroke rate of 26% over 2 years in the medical arm.[70] (Table 6)
   b) The elevated recurrent stroke rate (18% at 1 month) demonstrated in the Rochester, MN data compared with NASCET may be partly explained by the thorough screening and careful selection of included patients (i.e selection bias), whereas the population-based county data represent an unbiased sample.

Table 6. Summary of Studies indicating the natural history of symptomatic carotid stenosis

Study/Trial	Population	Risk
NASCET [66,70,71]	stenosis < 50% 50-69%	Ipsilateral stroke rate over 5 years 18.7% (3% per year) 22% (4% per year)
	stenosis 70-99% Medical Surgical	Ipsilateral stroke risk over 2 years 26% (13% per year) 9% (4% per year)
*ECST [72] 3024 patients	Any degree of stenosis Medical Surgical	Aggregate risk[‡] over 3 years 26.5% (8.8% per year) 14.9% (4.9% per year)
[†]Veteran Affairs Cooperative Study [73] 189 patients	stenosis $\geq$ 50% Medical Surgical stenosis $\geq$ 70% Medical Surgical	Ipsilateral stroke/TIA over 1 year 19.4% per year 7.7% per year 25.6% per year 7.9% per year

[†]Stopped prematurely, [‡]major stroke or death, **stroke or death

2) Degree of stenosis- In symptomatic carotid stenosis, the degree of stenosis significantly impacts the rate of recurrent ipsilateral stroke with higher risk corresponding to higher degrees of stenosis.

   a) In a re-analysis of the medical arm of the NASCET trial, the five-year rate of ipsilateral stroke in the symptomatic group with <50% extracranial stenosis was 18.7%. [70]

   b) This risk steadily climbed with increasing stenosis, with a risk of 20.2% in the 50-59% stenosis group, 25.8% in the 60-74% stenosis group, and 27.1% in the 75-94% stenosis group.[66]

   c) The risk of ipsilateral stroke in carotid stenosis has a U-shape curve, with risk peaking at a high degree of stenosis with subsequent decrease in near-occlusion and occlusion; the subset with 95-99% stenosis had a slightly lower risk of stroke at 17.2%.[66]

3) Symptomatic Carotid stenosis and Carotid endarterectomy (CEA)

   a) Benefit of carotid endarterectomy (CEA) over medical management in treatment of selected patients with carotid

stenosis shown by 2 Class 1 studies (NASCET and ECST).
A 3rd study (VACS) was stopped prematurely after the
NASCET and ECST results were announced
b) Difference between NASCET and ECST- method of
angiographic measurement (Figure 2)
   (i) NASCET calculated degree of stenosis using site of
   maximal narrowing as the numerator divided by the
   distal ICA diameter where the vessel walls became
   parallel and beyond any area of post stenotic
   dilatation.
   (ii) ECST calculated the degree of stenosis using the
   diameter at the site of maximal narrowing divided by
   the estimated diameter of the normal carotid bulb.
   (iii) NACET 70% stenosis corresponds to an 82% ECST
   stenosis
   (iv) In the original CEA trials, statins were not in
   widespread use and only a minority of patients was
   aggressively treated with lipid lowering agents
c) North American Symptomatic Carotid Endarterectomy
Trial (NASCET) [66]
   (i) Results showed a significant benefit of CEA in
   patients with 70-99% symptomatic stenosis
      1) 2 year ipsilateral stroke risk was 26% in
      medically treated patients and 9% in CEA group
      (p<0.001)

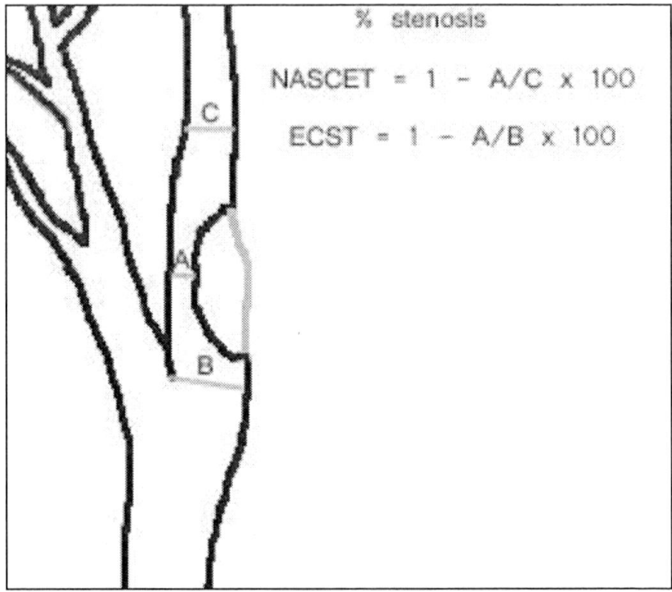

Figure 2. Measurement of carotid stenosis.

        2) Absolute risk reduction was 17%
        3) NNT was 6 at 2 years
   (ii) In the 50-69% symptomatic stenosis
        1) 5 year ipsilateral stroke rate was 15.7% in CEA group and 22.2% in medical group.
        2) In post-hoc analyses, the benefit was heterogenous. There was no benefit shown for CEA in women.
   (iii) In < 50% symptomatic stenosis
        1) No significant difference, a year ipsilateral stroke rate of 14.9% CEA vs 18.7% medical therapy group (p=0.16)
   (iv) There was a greater benefit from CEA in men compared to women. For prevention of an ipsilateral stroke, the NNT was 12 for men and 67 for women.
  d) European Carotid Surgery Trial (ECST) [72]
   (i) randomised controlled trial enrolled 3024 patients.
   (ii) any age, with some degree of carotid stenosis, who within the previous 6 months had had a transient or

mild symptomatic ischemic vascular event in the distribution of carotid arteries.

(iii) 1811 (60%) patients to surgery and 1213 (40%) to control (surgery to be avoided for as long as possible).

(iv) Outcome (major stroke or death) occurred in 669 (37·0%) surgery-group and 442 (36·5%) control-group.

(v) The risk of major ischemic stroke ipsilateral to the unoperated symptomatic carotid artery increased with severity of stenosis

(vi) Risk of major stroke or death at 3 years was 26·5% for the control group and 14·9% for the surgery group, an absolute benefit of 11·6%.

(vii) Conclusion: CEA is indicated for most patients with a recent non disabling carotid-territory ischaemic event when the symptomatic stenosis is > 80%.

e) Veterans Affairs Cooperative Studies Program 309 Trial (VACS) [73]

(i) Men with ischemic symptoms within 120 days of onset of symptoms due to (>50%) ipsilateral internal carotid artery stenosis (TIA, transient monocular blindness or small strokes)

(ii) Prospective, randomized, multicenter trial, 189 men randomized to CEA (n = 91) vs medical care (n = 98)

(iii) Endpoint- Cerebral infarction or crescendo transient ischemic attacks in the vascular distribution of the original symptoms or death within 30 days of randomization.

(iv) At a mean follow-up of 11.9 months, there was a significant reduction in stroke or crescendo TIAs in patients who received CEA (7.7%) compared with nonsurgical patients (19.4%), an absolute risk reduction of 11.7% (P = .011).

(v) The benefit of surgery was more profound in patients with internal carotid artery stenosis >70% (absolute risk reduction, 17.7%; P = .004)

f) Carotid Endarterectomy Trialists Collaboration (Rothwell) pooled analysis of the 3 symptomatic CEA trials [74]

(i) included 6,092 patients

(ii) Used NASCET definitions of stroke outcome events.

(iii) Benefit for CEA was shown for
1) 50-69% stenosis, ARR of 4.6% over 5 years (NNT 22)
2) 70% stenosis ARR of 16% over 5 years (NNT 6.3)
3) Near occlusion ARR of 5.6% over 2 years (p=0.19)
a) but only -1.7% over 5 years (p=0.9)
b) Near occlusion defined as angiographic collapsed ICA distal to stenosis, faster filling in the ECA compared to the ICA, & preferential filling of the intracranial circulation via collaterals
(iv) CEA not beneficial for symptomatic patients with 30-49% stenosis, and CEA harmful for symptomatic patients with < 30% stenosis
(v) Male sex (p = 0.003), age >75 (p = 0.03), and randomized within 2 weeks of the last symptomatic event (p = 0.009) were associated with greater CEA benefit [75]

g) In 2003, an estimated 117,000 inpatient CEA procedures were performed in the United States.[76]
(vi) Men have significantly higher surgery rates than women, and whites have significantly higher rates than blacks.
1) Data from the National Hospital Discharge Survey for 1980-1993 for people age $\geq$ 65 years demonstrated that CEA rates were 60% higher in men than women, and over four times higher in whites than blacks.[77]
2) disparity of CEA rates based upon gender and race may be partly explained by the higher prevalence of extracranial carotid occlusive disease in whites and males.

h) CEA Recommendations from AAN (Table 7)

Table 7. Carotid Endarterectomy Recommendations- American Academy of Neurology [78]

CEA is established as effective for recently symptomatic (within previous 6 months) patients with 70 to 99% ICA angiographic stenosis	Level A
CEA should not be considered for symptomatic patients with less than 50% stenosis	Level A
CEA may be considered for patients with 50 to 69% symptomatic stenosis but the clinician should consider additional clinical and angiographic variables	Level B Level C
It is recommended that the patient have at least a 5-year life expectancy and that the perioperative stroke/death rate should be <6% for symptomatic patients	Level A
Medical management is preferred to CEA for symptomatic patients with <50% stenosis	Level A
It is reasonable to consider CEA for patients between the ages of 40 and 75 years and with asymptomatic stenosis of 60 to 99% if the patient has an expected 5-year life expectancy and if the surgical stroke or death frequency can be reliably documented to be <3%	Level A
Women with 50 to 69% symptomatic stenosis did not show clear benefit in previous trials.	
In addition, patients with hemispheric TIA/stroke had greater benefit from CEA than patients with retinal ischemic events. Clinicians should also consider several radiologic factors in decision making about CEA..	Level C
For example, contralateral occlusion erases the small benefit of CEA in asymptomatic patients whereas in symptomatic patients, it is associated with increased operative risk but persistent benefit CEA for patients with angiographic near-occlusion in symptomatic patients is associated with a trend toward benefit at 2 years but not associated with a clear long-term benefit. Patients operated on within 2 weeks of their last TIA or mild stroke derive greater benefit from CE	
Symptomatic and asymptomatic patients undergoing CEA should be given aspirin (81 or 325 mg/day) prior to surgery and for at least 3 months following surgery to reduce the combined endpoint of stroke, myocardial infarction, and death	Level A
For patients with severe stenosis and a recent TIA or nondisabling stroke, CEA should be performed without delay, preferably within 2 weeks of the patient's last symptomatic event	Level C
There is insufficient evidence to support or refute the performance of CE within 4 to 6 weeks of a recent moderate to severe stroke	Level U

Carotid Stenting Studies

1) Stenting and Angioplasty with Protection in Patients at High Risk for Endarterectomy (SAPPHIRE) study [79]
   a) Compared high-risk patients CEA vs CAS
   b) 334 patients randomized
   c) Stopped because of slow enrollment
   d) No difference in long-term outcomes between CAS and CEA
2) CAVATAS (Carotid and Vertebral Artery Transluminal Angioplasty Study) [79]
   a) 504 pts
   b) Combine stroke or death rate at 30 days was Similar between 2 groups (10%)
3) Endarterectomy versus Angioplasty in Patients with Symptomatic Severe Carotid Stenosis (EVA-3S) [81]
   a) 527 pts randomized with >60% symptomatic carotid stenosis
   b) Stopped early in 2005 due to safety and futility-- higher 30 day rates of stroke and adverse events in the CAS arm
4) SPACE trial [82]
   a) Noninferiority study comparing CAS to CEA in symptomatic patients with high-grade (>70%) carotid artery stenosis
   b) 1713 patients
   c) study terminated because of inability to enroll
   d) Failure to prove noninferiority of CAS
5) Carotid Revascularization Endarterectomy vs Stent Trial (CREST) [83]
   a) CAS vs CEA in both symptomatic (>50%) and asymptomatic patients (60%)
   b) 2502 pts followed for mean 2.5 years
   c) no signicant different in primary events (stroke, MI or death) between 2 arms (7.2% CAS vs 6.8% CEA)
   d) Stroke more frequent with CAS and MI more likely after CEA
   e) Stenting tended to have greater efficacy in younger patients, age < 70
6) With the current evidence, Carotid stenting has no role in asymptomatic carotid stenosis.

7) Carotid stenting should be considered in patients with symptomatic carotid stenosis who are considered high surgical risk.

Carotid Occlusion

1) Incidence -The age and sex adjusted annual incidence of symptomatic carotid occlusion in Olmsted County, MN is 6 per 100,000 persons.[84]
2) Asymptomatic ICA occlusion
   a) considerably less risk of subsequent stroke than symptomatic carotid occlusion
   b) Natural history data on asymptomatic carotid occlusion can be derived from the NASCET trial, which demonstrated a 1.9% annual stroke risk in the territory of an asymptomatic occluded carotid artery.[66]
   c) Annual stroke rate in asymptomatic carotid occlusion is less than 2%.
3) Symptomatic ICA occlusion
   a) risk of recurrent cerebral infarction after symptomatic carotid occlusion is initially high at 30 days (8%), and then becomes relatively stable by 1 year (10%).[84]
   b) Extracranial to Intracranial Bypass Trial [11]
      (i) 1377 patients with symptomatic carotid atherosclerotic disease randomized to medical versus bypass surgery followed for an average of 56 months
      (ii) In the medical group of 714 patients, 59% were internal carotid artery occlusions. At the end of one year, 13.8% of these medical patients suffered stroke or death
      (iii) Final outcome included a 20% fatality rate in the medical arm, of which 6.6% of deaths were attributable to myocardial infarction or other cardiovascular etiologies
   c) High-risk subsets in symptomatic carotid occlusion
      (i) cerebral hemodynamic failure, as defined by increased oxygen extraction on positron emission tomography (PET) distal to a symptomatic carotid artery occlusion, was evaluated in 81 patients with an average follow-

up of 31.5 months.[85] Ipsilateral stroke occurred in 11 of 39 patients with hemodynamic failure and in only 2 of 42 patients without hemodynamic failure. The age-adjusted relative risk of ipsilateral stroke was approximately 7 times higher in hemodynamic failure, suggesting that PET may be a useful tool in identifying a subgroup of patients with symptomatic carotid occlusion at the highest risk for recurrent stroke [85]

(ii) Whether treatment of these high-risk patients with bypass will lead to a reduced risk of stroke is subject to ongoing study. Carotid Occlusion Surgery Study (COSS) is an NIH-funded, randomized clinical trial to determine if extracranial-intracranial (EC/IC) bypass surgery can reduce subsequent ipsilateral ischemic stroke (fatal and non-fatal) at two years. Eligible participants must have internal carotid artery occlusion producing hemispheric symptoms within the previous 120 days and ipsilateral increased oxygen extraction fraction (OEF) measured by positron emission tomography (PET).

Cardiac issues and Carotid Disease

1) Carotid disease as a marker for systemic atherosclerosis
   a) Coronary artery disease and extracranial carotid disease tends to coexist, as reflected by the high rate of myocardial infarction in patients with extracranial carotid disease
   b) The Mayo Asymptomatic Carotid Endarterectomy (MACE) Study [69]
      (i) illustrated the high incidence of coexistent coronary artery disease in patients with carotid stenosis when it was stopped prematurely due to a 26% rate of myocardial infarction in the surgical arm, likely due to withholding of aspirin in this group
   c) Patients with significant extracranial carotid atherosclerosis not only have a high incidence of coronary artery disease, but also accompanying peripheral vascular disease. A relatively high prevalence (almost one-third) of

extracranial carotid atherosclerotic disease (ranging from mild stenosis to occlusion) is seen in symptomatic peripheral vascular disease patients screened with ultrasound.[59,86]

d) The concomitant risk of coronary heart disease and cerebrovascular disease implies that both coronary heart disease and ischemic stroke are caused by the same "type" of atherosclerotic disease. However, inconsistent with this theory is the paradoxically high risk of stroke observed in certain populations with low risk of coronary heart disease.

   (i) "paradox" of high risk of stroke in populations with low risk of coronary heart disease was notably first observed in the Japanese population. [42,87,88]

   (ii) Stroke, unlike coronary artery disease, is a heterogeneous disorder comprised of various distinctive subtypes, of which extracranial carotid atherosclerosis accounts for only a fraction. This may partly explain the dichotomy, since blacks and Asians have more intracranial atherosclerotic disease, while whites have more extracranial disease, a marker of coronary atherosclerosis [6,8,10]

2) Carotid occlusive atherosclerosis in the setting of coronary artery bypass grafting (CABG)

   a) Since coronary and carotid disease tends to coexist, the occurrence of carotid disease in the setting of coronary artery bypass surgery (CABG) is not uncommon.

   b) Estimates indicate that 91% of CABG patients have no occlusive carotid disease, 5.5% have unilateral 50–99% stenosis, 2% have bilateral 50–99% stenoses, and 1.5% have carotid occlusion [89]

   c) In 2003, an estimated 467,000 coronary artery bypass surgeries were performed on 268,000 patients in the United States.[76] The overall risk of stroke following coronary artery bypass is low at 1.5-2% [89] but coexistent carotid stenosis or occlusion can predispose patients to a higher risk.[90]

   d) Influenced by NASCET data demonstrating a clear benefit of surgical treatment for symptomatic high-grade carotid stenosis, most centers currently accept a standard policy of CABG with prophylactic endarterectomy or carotid angioplasty/stenting (staged or synchronous) in patients with symptomatic carotid disease.

e) The risk of peri-operative stroke in the setting of carotid occlusion and CABG has a variable range, depending upon the study reviewed. D

f) Based upon aggregate data, the highest peri-operative stroke risk is observed in CABG patients with known carotid occlusion (11.5%) compared with stenosis $\geq$50% (6.7%) and no significant carotid disease (1.9%).[89] (Table 8).

Table 8. Data on carotid occlusion and CABG from selected studies.

	stroke/overall CABG (%)	%ICAO	stroke/CABG & ICAO (%)
Dashe [90]	22/1022 (2.2%)	2.4%	[†]2/25 (8%)
Furlan [91]	*	*	[†]4/49 (2%)
Tunio [92]	60/3344 (1.8%)	1.8%	4/61 (6.5%)
Ricotta [93]	29/1779 (1.6%)	1.7%	0/31 (0%)
Schwartz [94]	12/582 (2.1%)	3.6%	[†]1/21 (4.7%)
Mickleborough [95]	19/1631 (1.2%)	1.9%	[‡]6/31 (19.3%)

*not applicable, [†]ipsilateral, [‡]one contralateral, ICAO= internal carotid occlusion, CABG= coronary artery bypass grafting surgery.

Chapter Keypoints

- Whites are more likely to have extracranial carotid atherosclerosis, whereas intracranial atherosclerosis (ICAS) is more prevalent in Hispanic, Asians, and Blacks.
- Stroke recurrence rate for symptomatic LAA may be as high as 18% at 1-month
- Annual ipsilateral stroke risk for asymptomatic ICAS is approximately 1.4-3.5%.
- Annual ipsilateral stroke rate for symptomatic ICAS is approximately 12%
- Unlike asymptomatic ICAS, the stroke risk in symptomatic ICAS is not uniformly distributed over time, but is much higher during the acute period after an event.

- Stroke rate is increased in subgroup of patients with certain features, such as high-grade stenosis, recent event, and female gender
- Other factors such as radiographic progression of stenosis, type of qualifying event, and location of stenosis, have been considered possible risk factors of recurrent stroke
- In patients with certain high risk features (stenosis > 70%, within 30 days of the qualifying event), the 1 year ipsilateral stroke rate may be as high as 29%.
- patients with symptomatic ICAS, Aspirin use is recommended in preference to warfarin
- Extracranial carotid stenosis prevalence ranges from 3- 20%, depending upon the population studied.
- Significant modifiable risk factors for carotid atherosclerosis are duration of cigarette smoking, and duration and severity of hypertension and diabetes
- Annual stroke rate for people with asymptomatic extracranial carotid stenosis is approximately 2%.
- Annual risk of recurrent stroke at after symptomatic carotid occlusion is 8-10%, compared to an annual stroke rate in asymptomatic carotid occlusion of less than 2%.
- Carotid artery stenosis is an important marker of generalized atherosclerosis, especially coronary artery disease.
- Presence of significant carotid stenosis predisposes patients to a higher risk of peri-operative stroke following coronary artery bypass surgery (approximately 6%).

References

[1] Solberg LA, McGarry PA, Moossy J, et al. *Distribution of cerebral atherosclerosis by geographic location, race, and sex.* Lab Invest 1968;18:144–152

[2] Sacco RL, Kargman DE, Gu Q, Zamanillo MC. *Race-ethnicity and determinants of intracranial atherosclerotic cerebral infarction. The Northern Manhattan Stroke Study. Stroke. 1995;26:14-20.*

[3] Petty GW, Brown RD Jr, Whisnant JP, Sicks JD, O'Fallon WM, Wiebers DO. *Ischemic stroke subtypes: a population-based study of functional outcome, survival, and recurrence. Stroke. 2003;31:1062-8.*

[4]   Gorelick PB. *Distribution of atherosclerotic cerebrovascular lesions. Effects of age, race, and sex.* Stroke. 1993;24:I16-9 .

[5]   Gorelick PB, Caplan LR, Langenberg P, Hier DB, Pessin M, Patel D, Taber J. *Clinical and angiographic comparison of asymptomatic occlusive cerebrovascular disease. Neurology.1988;38:852-8.*

[6]   Gorelick PB, Caplan LR, Hier DB, Parker SL, Patel D. *Racial differences in the distribution of anterior circulation occlusive disease.* Neurology. 1984;34:54–59.

[7]   Solberg LA, McGarry PA. *Cerebral atherosclerosis in Negroes an.d Caucasians.* Atherosclerosis 1972; 16:141–154.

[8]   Feldmann E, Daneault N, Kwan E, et al. *Chinese–White differences in the distribution of occlusive cerebrovascular disease.* Neurology 1990;40:1541–1545.

[9]   Lynch GF, Gorelick PB. *Stroke in African Americans. Neurologic Clinics. 2000;18:273-90.*

[10]   Sacco RL, Boden-Albala B, Abel G, Lin IF, Elkind M, Hauser WA, Paik MC, Shea S. *Race-ethnic disparities in the impact of stroke risk factors: the northern Manhattan stroke study. Stroke. 2001;32:1725-31.*

[11]   The EC/IC Bypass Study Group. *Failure of extracranial-intracranial arterial bypass to reduce the risk of ischemic stroke: results of an international randomized trial.* N Engl J Med. 1985;313:1191-2000.

[12]   Kern R, Steinke W, Daffertshofer M, Prager R, Hennerici M. *Stroke recurrences in patients with symptomatic vs asymptomatic middle cerebral artery disease.* Neurology. 2005;65:859-864.

[13]   Nahab F, Cotsonis G, Lynn M, Feldmann E, Chaturvedi S, Hemphill JC, Zweifler R, Johnston K, Bonovich D, Kasner S, Chimowitz M and for the WASID Study Group. *Prevalence and Prognosis of Coexistent Asymptomatic Intracranial Stenosis.* Stroke. 2008;39;1039-1041.

[14]   Kremer C, Schaettin T, Georgiadis D, Baumgartner RW. *Prognosis of asymptomatic stenosis of the middle cerebral artery.* J Neurol Neurosurg Psychiatry. 2004;75:1300-1303.

[15]   Craig DR, Meguro K, Watridge C, Robertson JT, Barnett HJ, Fox AJ. *Intracranial internal carotid artery stenosis.* Stroke. 1982;13:825–828.

[16]   Marzewski DJ, Furlan AJ, St Louis P, Little JR, Modic MT, Williams G. *Intracranial internal carotid artery stenosis: longterm prognosis.* Stroke. 1982;13:821-824.

[17] Moufarrij NA, Little JR, Furlan AJ, Leatherman JR, Williams GW. *Basilar and distal vertebral artery stenosis: long-term follow-up.* Stroke.1986;17:938-942.

[18] The WASID study group. *Prognosis of patients with symptomatic vertebral or basilar artery stenosis. The warfarin-aspirin symptomatic intracranial disease (WASID) study group.* Stroke. 1998;29:1389 - 1392.

[19] Chimowitz MI, Lynn MJ, Howlett-Smith H, Stern BJ, Hertzberg VS, Frankel MR, Levine SR, Chaturvedi S, Kasner SE, Benesch CG, Sila CA, Jovin TG, Romano JG. *Warfarin-Aspirin Symptomatic Intracranial Disease Trial Investigators. Comparison of warfarin and aspirin for symptomatic intracranial arterial stenosis. New England Journal of Medicine. 2005;352:1305-16.*

[20] Bogousslavsky J, Barnett HJ, Fox AJ, Hachinski VC, Taylor W. *Atherosclerotic disease of the middle cerebral artery.* Stroke. 1986;17:1112-1120.

[21] Corston RN, Kendall BE, Marshall J. *Prognosis in middle cerebral artery stenosis.* Stroke. 1984;15:237-241.

[22] Mazighi M, Tanasescu R, Ducrocq X, Vicaut E, Bracard S, Houdart E, Woimant F. *Prospective study of symptomatic atherothrombotic intracranial stenoses: The GESICA Study.* Neurology. 2006; 66:1187-1191.

[23] Thijs VN, Albers GW. *Symptomatic intracranial atherosclerosis Outcome of patients who fail antithrombotic therapy.* Neurology. 2000;55:490-497.

[24] Kwon SU, Cho YJ, Koo JS, Bae HJ, Lee YS, Hong KS, Lee JH, Kim JS. *Cilostazol Prevents the Progression of the Symptomatic Intracranial Arterial Stenosis: The Multicenter Double-Blind Placebo-Controlled Trial of Cilostazol in Symptomatic Intracranial Arterial Stenosis.* Stroke 2005;36;782-786.

[25] Famakin BM, Chimowitz MI, Lynn MJ, Stern BJ, George MG, and for the WASID Trial Investigators. *Causes and Severity of Ischemic Stroke in Patients With Symptomatic Intracranial Arterial Stenosis.* Stroke. 2009;40:1999-2003.

[26] Kasner SE, Chimowitz MI, Lynn MJ, Howlett-Smith H, Stern BJ, Hertzberg VS, Frankel MR, Levine SR, Chaturvedi S, Benesch CG, Sila CA, Jovin TG, Romano JG, Cloft HJ. *Warfarin Aspirin Symptomatic Intracranial Disease Trial Investigators. Predictors of ischemic stroke in the territory of a symptomatic intracranial arterial stenosis.* Circulation. 2006;113:555-563.

[27] Petty GW, Brown RD Jr, Whisnant JP, Sicks JD, O'Fallon WM, Wiebers DO. *Ischemic stroke subtypes: a population-based study of incidence and risk factors*. Stroke. *1999;30:2513-6.*

[28] Williams JE, Chimowitz MI, Cotsonis GA, Lynn MJ, Waddy SP and for the WASID Investigators. *Gender Differences in Outcomes Among Patients With Symptomatic Intracranial Arterial Stenosis*. Stroke. 2007;38;2055-2062.

[29] Akins PT, Pilgram TK, Cross DT, Moran CJ. *Natural History of Stenosis from Intracranial Atherosclerosis by Serial Angiography*. Stroke. 1998;29;433-438

[30] Arenillas JF, Molina CA, Montaner J, Abilleira S, González-Sánchez MA, Álvarez-Sabín J. *Progression and Clinical Recurrence of Symptomatic Middle Cerebral Artery Stenosis: A Long-Term Follow-Up Transcranial Doppler Ultrasound Study*. Stroke. 2001;32;2898-2904.

[31] Flossmann E, Rothwell PM. *Prognosis of vertebrobasilar transient ischaemic attack and minor stroke*. Brain. 2003;126:1940-54.

[32] Marquardt L, Kuker W, Chandratheva A, Geraghty O, Rothwell PM. *Incidence and prognosis of >50% symptomatic vertebral or basilar artery stenosis: prospective population-based study*. Brain 2009:132;982-988.

[33] The WASID study group. *Prognosis of patients with symptomatic vertebral or basilar artery stenosis. The warfarin-aspirin symptomatic intracranial disease (WASID) study group*. Stroke. 1998;29:1389 - 1392.

[34] Kasner SE, Lynn MJ, Chimowitz MI, Frankel MR, Howlett-Smith H, Hertzberg VS, Chaturvedi S, Levine SR, Stern BJ, Benesch CG, Jovin TG, Sila CA, Romano JG and *for the Warfarin Aspirin Symptomatic Intracranial Disease (WASID) Trial Investigators. Warfarin vs aspirin for symptomatic intracranial stenosis: Subgroup analyses from WASID*. Neurology. 2006;67;1275-1278.

[35] Chaturvedi S, Turan TN, Lynn MJ, et al. *Risk factor status and vascular events in patients with symptomatic intracranial stenosis*. Neurology. 2007;69:2063-8.

[36] Turan TN, Cotsonis G, Lynn MJ, Chaturvedi S, Chimowitz M, *for the Warfarin-Aspirin Symptomatic Intracranial Disease (WASID) Trial Investigators. Relationship Between Blood Pressure and Stroke Recurrence in Patients With Intracranial Arterial Stenosis*. Circulation 2007;115;2969-2975.

[37] McGill HC, Arias-Stella J, Carbonell LM, Correa P, DeVeyra EA, Donoso S et al. *General findings of the International Atherosclerosis Project*. Lab Invest. 1968;18:498-512.

[38] Whisnant JP, Homer D, Ingall TJ, Baker HL Jr, O'Fallon WM, Wiebers DO. *Duration of cigarette smoking is the strongest predictor of severe extracranial carotid artery atherosclerosis*. Stroke 1990;21:707-14.

[39] Wang TJ, Nam BH, D'Agostino RB, Wolf PA, Lloyd-Jones DM, MacRae CA, Wilson PW, Polak JF, O'Donnell CJ. *Carotid intima-media thickness is associated with premature parental coronary heart disease: the Framingham Heart Study. Circulation. 2003;108:572-6.*

[40] O'Leary DH, Polak JF, Kronmal RA, Kittner SJ, Bond MG, Wolfson SK Jr, Bommer W, Price TR, Gardin JM, Savage PJ. *Distribution and correlates of sonographically detected carotid artery disease in the Cardiovascular Health Study. The CHS Collaborative Research Group. Stroke. 1992;23:1752-60.*

[41] Wilson PW, Hoeg JM, D'Agostino RB, Silbershatz H, Belanger AM, Poehlmann H, O'Leary D, Wolf PA. *Cumulative effects of high cholesterol levels, high blood pressure, and cigarette smoking on carotid stenosis. New England Journal of Medicine. 1997;337:516-22*

[42] Fine-Edelstein JS, Wolf PA, O'Leary DH, Poehlman H, Belanger AJ, Kase CS, D'Agostino RB. *Precursors of extracranial carotid atherosclerosis in the Framingham Study. Neurology.1994;44:1046-50.*

[43] Roederer GO, Langlois YE, Jager KA, et al. *The natural history of carotid arterial disease in asymptomatic patients with cervical bruits.* Stroke 1984;15:605-13.

[44] Whisnant JP, Homer D, Ingall TJ, Baker HL Jr, O'Fallon WM, Wiebers DO. *Duration of cigarette smoking is the strongest predictor of severe extracranial carotid artery atherosclerosis*. Stroke. 1990;21:707-14.

[45] Ingall TJ, Homer D, Baker HL Jr, Kottke BA, O'Fallon WM, Whisnant JP. *Predictors of intracranial carotid artery atherosclerosis. Duration of cigarette smoking and hypertension are more powerful than serum lipid levels.* Archives of Neurology. 1991;48:687-91.

[46] Amarenco P, Labreuche J, Lavallee P, Touboul PJ. *Statins in stroke prevention and carotid atherosclerosis: systematic review and up-to-date meta-analysis.* Stroke. 2004;35:2902-9.

[47] Kang S, Wu Y, Li X. *Effects of statin therapy on the progression of carotid atherosclerosis: a systematic review and meta-analysis.* Atherosclerosis. *2004;177:433-42.*

[48] Engstrom G, Jerntrop I, Pessah-Rasmussen H, Hedblad B, Berglund G, Janzon L. *Geographic distribution of stroke incidence within an urban population: relations to socio-economic circumstances and prevalence of cardiovascular risk factors.* Stroke. 2001;32:1098-1103.

[49] Jakovljevic D, Sarti C, Sivenius J et al. *Socioeconomic status and ischaemic stroke: The FINOMICA Stroke Register.* Stroke 2001; 32:14926.

[50] Lynch J, Kaplan GA, Salonen R, Cohen RD, Salonen JT. *Socioeconomic status and carotid atherosclerosis. Circulation. 1995;92:1786-92.*

[51] MacKenzie R, Nimmo F, Bachoo P, Alozairi O, Brittenden J. *The relationship between socio-economic status, geography, symptomatic carotid territory disease and carotid endarterectomy. European Journal of Vascular & Endovascular Surgery. 2003;26:145-9.*

[52] Momjian-Mayor I, Baron JC. *The pathophysiology of watershed infarction in internal carotid artery disease: review of cerebral perfusion studies.* Stroke 2005;36:567-77.

[53] Siebler M, Sitzer M, Steinmetz H. *Detection of intracranial emboli in patients with symptomatic extracranial carotid artery disease. Stroke. 1992;23:1652–*1654.

[54] Markus H. *Transcranial doppler detection of circulating cerebral emboli. A review. Stroke.* 1993;24:1246–1250.

[55] O'Leary DH, Polak JF, Kronmal RA, Kittner SJ, Bond MG, Wolfson SK Jr, Bommer W, Price TR, Gardin JM, Savage PJ. *Distribution and correlates of sonographically detected carotid artery disease in the Cardiovascular Health Study. The CHS Collaborative Research Group. Stroke. 1992;23:1752-60.*

[56] Jungquist G, Hanson BS, Isacsson SO, Janzon L, Steen B, Lindell SE. *Risk factors for carotid artery stenosis: an epidemiological study of men aged 69 years.* J Clin Epidemiol 1991;44:347-5386[JJJ] Furlan AJ, Craciun AR. *Risk of stroke during coronary artery bypass graft surgery in patients with internal artery disease documented by angiography.* Stroke 1985;16:797-799.

[57] Hillen T, Nieczaj R, Munzberg H, Schaub R, Borchelt M, Steinhagen-Thiessen E. *Carotid atherosclerosis, vascular risk profile and mortality in a population-based sample of functionally healthy elderly subjects: the Berlin ageing study. Journal of Internal Medicine. 2000;247:679-88.*

[58] Wolf PA, Kannel WB, Sorlie P, McNamara P, *Asymptomatic carotid bruit and risk of stroke. The Framingham study. JAMA.1981;245:1442-5.*

[59] Hennerici M, Aulich A, Sandmann W, Freund H-J. *Incidence of asymptomatic extracranial arterial disease.* Stroke. 1981;12:750-758.

[60] Ingall TJ, Homer D, Whisnant JP, Baker HL Jr, O'Fallon WM. *Predictive value of carotid bruit for carotid atherosclerosis.* Archives of Neurology.1989;46:418-22.

[61] Yin D, Carpenter JP. *Cost-effectiveness of screening for asymptomatic carotid stenosis. Journal of Vascular Surgery. 1998;27(2):245-55.*

[62] Derdeyn CP, Powers WJ. *Cost-effectiveness of screening for asymptomatic carotid atherosclerotic disease. Stroke.1996;27:1944-50.*

[63] Derdeyn CP, Powers WJ, Moran CJ, Cross DT, Allen BT. *Role of Doppler US in screening for carotid atherosclerotic disease.* Radiology. 1995;197:635-43.

[64] Executive Committee for the Asymptomatic Carotid Atherosclerosis Study. *Endarterectomy for asymptomatic carotid artery stenosis.* JAMA 1995;273:1421-8.

[65] MRC Asymptomatic Carotid Surgery Trial (ACST) *Collaborative Group. Prevention of disabling and fatal strokes by successful carotid endarterectomy in patients without recent neurological symptoms: randomized controlled trial.* Lancet 2004;363:1491–1502.

[66] Inzitari D, Eliasziw M, Gates P, Sharpe BL, Chan RK, Meldrum HE, Barnett HJ. *The causes and risk of stroke in patients with asymptomatic internal-carotid-artery stenosis. North American Symptomatic Carotid Endarterectomy Trial Collaborators. New England Journal of Medicine. 2000;342:1693-700.*

[67] Hobson RW, Weiss DG, Fields WS, Goldstone J, Moore WS, Towne JB, Wright CB, *for the Veterans Affairs Cooperative Study Group. Efficacy of carotid endarterectomy for asymptomatic carotid stenosis.* N Engl J Med. 1993;328:221–227.

[68] The CASANOVA Study Group. *The Carotid surgery versus medical therapy in asymptomatic carotid stenosis.* Stroke. 1991;1229-1235.

[69] Mayo Asymptomatic Carotid Endarterectomy Study Group. *Effectiveness of carotid endarterectomy for asymptomatic carotid stenosis: design of a clinical trial.* Mayo Clin Proc 1992;64:897–904.

[70] Barnett HJM, Taylor DW, Eliasziw M, Fox AJ, Ferguson GG, Haynes RB, Rankin RN, Clagett GP, Hachinski VC, Sackett DL, Thorpe KE, Meldrum HE, Spence JD. *Benefit of carotid endarterectomy in patients with symptomatic moderate or severe stenosis.* N Engl J Med 1998;339:1415–1425.

[71] North American Symptomatic Carotid Endarterectomy Trial Collaborators. *Beneficial effect of carotid endarterectomy in symptomatic patients with high-grade carotid stenosis.* N Engl J Med 1991;325:445-53.

[72] European Carotid Surgery Trialists' Collaborative Group. *Randomised trial of endarterectomy for recently symptomatic carotid stenosis: final results of the MRC European Carotid Surgery Trial (ECST).* Lancet 1998;351:1379–1387.

[73] Mayberg MR, Wilson SE, Yatsu F, Weiss DG, Messina L, Hershey LA, Colling C, Eskridge J, Deykin D, Winn HR. *Carotid endarterectomy and prevention of cerebral ischemia in symptomatic carotid stenosis. Veterans Affairs Cooperative Studies Program 309 Trialist Group.* JAMA 1991;266:3289–3294.

[74] Rothwell PM, Eliasziw M, Gutnikov SA, et al. *Analysis of pooled data from the randomised controlled trials of endarterectomy for symptomatic carotid stenosis.* Lancet 2003; 361: 107–16.

[75] Rothwell PM, Eliasziw M, Gutnikov SA, Warlow CP, Barnett HJM, for the Carotid Endarterectomy Trialists Collaboration. *Endarterectomy for symptomatic carotid stenosis in relation to clinical subgroups and timing of surgery.* Lancet. 2004;363:915–924.

[76] Thom T, Haase N, Rosamond W, Howard VJ, Rumsfeld J, Manolio T, Zheng ZJ, Flegal K, O'Donnell C, Kittner S, Lloyd-Jones D, Goff DC Jr, Hong Y, Adams R, Friday G, Furie K, Gorelick P, Kissela B, Marler J, Meigs J, Roger V, Sidney S, Sorlie P, Steinberger J, Wasserthiel-Smoller S, Wilson M, Wolf P. *American Heart Association Statistics Committee and Stroke Statistics Subcommittee. Heart disease and stroke statistics--2006 update: a report from the American Heart Association Statistics Committee and Stroke Statistics Subcommittee. Circulation. 2006;113:e85-151.*

[77] Gillum RF. *Epidemiology of carotid endarterectomy and cerebral arteriography in the United States. Stroke.* 1995;26:1724-1728.

[78] Chaturvedi S, Bruno A, Feasby T, Holloway R, Benavente O, Cohen SN, Cote R, Hess D, Saver J, Spence JD, Stern B, Wilterdink J. *Carotid Endarterectomy - An evidence-based review- Report of the Therapeutics and Technology Assessment Subcommittee of the American Academy of Neurology.* Neurology. 2005;65:794–801.

[79] Yadav JS, Wholey MH, Kuntz RE, et al. *Protected carotidartery stenting versus endarterectomy in high-risk patients.* N Engl J Med 2004;351:1493-501.

[80] CAVATAS Investigators. *Endovascular versus surgical treatment in patients with carotid stenosis in the Carotid and Vertebral Artery Transluminal Angioplasty Study (CAVATAS): a randomised trial.* Lancet 2001;357:1729-37.

[81] Mas J-L, Chatellier G, Beyssen B, et al. *Endarterectomy versus stenting in patients with symptomatic severe carotid stenosis.* N Engl J Med 2006;355:1660

[82] Ringleb PA, Allenberg J, Brückmann H, et al. 30 *Day results from the SPACE trial of stent-protected angioplasty versus carotid endarterectomy in symptomatic patients: a randomized non-inferiority trial.*Lancet 2006;368:1238.

[83] Brott TG, Hobson RW II, Howard G, et al. *Stenting versus endarterectomy for treatment of carotid-artery stenosis.* N Engl J Med 2010;363:11-23.

[84] Flaherty ML, Flemming KD, McClelland R, Jorgensen NW, Brown RD Jr. Population-based study of symptomatic internal carotid artery *occlusion: incidence and long-term follow-up. Stroke. 2004;35:e349-52*

[85] Grubb RL Jr, Derdeyn CP, Fritsch SM, Carpenter DA, Yundt KD, Videen TO, Spitznagel EL, Powers WJ. *Importance of hemodynamic factors in the prognosis of symptomatic carotid occlusion.* JAMA. *1998;280:1055-60.*

[86] Pilcher JM, Danaher J, Khaw KT. *The prevalence of asymptomatic carotid artery disease in patients with peripheral vascular disease. Clinical Radiology. 2000;55:56-61.*

[87] Kuller L, Reisler DM. *An explanation for variations in distribution of stroke and arteriosclerotic heart disease among populations and racial groups.* American journal of epidemiology. 1971;93:1-9.

[88] Reed DM. *The paradox of high risk of stroke in populations with low risk of coronary heart disease.* Am J Epidemiol 1990;131:579–588.

[89] Naylor AR, Mehta Z, Rothwell PM, Bell PR. *Carotid Artery disease and stroke during coronary artery bypass: a critical review of the literature.* Eur J Vasc Endovasc Surg. 2002;4:283-94.

[90] Dashe JF, Pessin MS, Murphy RE and Payne DD. *Carotid occlusive disease and stroke risk in coronary artery bypass graft surgery.* Neurol. 1997;49: 678–686.

[91] Furlan AJ, Craciun AR. Risk of stroke during coronary artery bypass graft surgery in patients with internal artery disease documented by angiography. Stroke. 1985;16:797-799.

[92] Tunio AM, Hingorani A, Ascher E. *Impact of an occluded internal carotid artery on the mortality and morbidity of patients undergoing coronary artery bypass grafting.* Am J Surg. 1999;178:201-5.

[93] Ricotta JJ, Faggiolii GL, Castilone A, Hassett JM. *Risk factors for stroke after cardiac surgery: Buffalo Cardiac–Cerebral Study Group.* J Vasc Surg 1995;21:359–364.

[94] Schwartz LB, Bridgman AH, Kieffer RW, *Asymptomatic carotid artery stenosis and stroke in patients undergoing cardiopulmonary bypass.* J Vasc Surg. 1995;21:146–153.

[95] Mickleborough LL, Walker PM and Takagi Y. *Risk factors for stroke in patients undergoing coronary artery bypass.* J Thorac Cardiovasc Surg. 1996; 112:1250–1259.

In: Handbook of Stroke and Neurocritical Care   ISBN: 978-61324-786-0
Editor: V. H. Lee   © 2012 Nova Science Publishers, Inc.

Chapter IV

Small Vessel Disease Occlusion

Vivien H. Lee

Department of Neurological Sciences,
Section of Stroke and Neurocritical care,
Rush University Medical Center, Chicago, IL, USA

1) subcortical infarcts that results from occlusion of a single penetrating artery
2) also known as Lacunar infarcts
   a) "lacune" = lake
3) Epidemiology
   a) SVD has best functional outcome, 82% had good functional outcome (defined as mRS of 1 or 2) at 1 year [1]
   b) SVD has lowest recurrence rate and highest survival [1,2,3,4]
   c) Study
      (i) SVD had lower baseline NIHSS, lower mortalitied, and no symptomatic ICH, Better outcomes in SVD even after adjusting for baseline NIHSS [5]
   d) Clinical Lacunar syndromes had an overall positive predictive value (PPV) of 87% for detecting radiologic

lacune, and was best for pure sensory and ataxic hemiparesis [6]

   e) Pure motore hemiparesis and senosorimotor stroke are poorly predicate of lacunar stroke [7]
4) Pathophysiology
   a) Autopsy findings of small cavitations, Typically < 15mm diameter
   b) Lipohyalinosis (fibrinoid degeneration)
   c) Penetrating vessels (Figure 1)
       (i) Arterioles
            1) terminal arterial vessels (i.e., immediately preceding a capillary bed)
            2) 90° angle into cortex
            3) only a single layer of smooth muscle cells (aterioles lack elastic lamina) and therefore are preferentially damaged from hypertension
       (ii) Lenticulostriate branches of MCA
       (iii) penetrating arteries from AchA
       (iv) Thalmogeniculate penetrators from PCAs
       (v) Paramedian perforators from basilar

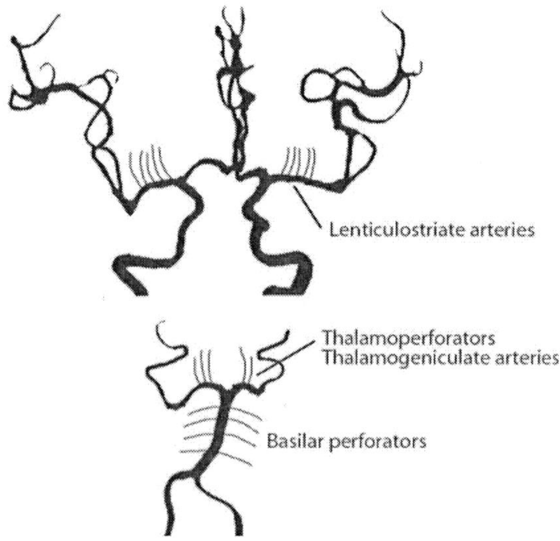

Figure 1. Perforator arteries affected in lacunar infarcts.

5) Typical locations of lacunar infarcts (figure 2)

a) Basal ganglia
   (i) Putamen
   (ii) Globus pallidus
   (iii) Thalamus
   (iv) Caudate
b) Subcortical white matter (internal capsule and corona radiate)
c) Pons
d) Cerebellum

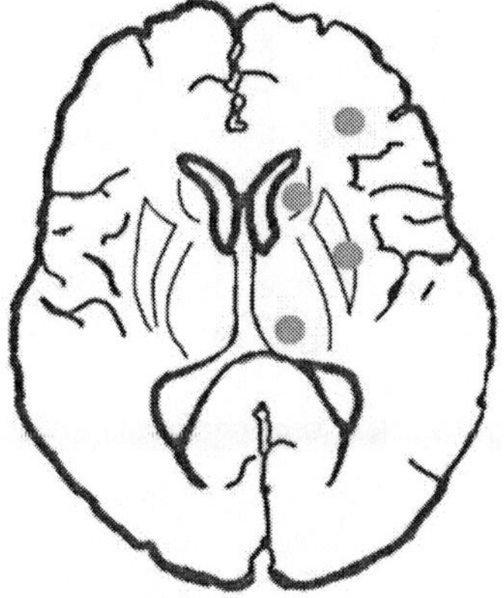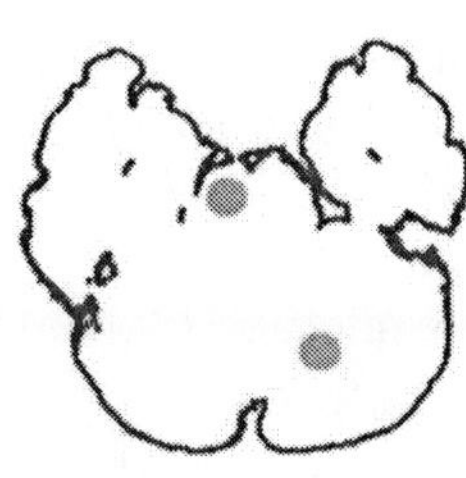

Figure 2. Typical Location of lacunar infarcts.

6) Clinical lacunar syndrome
   a) Lack of cortical symptoms (visual fields)
   b) Clinically can stutter before completing (capsular warning syndrome)
7) Classical Lacunar syndromes, described by Miller Fisher [8,9,10] [JKL]
   a) Pure motor – pons/internal capsule
      (i) "capsular warning syndrome" – hemiplegic TIAs preceding the event
   b) Pure sensory- thalalmus
   c) Sensorimotor- thalamocapsular
   d) Clumsy hand dysarthria- pons
   e) Ataxic hemiparesis – internal capsule, midbrain, pons
8) Mega lacunars
   a) Large deep infarcts (> 15mm)

b) Misnomer as most are really not lacunes, but typically are large artery or cardioembolic
c) May be due to an embolus initially arrested in the MCA stem and affected multiple lenticulostriate branches
d) Due to parent artery (MCA, basilar artery) atheroma that occludes the origin of the penetrator artery

References

[1] Petty GW, Brown RD Jr, Whisnant JP, Sicks JD, O'Fallon WM, Wiebers DO. Ischemic stroke subtypes: a population-based study of functional outcome, survival, and recurrence. *Stroke.* 2003;31:1062-8.

[2] Kolominsky-Rabas PL, Weber M, Gefeller O, Neundoerfer B,Heuschmann PU. Epidemiology of Ischemic Stroke Subtypes According to TOAST Criteria. Incidence, Recurrence, and Long-Term Survival in Ischemic Stroke Subtypes: A Population-Based Study. *Stroke.* 2001;32:2735-2740.

[3] Woo D, Gebel J, Miller R, Kothari R, Brott T, Khoury J, Salisbury S, Shukla R, Pancioli A, Jauch E, Broderick J. Incidence rates of first-ever ischemic stroke subtypes among blacks: a population-based study. *Stroke.*1999;30:2517-2522.

[4] Sacco RL, Shi T, Zamanillo MC, Kargman DE. Predictors of mortality and recurrence after hospitalized cerebral infarction in an urban community: the Northern Manhattan Stroke Study. *Neurology.* 1994;44:626–634.

[5] Mustanoja S, Meretoja A, Putaala J, Viitanen V, Curtze S, Atula S, Artto V, Happola O, Kaste M, and for the Helsinki Stroke Thrombolysis Registry Group. Outcome by Stroke Etiology in Patients Receiving Thrombolytic Treatment: Descriptive Subtype Analysis. *Stroke.* 2011;42:102–106.

[6] Gan R, Sacco RL, Kargman DE, et al: Testing the validity of the lacunar hypothesis: The Northern Manhattan Stroke Study experience. *Neurology* 1997. 48:1204-1211

[7] Toni D, Del Duca R, Fiorelli M, Sacchetti ML, Bastianello S, Giubilei F, Martinazzo C, Argentino C. Pure motor hemiparesis and sensorimotor stroke. Accuracy of very early clinical diagnosis of lacunar strokes. *Stroke.* 1994 Jan;25(1):92-6.

[8]   Fisher CM. Pure sensory stroke involving face, arm and leg. *Neurology.* 1965; 15: 76–80.

[9]   Fisher CM. Ataxic hemiparesis. *Arch. Neurol.* 1978; 35: 126–128.

[10] Fisher CM. *A lacunar stroke: the dysarthria–clumsy hand syndrome.*

In: Handbook of Stroke and Neurocritical Care   ISBN: 978-61324-786-0
Editor: V. H. Lee   © 2012 Nova Science Publishers, Inc.

Chapter V

Ischemic Stroke - Cardioembolic

Marc Lazzaro
Department of Neurological Sciences,
Section of Stroke and Neurocritical care,
Rush University Medical Center, Chicago, IL, USA

1) Background
   a) The category of cardioembolic stroke includes arterial occlusions presumed to be due to an embolus arising from the heart.(1) Many patients with a potential cardioembolic source for ischemic stroke (IS) have concomitant cerebrovascular disease, making the distinction between etiologies challenging (Table 1).
   b) Stroke from a cardiac source accounts for up to 29% of ischemic strokes.[2-4]
   c) Previous studies have categorized cardioembolic sources as high-risk or low-risk based on the propensity for embolism (Table 2).[1] A patient with a stroke and a finding of a medium-risk cardiac source without other source of embolism may be considered a possible cardioembolic stroke.
   d) Clinical and radiographic characteristics of cardioembolic stroke vary and may be similar to those found in large artery atherosclerosis. Involvement of more than one

vascular territory and evidence of systemic embolism support a cardiogenic etiology.

e) Features on initial CT scan have been associated with cardioembolic stroke, however the predictive value of these findings is low.[5]

(i) High-risk patients were more likely to have infarcts involving one-half of the lobe or larger or infarcts involving both superficial or deep structures.

(ii) Deep, small infarcts had a negative association with the presence of a cardiac source of embolism.

f) A cardioembolic etiology is often considered in non-lacunar infarcts in the absence of intracranial arterial disease and in the presence of multiple infarcts.

g) Older age has been strongly associated with cardioembolic subtype of stroke in population-based studies.[3, 6] This has been attributed to the increased prevalence of atrial fibrillation with age.[7, 8]

h) Common causes of cardioembolic stroke include atrial fibrillation, coronary artery disease, valvular heart disease, mitral annulus calcification, and cardiomyopathy.[4]

i) Cardiogenic stroke carries a high rate of recurrence and therefore the impact of change in management warrants aggressive evaluation for a cardiac etiology in suspected cases.

j) conversion of cardioembolic ischemic stroke is a serious complication necessitating careful decision making in choosing the appropriate antithrombotic therapy.

Table 1. Features suggestive of cardioembolic stroke

Clinical Features
Cortical or cerebellar dysfunction (vs. lacunar syndrome)
Diagnostic Testing
Radiographic findings of cortical, cerebellar, brain stem, or subcortical infarct >1.5 cm
Multiple vascular territories involved
Systemic signs of cardioembolism
Absence of large artery source of embolism

Table 2. TOAST Classification of High-Risk and Medium-Risk Cardioembolic Sources [1]

High-Risk Sources
Mechanical prosthetic valve
Mitral stenosis with atrial fibrillation
Atrial fibrillation (other than lone Afib)
Left atrial/atrial appendage thrombus
Sick sinus syndrome
Recent myocardial infaraction (<4 weeks)
Left ventricular thrombus
Dilated cardiomyopathy
Akinetic Left ventricular segment
Atrial myxoma
Infective endocarditis
Medium-Risk Sources
Mitral valve prolapse
Mitral annulus calcification
Mitral stenosis without Afib
Left atrial turbulence (smoke)
Atrial septal aneurysm
Patent foramen ovale
Atrial flutter
Lone atrial fibrillation
Bioprosthetic cardiac valve
Nonbacterial thrombotic endocarditis
Congestive heart failure
Hypokinetic left ventricular segment
Myocardial infarction (>4 weeks, <6 months)

2) Pathophysiology
- a) An embolism travels from the heart and may become lodged in neck or brain blood vessels causing arterial occlusion. Thromboembolism may lead to large artery occlusion or multifocal distal occlusions. Spontaneous recanalization of a large artery occlusion may also lead to distal showering of emboli causing a more diffuse or multifocal pattern of ischemia.
- b) The embolus pathology varies depending on the cardiogenic subtype.
    - (i) Thrombotic embolism
        - 1) Usually "red thrombus," composed of platelet and fibrin network, whereas artery-to-artery embolus is more commonly thought to be "white

thrombus," composed primarily of platelet aggregates.[9]

    (ii) Infective embolism (bacterial) (Figure 1)

    (iii) Tumor embolism (myxoma)

    (iv) Calcification

c) Commonly results in "embolic pattern" with multiple similarly aged ischemic lesions in different vascular territories, less likely to be lacunar appearing (Figure 2,3).

d) May appear to have large artery occlusion (ie. hyperdense MCA sign on CT). Initial CT scan in patients with acute stroke may suggest presence of an underlying cardioembolic source such as:

    (i) infarcts involving ½ lobe or larger and infarcts involving both superficial and deep structures, or may suggest against cardioembolic stroke by presence of deep small infarcts, however the predictive value is limited.[5]

e) Hemorrhagic conversion occurs at a high rate with cardioembolic stroke, which may be related to spontaneous recanalization of a transiently occluded large artery resulting in high flow reperfusion of ischemic tissue.

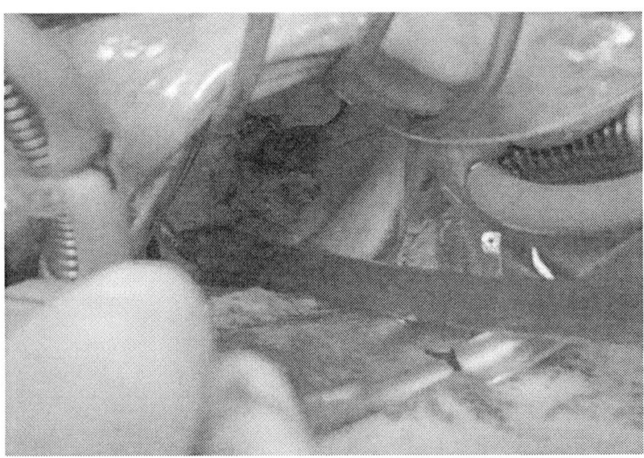

Figure 1. Intraoperative image of a mitral valve vegetation in a patient with gram positive bacterial endocarditis.

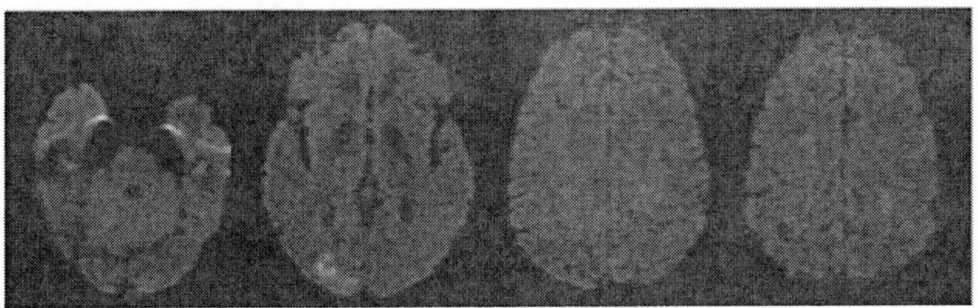

Figure 2. Diffusion weighted MRI sequence showing infarcts in multiple territories in a patient with bacterial endocarditis.

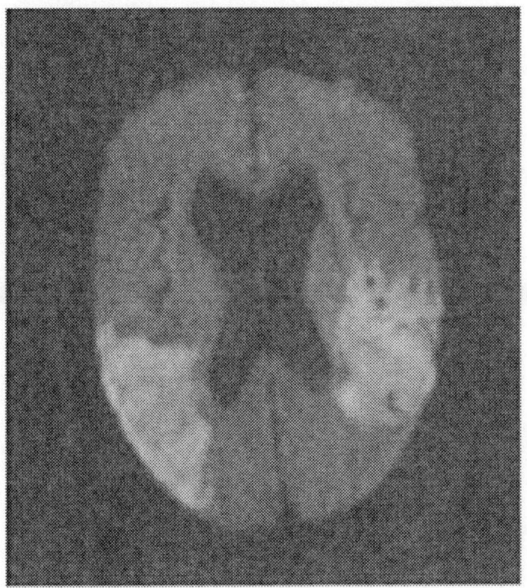

Figure 3. Diffusion weighted MRI sequence showing bilateral MCA distribution infarcts in a patient with cardioembolic source of stroke.

3) Clinical Presentation
    a) The clinical presentation of cardioembolic stroke varies widely and includes sudden focal neurological deficit. Presentation may include acute large artery occlusion with the accompanying large artery syndrome (ie MCA syndrome). Emboli to distal branches may lead to more variable clinical findings.
    b) Exam findings in cardioembolic stroke may vary:

(i) Data from case series suggest rapidity and loss of consciousness at onset were associated with cardiogenic stroke.[10]

(ii) An analysis of 1,290 patients from the NINDS Stroke Data Bank showed that diminished level of consciousness, visual field deficit, neglect, and aphasia were significantly associated with an increasing risk of having a cardiac source of embolism.[11]

(iii) Concurrent systemic embolism, including acute arterial occlusion in an extremity or mesenteric vasculature and retinal embolism may be a supportive exam findings, however this is a rare associated finding (2.3%).[4] Among patients with atrial fibrillation, systemic embolism is less common than cerebral embolism,[12] and may often be asymptomatic due to protection in the limbs and viscera from collateral circulation.[13]

Categories of Cardioembolic Stroke

1) Dysrhythmias
   a) Atrial fibrillation
   b) Sick sinus syndrome
2) Structural
   a) Myocardial infarction
   b) Cardiomyopathy
   c) Valvular
   d) Wall Defects
   e) Mass Lesions
3) Endocarditis
   a) Non-infectious
   b) Infectious
4) Aortic Atheroma

Dysrhythmias

1) Atrial fibrillation (AF)
   a) AF has been considered the most important single cause of ischemic stroke in the elderly and is responsible for about 10% of all ischemic strokes.[14]
   b) The prevalence of AF increases with age, occurring in nearly 9% of people over the age of 80 years.[15]
   c) Thrombogenesis in AF is multifactorial and is likely due to stasis in a poorly contractile left atrium in the setting of a prothrombotic or hypercoagulable state.[16]
   d) Paroxysmal AF is recognized as having comparable risk of stroke to persistent or permanent AF and oral anticoagulation is recommended in these patients.[17]
   e) Evaluation should include electrocardiogram as well as inpatient continuous cardiac telemetry and Holter monitoring. Holter monitoring may be superior to continuous cardiac telemetry in detecting paroxysmal and persistent atrial fibrillation.[18]
      (i) Transthoracic and transesophageal echocardiography are necessary to evaluate for cardiac thrombus.
      (ii) In TTE, There is limited visualization of the left atrium and left atrial appendage due to anatomic positioning.
      (iii) The yield of TTE is variable as a screening method in patients with IS and increases in patients with known heart disease or arrhythmia.[19]
      (iv) TEE Allows better visualization of heart structures and identification of embolic source with a higher diagnostic yield than TTE due to ability to visualize the left atrium and left atrial appendage that may harbor embolic source.[20]
      (v) In high-risk patients with AF, transesophageal echocardiography findings associated with increased risk of thromboembolism are dense spontaneous echocardiographic contrast ("smoke"), thrombus in the atrial appendage, and aortic plaque.[21]
      (vi) Spontaneous echo contrast or "smoke" refers to stasis of blood flow in the atrial appendage seen on TEE that appears as smoke-like echoes.

f)   Management

(i) Adjusted-dose warfarin is superior to aspirin in preventing recurrent stroke in patients with Afib and appears to be relatively safe (annual rate of bleeding of about 1.3%).[22]

(ii) Goal INR is between 2.0 and 3.0.

(iii) A summary of several large randomized controlled trials of management of patients with atrial fibrillation is presented in table 3. Warfarin is superior to aspirin and aspirin plus clopidogrel for stroke prevention in atrial fibrillation. Additionally, adjusted dose warfarin (INR 2.0 – 3.0) is better than low-intensity fixed dose warfarin (INR 1.2 – 1.5). ASA and clopidogrel combination therapy is a reasonable alternative to warfarin in patients with AF and in whom anticoagulation is contraindicated.[23]

(iv) There is no evidence that addition of an antiplatelet agent to anticoagulation will further reduce the risk of recurrent stroke in patients with AF.

(v) Rate control does not offer thromboembolism reduction when compared to rhythm control (2.9 – 7.9% vs 0 to 0.5%).[24]

(vi) The ideal time to initiation of anticoagulation following stroke is not well known. Current AHA guidelines recommend initiating oral anticoagulation within 2 weeks of an ischemic stroke or TIA, unless large infarcts or uncontrolled hypertension necessitates further delay.[25]

Table 3. Selected trials of stroke prevention in non-valvular atrial fibrillation

Trial	AFASAK[26]	SPAF(27)	EAFT[22]	SPAF II[28]	SPAF III[29]	ACTIVE[(30]	ACTIVE A[23]
Year	1989	1991	1993	1994	1996	2006	2009
Mean age	74	67	71	$\leq 75 = 64$ $>75 = 80$	67	70	71
n	1007	1330	1007	1100	1044	6706	7554
Target INR	$2.8 - 4.2$	$2.0 - 3.5$	$2.5 - 4.0$	$2.0 - 4.5$	Low intensity: 1.2-1.5 Adjusted dose: 2.0-3.0	$2.0 - 3.0$	------
Design	Placebo vs ASA	Placebo vs warfarin	Placebo vs ASA	Warfarin vs ASA	Low-intensity fixed dose warfarin plus ASA vs adjusted dose warfarin	Warfarin vs ASA + clopidogrel (75mg/d)	ASA + clopidogrel (75mg/d) vs ASA + placebo
ASA(mg/d)	75	325	300	325	325	75-100	325
Primary endpoint	TIA, minor stroke, disabling stroke, fatal stroke, peripheral embolism	Ischemic stroke, systemic embolism	Ischemic stroke, systemic embolism, cerebral hemorrhage, vascular death, myocardial infarction	Ischemic stroke, systemic thrombo-embolism	Ischemic stroke, systemic thrombo-embolism	Stroke, systemic embolism, MI, vascular death	Stroke, systemic embolism, MI, vascular death
Remarks	Warfarin is superior to ASA or placebo.	Warfarin is superior to ASA or placebo	Warfarin is superior to ASA	Warfarin benefit was lost due to hemorrhage, especially in those over 75 years of age.	Adjusted dose warfarin is better than low-intensity fixed dose warfarin plus ASA	Warfarin is superior to ASA plus clopidogrel	ASA plus clopidogrel is a reasonable alternative in patients who are ineligible for warfarin therapy.

AFASKA: Atrial fibrillation aspirin anticoagulation study; SPAF: Stroke prevention in atrial fibrillation study; EAFT: European atrial fibrillation trial; ACTIVE: Atrial fibrillation clopidogrel trial with irbesartan for prevention of vascular events; ASA: aspirin; INR: international normalized ratio.

(vii) There is no evidence to support escalating the INR goal in patients with Afib who present with recurrent ischemic stroke or TIA despite therapeutic anticoagulation. This will carry an increased bleeding risk.

2) Sick sinus syndrome (SSS)
   a) Sick Sinus Syndrome is characterized by unexplained bradycardia or sinus arrest without associated supraventricular tachyarrhythmias.[32] Bradycardia may be due to disordered impulse generation within the sinus node or impaired conduction from sinus node to atrium. When complicating supraventricular arrhythmias are present, it may be called "bradycardia-tachycardia syndrome."
   b) SSS is more common among the elderly and is one of the most common indications for cardiac pacemaker implantation.
   c) Symptoms include syncope, light-headedness, and palpitations.[33]
   d) Stroke has been reported as high as 14.3% in patients with SSS.[32]
   e) Atrial fibrillation has been reported in up to 35% of paced patients with SSS.[34]
   f) Evaluation is focused on cardiac rhythm diagnostics and may include EKG or longer-term monitoring with Holter or extended duration event monitoring.
   g) Management
   (i) Cardiac pacemaker implantation does not seem to be protective of ischemic stroke, however patients who convert to atrial fibrillation may be at high-risk for stroke.[35]
   (ii) There are no prospective, randomized trials demonstrating aspirin or anticoagulation use in sick sinus syndrome. Aspirin therapy is appropriate for secondary stroke prevention. Aggressive pursuit of underlying atrial fibrillation should be considered.

3) Rhythm evaluation
   a) Diagnostic testing for rhythm abnormalities will depend on the degree of suspicion of an underlying rhythm abnormality.

b) Electrocardiogram offers fast, inexpensive, and reliable evaluation of the cardiac rhythm. Disadvantages include brief recording time.

c) Cardiac telemetry includes remote cardiac monitoring during inpatient hospitalization that allows for continuous monitoring and real-time notification of considerable rhythm abnormalities. The major role for continuous cardiac telemetry is detection of malignant ventricular arrhythmias, marked changes in heart rate, or prolonged rhythm disturbances. Disadvantages include computer interpretation for rhythm abnormalities. Cardiac telemetry monitors often require a change in rate to alarm and therefore subtle arrhythmias may be missed.

d) Holter monitoring commonly involves a 24- or 48-hour period of cardiac rhythm recording that is reviewed by a cardiologist. Disadvantages include delay in time for interpretation.

e) 30-day event monitoring allows for extended duration recording. Abnormal rhythm periods are detected automatically or recorded after initiation of recording by patient after symptoms. Disadvantages include extended duration of wearing monitor.

f) Implantable recorder utilizes a small implantable device that records abnormal cardiac rhythm episodes and may be used for extended duration recording for months to years. Disadvantages include the necessity of a minor procedure.

Table 4. CHADS2 Score

	Condition	Points
C	Congestive Heart Failure	1
H	Hypertension (>160 mmHg) or treated HTN	1
A	Age >75 years	1
D	Diabetes Mellitus	1
S2	Prior Stroke or TIA	2

Table 5. Annual stroke risk based on CHADS2 score [31]

CHADS2 Score	Stroke Risk %	95% CI
0	1.9	1.2 – 3.0
1	2.8	2.0 – 3.8
2	4.0	3.1 – 5.1
3	5.9	4.6 – 7.3
4	8.5	6.3 – 11.1
5	12.5	8.2 – 17.5
6	18.2	10.5 – 27.4

Structural

1) Myocardial infarction
    a) Myocardial infarction (MI) can result in hypokinetic or akinetic cardiac walls, which may be susceptible to thrombus formation. Ischemic stroke is more common among patients with MI who have an associated left ventricular (LV) thrombus than in those patients without a LV thrombus.
    b) Evaluation- Echocardiography should be performed in patients with MI and IS to evaluate for thrombus.
    c) Management
        (i) In the presence of thrombus, patients can be treated with oral anticoagulation, goal INR 2.0 to 3.0, for at least 3 months and possibly up to 1 year. Termination of anticoagulation should be considered if repeat echocardiography shows evidence of thrombus resolution.[25]
        (ii) Low dose aspirin (81 mg daily) should be used concurrently for ischemic coronary artery disease during oral anticoagulant therapy.
2) Cardiomyopathy
    a) Cardiomyopathy may result from ischemia as the result of coronary artery disease, or may be nonischemic and related to genetic or acquired defects of myocardial cell metabolism. Cardiomyopathy can lead to reduced stroke

volume and left ventricular stasis that may lead to thrombogenesis and embolism.

b) Two large studies demonstrated an increased risk of stroke with reduced ejection fraction (EF), the Survival and Ventricular Enlargement (SAVE) study,[36] and the Studies of Left Ventricular Dysfunction (SOLVD) trial.[37]

   (i) SAVE trial

      1) The SAVE trial consisted of patients who had a myocardial infarction. Patients with EF of 29% to 35% (mean, 32%) had a stroke rate of 0.8% per year; the rate in patients with EF </= 28% (mean, 23%) was 1.7% per year (Table 6).

      2) Furthermore, patients with an EF <28% had a 5-year cumulative stroke risk of 8.1% compared with 4.1% for those with an EF >35%.

      3) There was an 18% increment in the risk of stroke for every 5% decline in EF.

   (ii) SOLVD trial- a retrospective study that showed a 58% increase in risk of thromboembolic events for every 10% decrease in EF among women (p = 0.01), however there was no significant increase in risk among men.

c) Evaluation

   (i) Echocardiography is useful in diagnosing cardiomyopathy and assessing cardiac function. Alternative modalities including cardiac MRI and cardiac CT may be considered.

d) Management

   (i) Retrospective data suggest that warfarin may reduce mortality and both initial and recurrent ischemic stroke rates in patients with impaired LV function, however no randomized clinical studies have demonstrated the efficacy of anticoagulation.

Table 6. SAVE Study stroke rate

EF 29 – 35%	0.8% per year
EF </= 28%	1.7% per year

(ii) AHA guidelines recommend considering warfarin (INR goal 2.0 to 3.0) or antiplatelet therapy for secondary stroke prevention in patients with dilated cardiomyopathy.[25] There is no recommendation for primary prevention of stroke in patients with a low ejection fraction. The conservative approach is use of single antiplatelet therapy, while a more aggressive approach is to initiate anticoagulation for patients with EF of < 30%. Additional factors such as spontaneous echo contrast ("smoke") on echocardiography may further suggest the need for anticoagulation.

3) Valvular Cardiac Disease

    a) Various heart valve conditions have been associated with ischemic stroke. Due to the high recurrence of thromboembolic events in patients with valvular disease, anticoagulation is commonly implemented. Evaluation of patients with valvular cardiac disease requires valve imaging with echocardiography or alternative imaging modalities such as cardiac MRI or cardiac CT.

    b) Rheumatic Mitral Valve Disease

        a) Rheumatic heart disease is a condition in which heart valves are damaged by the inflammatory disease known as rheumatic fever, which is the result of Group A Streptococcus pharyngitis. Recurrent embolism occurs in 30% to 65% of patients with rheumatic mitral valve disease.[25] Long-term anticoagulation has been shown to reduce the risk of systemic embolism in patients with rheumatic mitral valve disease.[38] Current AHA/ASA guidelines recommend:

        b) Warfarin long-term anticoagulation (target INR 2.5, range 2.0 – 3.0) for patients with ischemic stroke or TIA regardless of presence of atrial fibrillation.

        c) Addition of Aspirin 81 mg per day is suggested for patients with ischemic stroke or TIA with rheumatic mitral valve disease who have recurrent embolism despite warfarin anticoagulation.

    c) Mitral Valve Prolapse

        a) Mitral valve prolapse is a common form of valvular disease in adults with no clear link to thromboembolic phenomena. Single antiplatelet therapy is appropriate for secondary stroke prevention.[25]

d) Mitral Annular Calcification

    a) May lead to mitral stenosis and predispose to endocarditis and arrhythmias. A direct link to thromboembolic events is not clear. In addition to thromboembolism, fibrocalcific material may embolize from the calcified mitral annulus.[39] Distinguishing between thromboembolism and clacific material embolization is rarely possible, and therefore anticoagulation may be unjustified. Antithrombotic therapies have not been compared in randomized trials.

    b) AHA/ASA guidelines suggest:

        (i) Antiplatelet therapy for patients with ischemic stroke or TIA and mitral annular calcification

        (ii) Consider antiplatelet therapy or warfarin therapy for patients with mitral valve regurgitation caused by mitral annular calcification without atrial fibrillation.

e) Aortic Valve Disease

    a) Systemic calcific microembolism has been reported in an autopsy study of patients with calcific aortic stenosis, however most were clinically silent.[40] No randomized trials have compared antithrombotic therapies.

    b) AHA/ASA guidelines suggest:

        (i) In patients with aortic valve disease and ischemic stroke or TIA, but not atrial fibrillation, antiplatelet therapy may be considered.

f) Prosthetic Heart Valves

    a) Various prosthetic heart valves exist and all necessitate antithrombotic prophylaxis.

    b) AHA/ASA guidelines recommend:

        (i) Secondary stroke prevention for patients with modern mechanical prosthetic heart valves with oral anticoagulation (goal INR 3.0, range 2.5 to 3.5).

(ii) Aspirin 75 mg to 100 mg per day may be added in patients who have ischemic stroke or systemic embolism despite oral anticoagulation.

(iii) In patients with bioprosthetic heart valves with no other source of thromboembolism, oral anticoagulation may be considered.

4) Wall Defects

   a) Atrial Septal Aneurysm/Patent Foramen Ovale –see chapter 6.

   b) Ventricular Aneurysm

      a) Retrospective data from a series of 76 patients suggests a low incidence of systemic emboli with chronic ventricular aneurysm, and therefore the use of long-term anticoagulation is not recommended.[41]

   c) Hypokinetic wall segments

      a) Hypokinetic wall segments may develop following myocardial infarction. In the presence of an associated thrombus demonstrated on TTE, anticoagulation with warfarin and an INR range 2.0 – 3.0 should be maintained.

   d) Lipomatous Hypertrophy of the Interatrial Septum (LHIS)

      a) Lipomatous hypertrophy of the interatrial septum is characterized by accumulation of adipose tissue in the interatrial septum. A 2.2% incidence has been reported and LHIS has been typically associated with obesity and advanced age. Atrial arrhythmias have been reported in association with LHIS, however the exact mechanism is unclear. Arrhythmias may be due to associated atherosclerotic coronary artery disease or by disturbances in conducting pathways due to adipose deposition.[42]

      b) No guidelines have been established for the management of patients with ischemic stroke who have been found to have LHIS, however a thorough evaluation for underlying arrhythmia should be considered.

5) Mass Lesions

   a) Myxoma

      (i) Cardiac myxoma is considered a benign tumor with a female preponderance of 2:1 and usual age of onset between 30 and 60 years. Cases are often sporadic, but may be familial. Presentation may include obstructive symptoms such as syncope, systemic embolization, and constitutional symptoms.[43]

(ii) Stroke may be ischemic or hemorrhagic and may be recurrent.

(iii) Serum studies may identify elevation of ESR and C-reactive protein as well as anemia reflecting an inflammatory state.[44]

(iv) Evaluation

1) TEE has been reported as having 100% sensitivity for cardiac myxoma and is recommended over TTE in suspected cases.[45]

2) Cardiac MRI may provide useful information in guiding surgical resection, including size, attachment, and mobility.[46]

3) Myxomatous cerebral aneurysms that predispose to cerebral hemorrhage may be small and unidentified on non-invasive imaging modalities and therefore catheter cerebral angiography should be considered.[44]

4) Metastasized tumor fragments to the cerebral vasculature may enlarge causing vessel occlusion and delayed infarction.[47]

(v) Management

1) No guidelines exist for management of myxomas in stroke patients, however small series and case reports advise early surgical resection to prevent early recurrent stroke.[44, 48]

2) Timing of surgical resection is made on an individual basis and requires consideration of infarct size given the necessity of heparinization during surgery and the associated risk of hemorrhage.

3) Anticoagulation while awaiting definitive surgical treatment may not be effective if the embolus is myxomatous embolism rather than thrombus.

4) Tumor recurrence has been reported in up to 1 – 3% of sporadic cases, thought to be largely due to inadequate resection.[49] Annual

echocardiography surveillance imaging for the subsequent 3-4 years may be considered.
   b) Papillary fibroelastomas
      (i)   Papillary fibroelastomas are benign cardiac tumors characterized by collagen and elastin fronds covered with endothelial cells. It has been postulated that embolism from these structures is likely thrombotic rather than tumor fragmentation.[50]
      (ii) Due to limited data, the ideal therapy for secondary stroke prevention is not known, however early surgical excision has been advocated,[51] and anticoagulation while awaiting surgical excision has been proposed.[50]

Endocarditis

1) Non-infectious endocarditis
   a) Non-infectious endocarditis, or non-bacterial thrombotic endocarditis (NBTE), may occur in the setting of various systemic disorders including malignancy and autoimmune disorders. Formation of sterile thrombi on cardiac valves and the adjacent endocardium occurs with trauma to the valve or in a systemic hypercoagulable state.
   b) Evaluation
   c) Echocardiography is important in diagnosis and TEE should be considered over TTE for the detection of smaller vegetations.
   d) Management
   e) Randomized clinical trial data on NBTE treatment are lacking, and guidelines in ischemic stroke patients are not established, however the American College of Chest Physicians support use of anticoagulation in patients with NBTE and systemic thromboembolism[52]
2) Infectious Endocarditis
   a) In a series of 203 patients with infective endocarditis, stroke occurred in 21% of patients, and only 56% of those who underwent echocardiography were found to have vegetations.[53]

b)   Bacterial endocarditis predominantly involves the valves and may include small masses of microorganisms called vegetations (Figure 1).

c)   The pathophysiology of ischemic stroke in infective endocarditis is likely due to occlusive vegetation fragment microemboli, while a pyogenic arteritis may play a larger role in hemorrhagic stroke.

d)   Evaluation

1)   Blood cultures are essential in evaluation. Staphylococcus aureus is the most commonly associated organism with neurologic complications.[54, 55]

2)   Echocardiography is necessary and should be performed urgently. TEE is preferred over TTE for evaluation of valve vegetation.

3)   Brain imaging is important to differentiate ischemic and hemorrhagic lesions and characterize lesion size, which may be important in risk stratification if surgery is needed.

4)   Cerebral angiography should be performed if there is concern for mycotic aneurysms and should be considered prior to valve replacement surgery. Mycotic aneurysms rarely have been proven to be the cause of intracranial hemorrhage, only about 1% to 3% in patients with infective endocarditis.(56) Endovascular treatment may be considered for mycotic aneurysms that do not show regression despite antibiotic therapy to prevent perioperative rupture in patients undergoing valve replacement.[57]

e)   Management

1)   The cornerstone of medical management includes early initiation of antibiotic therapy.

2)   Infective endocarditis in the setting of a mechanical valve poses a therapeutic dilemma weighing the risk of hemorrhage from anticoagulation combined with antibiotic therapy against the high risk of clot formation on the artificial valve. Anticoagulation has not been shown to be beneficial in native valve endocarditis and increases the risk of hemorrhage. In

artificial valve endocarditis, the decision to resume anticoagulation must be individualized.

3) Surgical therapy must be individualized and may be necessary if there is persistent echocardiographic vegetation or multiple thromboembolic events despite antibiotic therapy, and ischemic stroke should not be considered a contraindication. Radiographic imaging to exclude a hemorrhagic component should be performed prior to surgery and aniographic evaluation for mycotic aneurysm should be considered prior to heparinization with surgery.

Aortic Atheroma

1) Among patients with ischemic stroke, the prevalence of ulcerated aortic arch plaques is up to 28%, and this rate is even higher (61%) in those with no known cause of stroke.[58]
2) Atheromatous lesions in the ascending aorta detected on TEE are associated with a risk of embolic stroke. Specifically, lesions 4mm or larger in thickness are more likely to be responsible for ischemic stroke.[59]
3) Evaluation
   a) Echocardiography with TEE is superior to TTE by providing higher resolution, better proximal aortic arch visualization, and more reliable interpretation.[60]
4) Management
   a) Randomized data evaluating antiplatelet, anticoagulation, and statin therapies in ischemic stroke patients with aortic atheroma and no other identifiable cause of stroke are lacking.
   b) Non-randomized observational data favors the use of anticoagulation for reducing thromboembolic events.[61]
   c) More aggressive therapies with anticoagulation may be warranted in aortic atheroma with thickness greater than 4 mm, plaque ulceration, and the finding of mobile components.

References

[1]   Adams HP, Jr., Bendixen BH, Kappelle LJ, Biller J, Love BB, Gordon DL, et al. *Classification of subtype of acute ischemic stroke. Definitions for use in a multicenter clinical trial. TOAST. Trial of Org 10172 in Acute Stroke Treatment.* Stroke. 1993 Jan;24(1):35-41.

[2]   Petty GW, Brown RD, Jr., Whisnant JP, Sicks JD, O'Fallon WM, Wiebers DO. *Ischemic stroke subtypes: a population-based study of incidence and risk factors.* Stroke. 1999 Dec;30(12):2513-6.

[3]   Bejot Y, Caillier M, Ben Salem D, Couvreur G, Rouaud O, Osseby GV, et al. *Ischaemic stroke subtypes and associated risk factors: a French population based study.* J Neurol Neurosurg Psychiatry. 2008 Dec;79(12):1344-8.

[4]   Caplan LR, Hier DB, D'Cruz I. *Cerebral embolism in the Michael Reese Stroke Registry.* Stroke. 1983 Jul-Aug;14(4):530-6.

[5]   Kittner SJ, Sharkness CM, Sloan MA, Price TR, Dambrosia JM, Tuhrim S, et al. *Features on initial computed tomography scan of infarcts with a cardiac source of embolism in the NINDS Stroke Data Bank.* Stroke. 1992 Dec;23(12):1748-51.

[6]   Schulz UG, Rothwell PM. *Differences in vascular risk factors between etiological subtypes of ischemic stroke: importance of population-based studies.* Stroke. 2003 Aug;34(8):2050-9.

[7]   Go AS, Hylek EM, Phillips KA, Chang Y, Henault LE, Selby JV, et al. *Prevalence of diagnosed atrial fibrillation in adults: national implications for rhythm management and stroke prevention: the AnTicoagulation and Risk Factors in Atrial Fibrillation (ATRIA) Study.* JAMA. 2001 May 9;285(18):2370-5.

[8]   Tsang TS, Petty GW, Barnes ME, O'Fallon WM, Bailey KR, Wiebers DO, et al. *The prevalence of atrial fibrillation in incident stroke cases and matched population controls in Rochester, Minnesota: changes over three decades.* J Am Coll Cardiol. 2003 Jul 2;42(1):93-100.

[9]   Gunning AJ, Pickering GW, Robb-Smith AH, Russell RR. *Mural Thrombosis of the Internal Carotid Artery and Subsequent Embolism.* Q J Med. 1964 Jan;33:155-95.

[10]   Ramirez-Lassepas M, Cipolle RJ, Bjork RJ, Kowitz J, Snyder BD, Weber JC, et al. *Can embolic stroke be diagnosed on the basis of neurologic clinical criteria?* Arch Neurol. 1987 Jan;44(1):87-9.

[11]   Kittner SJ, Sharkness CM, Sloan MA, Price TR, Dambrosia JM, Tuhrim S, et al. *Infarcts with a cardiac source of embolism in the*

NINDS Stroke Data Bank: neurologic examination. Neurology. 1992 Feb;42(2):299-302.

[12] Go AS, Hylek EM, Chang Y, Phillips KA, Henault LE, Capra AM, et al. *Anticoagulation therapy for stroke prevention in atrial fibrillation: how well do randomized trials translate into clinical practice?* JAMA. 2003 Nov 26;290(20):2685-92.

[13] Andersen LV, Vestergaard P, Deichgraeber P, Lindholt JS, Mortensen LS, Frost L. *Warfarin for the prevention of systemic embolism in patients with non-valvular atrial fibrillation: a meta-analysis.* Heart. 2008 Dec;94(12):1607-13.

[14] Lip GY, Edwards SJ. *Stroke prevention with aspirin, warfarin and ximelagatran in patients with non-valvular atrial fibrillation: a systematic review and meta-analysis.* Thromb Res. 2006;118(3):321-33.

[15] Kannel WB, Wolf PA, Benjamin EJ, Levy D. *Prevalence, incidence, prognosis, and predisposing conditions for atrial fibrillation: population-based estimates.* Am J Cardiol. 1998 Oct 16;82(8A):2N-9N.

[16] Watson T, Shantsila E, Lip GY. *Mechanisms of thrombogenesis in atrial fibrillation: Virchow's triad revisited.* Lancet. 2009 Jan 10;373(9658):155-66.

[17] Fuster V, Ryden LE, Asinger RW, Cannom DS, Crijns HJ, Frye RL, et al. ACC/AHA/ESC Guidelines for the Management of Patients With Atrial Fibrillation: Executive Summary A Report of the American College of Cardiology/American Heart Association Task Force on Practice Guidelines and the European Society of Cardiology Committee for Practice Guidelines and Policy Conferences (Committee to Develop Guidelines for the Management of Patients With Atrial Fibrillation) Developed in Collaboration With the North American Society of Pacing and Electrophysiology. Circulation. 2001 Oct 23;104(17):2118-50.

[18] Lazzaro MA, Krishnan K, Prabhakaran S. *Detection of Atrial Fibrillation with Concurrent Holter Monitoring and Continuous Cardiac Telemetry Following Ischemic Stroke and Transient Ischemic Attack.* J Stroke Cerebrovasc Dis. 2010 Jul 23.

[19] Donaldson RM, Emanuel RW, Earl CJ. *The role of two-dimensional echocardiography in the detection of potentially embolic intracardiac masses in patients with cerebral ischaemia.* J Neurol Neurosurg Psychiatry. 1981 Sep;44(9):803-9.

[20] Tegeler CH, Downes TR. *Cardiac imaging in stroke.* Stroke. 1991 Sep;22(9):1206-11.

[21] Transesophageal echocardiographic correlates of thromboembolism in high-risk patients with nonvalvular atrial fibrillation. *The Stroke Prevention in Atrial Fibrillation Investigators Committee on Echocardiography.* Ann Intern Med. 1998 Apr 15;128(8):639-47.

[22] Secondary prevention in non-rheumatic atrial fibrillation after transient ischaemic attack or minor stroke. *EAFT (European Atrial Fibrillation Trial) Study Group.* Lancet. 1993 Nov 20;342(8882):1255-62.

[23] Connolly SJ, Pogue J, Hart RG, Hohnloser SH, Pfeffer M, Chrolavicius S, et al. *Effect of clopidogrel added to aspirin in patients with atrial fibrillation.* N Engl J Med. 2009 May 14;360(20):2066-78.

[24] Sherman DG. *Stroke prevention in atrial fibrillation: pharmacological rate versus rhythm control.* Stroke. 2007 Feb;38(2 Suppl):615-7.

[25] Sacco RL, Adams R, Albers G, Alberts MJ, Benavente O, Furie K, et al. *Guidelines for prevention of stroke in patients with ischemic stroke or transient ischemic attack: a statement for healthcare professionals from the American Heart Association/American Stroke Association Council on Stroke: co-sponsored by the Council on Cardiovascular Radiology and Intervention: the American Academy of Neurology affirms the value of this guideline.* Stroke. 2006 Feb;37(2):577-617.

[26] Petersen P, Boysen G, Godtfredsen J, Andersen ED, Andersen B. *Placebo-controlled, randomised trial of warfarin and aspirin for prevention of thromboembolic complications in chronic atrial fibrillation. The Copenhagen AFASAK study.* Lancet. 1989 Jan 28;1(8631):175-9.

[27] *Stroke Prevention in Atrial Fibrillation Study. Final results.* Circulation. 1991 Aug;84(2):527-39.

[28] Ezekowitz MD, James KE. *Stroke Prevention in Atrial Fibrillation II Study.* Lancet. 1994 Jun 11;343(8911):1508-9.

[29] Adjusted-dose warfarin versus low-intensity, fixed-dose warfarin plus aspirin for high-risk patients with atrial fibrillation: *Stroke Prevention in Atrial Fibrillation III randomised clinical trial.* Lancet. 1996 Sep 7;348(9028):633-8.

[30] Connolly S, Pogue J, Hart R, Pfeffer M, Hohnloser S, Chrolavicius S, et al. *Clopidogrel plus aspirin versus oral anticoagulation for atrial fibrillation in the Atrial fibrillation Clopidogrel Trial with Irbesartan for prevention of Vascular Events (ACTIVE W): a randomised controlled trial.* Lancet. 2006 Jun 10;367(9526):1903-12.

[31] Gage BF, Waterman AD, Shannon W, Boechler M, Rich MW, Radford MJ. *Validation of clinical classification schemes for predicting stroke: results from the National Registry of Atrial Fibrillation.* JAMA. 2001 Jun 13;285(22):2864-70.

[32] Rubenstein JJ, Schulman CL, Yurchak PM, DeSanctis RW. *Clinical spectrum of the sick sinus syndrome.* Circulation. 1972 Jul;46(1):5-13.

[33] Radford DJ, Julian DG. *Sick sinus syndrome: experience of a cardiac pacemaker clinic.* Br Med J. 1974 Aug 24;3(5929):504-7.

[34] Andersen HR, Nielsen JC, Thomsen PE, Thuesen L, Mortensen PT, Vesterlund T, et al. *Long-term follow-up of patients from a randomised trial of atrial versus ventricular pacing for sick-sinus syndrome.* Lancet. 1997 Oct 25;350(9086):1210-6.

[35] Fisher M, Kase CS, Stelle B, Mills RM, Jr. *Ischemic stroke after cardiac pacemaker implantation in sick sinus syndrome.* Stroke. 1988 Jun;19(6):712-5.

[36] Pfeffer MA, Braunwald E, Moye LA, Basta L, Brown EJ, Jr., Cuddy TE, et al. *Effect of captopril on mortality and morbidity in patients with left ventricular dysfunction after myocardial infarction. Results of the survival and ventricular enlargement trial. The SAVE Investigators.* N Engl J Med. 1992 Sep 3;327(10):669-77.

[37] Loh E, Sutton MS, Wun CC, Rouleau JL, Flaker GC, Gottlieb SS, et al. *Ventricular dysfunction and the risk of stroke after myocardial infarction.* N Engl J Med. 1997 Jan 23;336(4):251-7.

[38] Fleming HA. *Anticoagulants in rheumatic heart-disease.* Lancet. 1971 Aug 28;2(7722):486.

[39] Nestico PF, Depace NL, Morganroth J, Kotler MN, Ross J. *Mitral annular calcification: clinical, pathophysiology, and echocardiographic review.* Am Heart J. 1984 May;107(5 Pt 1):989-96.

[40] Holley KE, Bahn RC, McGoon DC, Mankin HT. *Spontaneous Calcific Embolization Associated with Calcific Aortic Stenosis.* Circulation. 1963 Feb;27:197-202.

[41] Lapeyre AC, 3rd, Steele PM, Kazmier FJ, Chesebro JH, Vlietstra RE, Fuster V. *Systemic embolism in chronic left ventricular aneurysm: incidence and the role of anticoagulation.* J Am Coll Cardiol. 1985 Sep;6(3):534-8.

[42] Heyer CM, Kagel T, Lemburg SP, Bauer TT, Nicolas V. *Lipomatous hypertrophy of the interatrial septum: a prospective study of incidence, imaging findings, and clinical symptoms.* Chest. 2003 Dec;124(6):2068-73.

[43] Lee VH, Connolly HM, Brown RD, Jr. *Central nervous system manifestations of cardiac myxoma.* Arch Neurol. 2007 Aug;64(8):1115-20.

[44] O'Rourke F, Dean N, Mouradian MS, Akhtar N, Shuaib A. *Atrial myxoma as a cause of stroke: case report and discussion.* CMAJ. 2003 Nov 11;169(10):1049-51.

[45] Engberding R, Daniel WG, Erbel R, Kasper W, Lestuzzi C, Curtius JM, et al. *Diagnosis of heart tumours by transoesophageal echocardiography: a multicentre study in 154 patients. European Cooperative Study Group.* Eur Heart J. 1993 Sep;14(9):1223-8.

[46] Reddy DB, Jena A, Venugopal P. *Magnetic resonance imaging (MRI) in evaluation of left atrial masses: an in vitro and in vivo study.* J Cardiovasc Surg (Torino). 1994 Aug;35(4):289-94.

[47] Price DL, Harris JL, New PF, Cantu RC. *Cardiac myxoma. A clinicopathologic and angiographic study.* Arch Neurol. 1970 Dec;23(6):558-67.

[48] Namboodiri KK, Chaliha MS, Manoj RK, Grover A. *Central nervous embolism as an usual presentation of left atrial myxoma.* J Postgrad Med. 2004 Apr-Jun;50(2):151.

[49] McCarthy PM, Piehler JM, Schaff HV, Pluth JR, Orszulak TA, Vidaillet HJ, Jr., et al. *The significance of multiple, recurrent, and "complex" cardiac myxomas.* J Thorac Cardiovasc Surg. 1986 Mar;91(3):389-96.

[50] Veinot JP. *Fibroelastoma and embolic stroke.* Circulation. 1999 May 25;99(20):2709-12.

[51] Zurru MC, Romano M, Patrucco L, Cristiano E, Milei J. *Embolic stroke secondary to cardiac papillary fibroelastoma.* Neurologist. 2008 Mar;14(2):128-30.

[52] Salem DN, Stein PD, Al-Ahmad A, Bussey HI, Horstkotte D, Miller N, et al. *Antithrombotic therapy in valvular heart disease--native and prosthetic: the Seventh ACCP Conference on Antithrombotic and Thrombolytic Therapy.* Chest. 2004 Sep;126(3 Suppl):457S-82S.

[53] Hart RG, Foster JW, Luther MF, Kanter MC. *Stroke in infective endocarditis.* Stroke. 1990 May;21(5):695-700.

[54] Heiro M, Nikoskelainen J, Engblom E, Kotilainen E, Marttila R, Kotilainen P. *Neurologic manifestations of infective endocarditis: a 17-year experience in a teaching hospital in Finland.* Arch Intern Med. 2000 Oct 9;160(18):2781-7.

[55] Patel FM, Das A, Banerjee AK. *Neuropathological complications of infective endocarditis : study of autopsy material.* Neurol India. 2001 Mar;49(1):41-6.

[56] Hart RG, Kagan-Hallet K, Joerns SE. *Mechanisms of intracranial hemorrhage in infective endocarditis.* Stroke. 1987 Nov-Dec;18(6):1048-56.

[57] Erdogan HB, Erentug V, Bozbuga N, Goksedef D, Akinci E, Yakut C. *Endovascular treatment of intracerebral mycotic aneurysm before surgical treatment of infective endocarditis.* Tex Heart Inst J. 2004;31(2):165-7.

[58] Amarenco P, Duyckaerts C, Tzourio C, Henin D, Bousser MG, Hauw JJ. *The prevalence of ulcerated plaques in the aortic arch in patients with stroke.* N Engl J Med. 1992 Jan 23;326(4):221-5.

[59] Amarenco P, Cohen A, Tzourio C, Bertrand B, Hommel M, Besson G, et al. *Atherosclerotic disease of the aortic arch and the risk of ischemic stroke.* N Engl J Med. 1994 Dec 1;331(22):1474-9.

[60] Thenappan T, Ali Raza J, Movahed A. *Aortic atheromas: current concepts and controversies-a review of the literature.* Echocardiography. 2008 Feb;25(2):198-207.

[61] Ferrari E, Vidal R, Chevallier T, Baudouy M. *Atherosclerosis of the thoracic aorta and aortic debris as a marker of poor prognosis: benefit of oral anticoagulants.* J Am Coll Cardiol. 1999 Apr;33(5):1317-22.

In: Handbook of Stroke and Neurocritical Care   ISBN: 978-61324-786-0
Editor: V. H. Lee   © 2012 Nova Science Publishers, Inc.

Chapter VI

Ischemic Stroke- Cryptogenic

Shyam Prabhakaran
Department of Neurological Sciences,
Section of Stroke and Neurocritical care,
Rush University Medical Center, Chicago, IL, USA

Key Points

1) Upto 40% of all ischemic strokes are classified as cryptogenic
2) Important novel risk factors may underlie cryptogenic stroke including paroxysmal atrial fibrillation, cardiac anomalies such as patent foramen ovale, subclinical atherosclerotic lesions in the aortic arch or large craniocervical arteries, and prothrombotic states
3) An exhaustive search for these potential causes should be considered in all patients before classifying as cryptogenic stroke
4) The short-term risk of recurrent stroke following cryptogenic stroke is intermediate between large artery (high risk) and small artery (low risk) ischemic stroke subtypes
5) Antiplatelet therapy is the mainstay of stroke prevention as empiric anticoagulation has not been shown to be superior to aspirin alone

Introduction

1) Cryptogenic stroke is defined as brain infarction that is not attributable to a source of definite cardioembolism, large artery atherosclerosis, or small artery disease despite extensive vascular, cardiac, and serologic work-up.
2) In modern registries, it represents approximately 30-40% of all ischemic strokes. [1,2]
3) Single or multiple superficial hemispheric infarcts occur in the majority of presentations with final diagnosis of cryptogenic stroke although large subcortical infarcts are also reported. [1]
4) Cortical symptoms and signs are common at presentation while lacunar syndromes are less common.[1]

Etiologies

1) With the exception of a lower prevalence of hypertension, [3] traditional risk factors do not appear to more or less common in patients with cryptogenic stroke.
2) Several mechanisms may explain cryptogenic stroke
    a) Paradoxical or occult embolism
        (i) Repeat of angiography in patients with cortical infarcts often find recanalization thrombus, consistent with occult embolism [1]
        (ii) Patients with atrial or ventricular septal defects or rarely pulmonary arteriovenous malformations may have venous sources of embolism that pass through the shunt and result in arterial occlusions [4]
        (iii) Screening for atrial septal defects is reasonable and if found, lower extremity and pelvic venous imaging (Doppler or MRV) is reasonable following cryptogenic stroke [5,6]
        (iv) Transcranial Doppler with agitated saline is also another method to detect right-left shunts
    b) Atrial septal anomalies and risk of stroke
        (i) Patent foramen ovale (PFO) are found in 25% of adults while atrial septal aneurysms (ASA) are less common (1-2%)

(ii) Right-left shunting can occur at rest, with Valsalva maneuvers, or chronic right-heart strain (i.e. pulmonary hypertension)

(iii) Presence of ASA and/or PFO may also predispose to atrial arrhythmias such as paroxysmal atrial fibrillation [7]

(iv) Case-control, prospective, and population-based studies suggest PFO alone is not a risk factor for stroke or recurrent stroke following cryptogenic first-time stroke [8]; however, the relationship may be stronger in young cryptogenic stroke patients (age < 55 years).

(v) 1 study found that presence of PFO and ASA was independent risk factor recurrent stroke (HR 4.2, 15.2% vs. 4.2% risk at 4 years) but 2 others have not (9, 10,11)

c) Paroxysmal atrial fibrillation

(i) May go undetected if cardiac monitoring is brief

(ii) Long-term monitoring studies suggest that upto 23% of cryptogenic stroke patients may have paroxysmal atrial fibrillation [12]

(iii) Long-term monitoring with 21-day mobile cardiac outpatient telemetry (MCOT) or event monitors is recommended in cryptogenic stroke patients if inpatient telemetry or 24-48hr Holter monitoring is unrevealing

d) Subclinical atherosclerosis

(i) Sub-stenotic atherosclerotic plaques in the major intracranial and extracranial arteries may cause cryptogenic strokes due to plaque instability, co-existing thrombosis and embolism [13]

(ii) Aortic arch disease, especially when associated with mobile thrombus, > 4mm in size, or ulceration is also associated with cryptogenic stroke

(iii) Craniocervical vascular imaging and transesophageal echocardiography are required in the work-up of cryptogenic stroke

e) Thrombophilia

(i) The battery of tests usually performed includes protein C and S activity, anti-thrombin III activity, lupus anticoagulant, B-2 glycoprotein Ab, cardiolipin Ab, factor VIII level, fibrinogen, homocysteine, lipoprotein "a", C-reactive protein, hemoglobin electrophoresis, and factor V Leiden, prothrombin gene, methyltetrahydrofolate (MTHFR) mutation analysis

    (ii) However, studies have not consistently shown that cryptogenic stroke patients are more likely than other stroke. [14]

    (iii) In young patients (< 45 years old) with no other risk factors or underlying etiology, a search for hypercoagulable state is reasonable.

f) Rare genetic conditions

    (i) Small publications suggest that Fabry disease may be found in 4% of patients with cryptogenic stroke, higher than expected in the population [15]

    (ii) Typically, Fabry disease presents with infarcts in the posterior circulation and dolichoectasia of the basilar artery; these can precede the systemic signs of cardiac and renal failure and skin and nerve changes

Diagnostic Tests

1) Intracranial and extracranial vascular imaging to exclude large artery stenosis due to atherosclerosis, vasculitis, or dissection

    a) MRA, CTA, TCD, Carotid Doppler, and/or angiography

        (i) Tests should be normal but subtle findings may include:

            1) Non-stenotic carotid plaques

            2) Multifocal irregularities intracranial circulation

2) Cardiac imaging to exclude structural abnormalities including PFO, ASA, atrial enlargement, thrombus, tumors, valvular lesions, and aortic arch disease

    a) Transthoracic and transesophageal echocardiography, cardiac MRI

        (i) Detected abnormalities in cryptogenic stroke include:

            1) PFO or other atrial septal defect

            2) Atrial septal aneurysm

            3) Aortic arch atheroma

      4) Atrial or appendage thrombus

      5) Spontaneous echo contrast

      6) Enlarged left atrium

      7) Valvular strands or excrescences

3) Telemetry to detect paroxysmal atrial fibrillation or flutter

    a) Continuous inpatient telemetry, Holter monitor (24-48 hour), serial EKGs, 21-day MCOT, or implantable loop monitors

4) Serologic and other tests

    a) Complete blood count, electrolytes, sedimentation rate, VDRL test, fasting lipid panel, hemoglobin A1c, homocysteine, lipoprotein 'a', c-reactive protein

    b) Protein C and S activity, anti-thrombin III activity, lupus anticoagulant, B-2 glycoprotein Ab, cardiolipin Ab, factor VIII level, fibrinogen, plasminogen activator inhibitor level, endogenous tissue plasminogen activator level, thrombin time, hemoglobin electrophoresis, and factor V Leiden, prothrombin gene, MTHFR mutation analysis

    c) Genetic testing for Fabry disease (alpha-galactosidase level)

    d) Lumbar puncture to exclude vasculitis

    e) Lower extremity Doppler and/or MRV pelvis for venous thrombosis

Prognosis and Management

1) Consider tPA in 4.5 hour window in eligible patients (see acute thrombolysis chapter)

2) Benefit from thrombolysis similar to other stroke subtypes

3) Better prognosis for functional recovery compared with other subtypes with 50-60% achieving mRS < 2 at long-term follow-up [16]

4) Antiplatelet therapy is the mainstay for secondary stroke prevention following cryptogenic stroke following complete diagnostic evaluation and exclusion of definite cardiac sources of embolism

    a) The Warfarin-Aspirin Recurrent Stroke Study (WARSS) compared aspirin and warfarin in the prevention of recurrent strokes following non-cardioembolic ischemic strokes and found the two were equivalent [17]

b) Aspirin, clopidogrel, or extended-release dipyridamole plus aspirin in monotherapy are all reasonable options for secondary prevention following cryptogenic stroke

5) Strategies addressing other risk factors such as hypertension, dyslipidemia, and smoking cessation are also integral to stroke prevention following cryptogenic stroke

6) Absent randomized controlled data to support PFO closure, current guidelines do not recommend endovascular or surgical closure; medical therapy as outlined above is the standard of care

7) Should recurrent strokes occur despite maximal medical management, endovascular or surgical treatment may be considered weighing risks and benefits with patient preferences

References

[1] Sacco RL, Ellenberg JH, Mohr JP, et al. *Infarcts of undetermined cause: theNINCDS Stroke Data Bank.* Ann Neurol 1989; 25:382.

[2] Petty GW, Brown RD, Whisnant JP, et al. *Ischemic stroke subtypes: a population-based study of incidence and risk factors.* Stroke 1999; 30-2513.

[3] Schulz UG, Rothwell PM. *Differences in vascular risk factors between etiological subtypes of ischemic stroke: importance of population-based studies.* Stroke 2003; 34:2050.

[4] Cerrato P, Imperiale D, Priano L, et al. *Transoesophageal echocardiography in patients without arterial or major cardiac sources of embolism: differences between subtypes.* Cerebrovasc Dis 2002; 13:174.

[5] Stollberger C, Slany J, Schuster I, et al. *The prevalence of deep venous thrombosis in patients with suspected paradoxical embolism.* Ann Intern Med 1993 Sep 15;119(6):461-5.

[6] Cramer SC, Rordorf G, Maki JH, et al. *Increased pelvic vein thrombi in cryptogenic stroke: results of the Paradoxical Emboli from Large*

Veins in Ischemic Stroke (PELVIS) study. Stroke 2004 Jan;35(1):46-50.

[7]   Djaiani G, Phillips-Bute B, Podgoreanu M, et al. *The association of patent foramen ovale and atrial fibrillation after coronary artery bypass graft surgery.* Anesth Analg. 2004 Mar;98(3):585-9.

[8]   Petty GW, Khandheria BK, Meissner I, et al. *Population-based study of the relationship between patent foramen ovale and cerebrovascular ischemic events.* Mayo Clin Proc. 2006 May;81(5):602-8.

[9]   Mas JL, Arquizan C, Lamy C, et al. *Recurrent cerebrovascular events associated with patent foramen ovale, atrial septal aneurysm, or both.* N Engl J Med 2001 Dec 13;345(24):1740-6.

[10]   Serena J, Marti-Fabregas J, Santamarina E, et al. *Recurrent stroke and massive right-to-left shunt: results from the prospective Spanish multicenter (CODICIA) study.* Stroke. 2008 Dec;39(12):3131-6.

[11]   Homma S, Sacco RL, Di Tullio MR, Sciacca RR, Mohr JP. *Effect of medical treatment in stroke patients with patent foramen ovale: patent foramen ovale in Cryptogenic Stroke Study.* Circulation 2002 Jun 4;105(22):2625-31.

[12]   Tayal AH, Tian M, Kelly KM, et al. *Atrial fibrillation detected by mobile cardiac outpatient telemetry in cryptogenic TIA or stroke.* Neurology 2008; 71:1696.

[13]   DiTullio MR, Sacco RL, Gersony D, et al. *Aortic atheromas and acute ischemic stroke: a transesophageal echocardiographic study in an ethnically mixed population.* Neurology 1996; 46:1560.

[14]   Belvis R, Santamaria A, Marti-Fabregas J, et al. *Diagnostic yield of prothrombotic state studies in cryptogenic stroke.* Acta Neurol Scand 2006; 114:250.

[15]   Rolfs A, Bottcher T, Zschiesche M, et al. *Prevalence of Fabry disease in patients with cryptogenic stroke: a prospective study.* Lancet 2005; 366:1794.

[16]   Petty GW, Brown RD, Whisnant JP, et al. *Ischemic stroke subtypes: a population-based study of functional outcomes, survival, and recurrence.* Stroke 2000; 31:1062.

[17]   Mohr JP, Thompson JLP, Lazar RM, et al. *A comparison of warfarin and aspirin for prevention of recurrent ischemic stroke.* N Engl J Med 2001; 345:1444.

In: Handbook of Stroke and Neurocritical Care   ISBN: 978-61324-786-0
Editor: V. H. Lee   © 2012 Nova Science Publishers, Inc.

Chapter VII

Ischemic Stroke - Other Rare Causes

Jim Conners
Department of Neurological Sciences,
Section of Stroke and Neurocritical care,
Rush University Medical Center, Chicago, IL, USA

Background

1) Account for 5% of all ischemic strokes
2) Major categories include infectious and inflammatory conditions, hereditary conditions, hematologic dyscrasias, and non-inflammatory disorders of the arterial wall
3) Infectious/inflammatory
4) Hereditory

Vasculitis- Primary CNS and Systemic Diseases

1) Primary CNS vasculitis
   a) Pathophysiology

        (i) Idiopathic and progressive infiltration of the CNS vasculature with mononuclear cells

        (ii) typically involves small and middle sized arteries as well as leptomeninges

        (iii) leads to ischemia, infarction and hemorrhage

   b) Signs and Symptoms

        (i) Ischemic stroke, SAH and IPH as well as seizures and cranial neuropathies can all be found making presentation highly variable

        (ii) Headache associated with subacute cognitive decline is most common presentation

   c) Diagnosis D

        (i) Essential to differentiate from other vasculitides (infectious and non-infectious) with serum and CSF studies

        (ii) CT or MRI may demonstrate a combination of both ischemic and hemorrhagic strokes

        (iii) Angiographic features include multifocal stenoses. Conventional angiography is gold standard but will be normal if disease is restricted to vessels <500μm.

        (iv) Brain biopsy gives definitive diagnosis. Ideal biopsy contains cortex, leptomeninges and cortical vessel

   d) Treatment

        (i) Immunosuppression with high dose IV steroids

        (ii) For clinically deteriorating patients, addition of cyclophosphamide, azathioprine or methotrexate has been advocated

2) Systemic vasculitic disorders

Other Inflammatory Conditions

1) Auto-immune connective tissue disorders

   a) Systemic Lupus Erythematosus- most common cause of stroke in SLE is cardioembolism due to;

Systemic vasculitis syndrome	Common presenting features	Cerebrovascular findings	Diagnosis	Primary treatment
Large Vessel Vasculitis				
Temporal Arteritis (Giant Cell Arteritis)	Patients >50 y/o, Headache, polymyalgia rheumatica, jaw or tongue claudication, scalp tenderness, fever, vision disturbances	Stroke and TIA related to vertebrobasilar & carotid involvement or aortic dissection	Age >50, new localized headache, elevated ESR or CRP. Biopsy for confirmation	High dose steroids-- begin immediately (prior to biopsy confirmation) if high suspicion to avoid potential visual loss
Takayasu's arteritis	Predominantly in young Asian women. Extremity claudication, athralgias, constitutional symptoms, renal ischemia	Narrowing, occlusion or dilation of aorta and craniocervical vessels lead to CNS ischemia	In correct clinical setting, angiography reveals tapered luminal narrowing with vessel wall thickening not due to other causes	Glucocorticoids are standard, angioplasty or bypass graft may be indicated
Medium Sized Vessel Vasculitis				
Polyarteritis Nodosa (PAN)	Systemic necrotizing vasculitis that affects almost any organ system but spares the lungs Idiopathic or secondary to connective tissue disease, chronic viral infection or leukemia	Ischemic stroke or ICH in 10% of patients More likely secondary to HTN from renal involvement than CNS vasculitis	No diagnostic lab test Need tissue biopsy of involved organ	Idiopathic PAN- Glucocorticoids +/- cyclophosphamide based on response and severity of illness Secondary PAN mandates treatment of primary disease state

Kawasaki disease	Predominantly self limited and occurs in childhood Fever, conjunctivitis, lymphadenopathy, rash, oral erythema and coronary artery aneurysms	Rarely presents with CNS vasculitis and subsequent stroke or encephalopathy	Fever > 5 days plus 4 of the following 5; Conjunctivitis, oral mucous membrane changes, extremity changes, polymorphous rash, cervical lymphadenopathy	High-dose aspirin and intravenous immune globulin
Small Vessel Vasculitis				
Microscopic polyangiitis	Pulmonary hemorrhage, glomerulonephritis	Headache and seizure most common CNS complication although ischemic and hemorrhagic strokes have been reported	ANCA (+) Tissue biopsy needed (absence of granulomatous inflammation helps differentiate from Wegener's Granulomatosis)	Glucocorticoids +/- cytotoxic agents
Churg-Strauss Syndrome	Necrotizing vasculitis, asthma, eosinophilia, granulomas	Rarely present with encephalopathy due to small diffuse ischemic infarcts	ANCA (+) Typical symptoms plus biopsy with extravascular eosinophils	Glucocorticoids +/- cytotoxic agents
Cogan's Syndrome	Interstitial keratitis and hearing loss Mean age of onset 25yrs.	Cerebrovascular involvement rare but includes ischemic stroke and CVST	No specific diagnostic test Diagnosis suggested by keratitis, acute hearing loss and negative work up for syphilis and other autoimmune conditions	Glucocorticoids

Libman-Sacks endocarditis, valvulopathy, and infective endocarditis. Other associated features include hypercoagulable states (lupus anticoagulant and anti-cardiolipin antibodies), accelerated atherosclerosis, and rarely cerebral vasculitis
   b) Rheumatoid arthritis- associated with accelerated atherosclerosis, as well as possible vasculitis, hypercoagulability and rare instances of dural rheumatoid involvement predisposing to venous sinus thrombosis
2) Behçet's Disease- classically characterized by oral aphthous ulcers, genital ulcers and uveitis however is a multisystemic inflammatory process
   a) Unclear etiology but current theory points to antigenic cross reactivity triggered by infection leading to an autoimmune response
   b) Most common in middle eastern and Japanese patients with mean age of onset 25-30 years
   c) Inflammatory lesions in the parenchyma make up 80% of neuro-Behçet's with the other 20% being neurovascular (Cerebral venous sinus thrombosis most common but can also see arterial occlusion, arterial malformations and aneurysms)
   d) Treatment consists of immunosuppression and anticoagulation if CVST
3) Sarcoidosis- rarely causes ischemic stroke although there are multiple possible mechanisms that need to be considered including;
   a) perivascular granulomatous inflammation causing small vessel thrombosis
   b) cardioembolism related to cardiomyopathy
   c) large vessel inflammation with thrombosis or compression from granulomas
   d) sinovenous infiltration leading to CVST
4) Sneddon's Syndrome- well delineated syndrome characterized by the association of TIA or stroke and widespread livedo racemosa, a purplish mottling of the skin
   a) typically affects middle aged women, with the first stroke often occurring before age 45

  b) trunk and/or buttocks livedo racemosa is noted in nearly all patients but it may also be located on limbs, face, hands, or feet

  c) unclear etiology though two main hypotheses are a hypercoagulable state and a small vessel vasculopathy

  d) 40%–50% of patients with Sneddon's syndrome are aPL-positive

5) Susac's syndrome- rare microangiopathy of unclear etiology with encephalopathy, branch retinal artery occlusions and sensorineural hearing loss.

  a) most patients are Caucasian women 20-40 yrs old

  b) MRI demonstrates multifocal T2 hyperintensities that enhance as well as characteristic black holes in the corpus callosum

  c) retinal angiography demonstrates multifocal fluorescence and branch retinal artery occlusions

  d) typically has a multiphasic course with spontaneous improvements although patients commonly left with long term sequelae

  e) empirical treatment with immunosuppressive agents

6) Kohlmeier-Degos syndrome (Malignant Atrophic Papulosis)- occlusive arteriopathy of unknown etiology.

  a) Most common in white males in 2nd and 3rd decades.

  b) Clinical findings include;

    (i) cutaneous lesions- initially pink macules that become papular with depressed porcelain white center

    (ii) GI lesions which are similar in appearance to skin lesions and lead to microvascular infarction and subsequent GI perforation

    (iii) CNS ischemia and infarction noted in parenchyma, cranial nerves and spinal roots

  c) If limited to cutaneous involvement, patients have normal life span however the systemic variant has a fatal outcome with no known treatment

Infectious Causes of Stroke

1) Background

a) Acute and chronic infections may lead to ischemic stroke through various mechanisms;

b) act as a trigger for thrombosis due to a procoagulant state and increased platelet reactivity

c) direct cerebrovascular involvement through vessel wall infiltration, inflammation/vasculitis, or occlusion

d) systemic effects leading to cerebral embolism

2) Bacterial Infections

a) Bacterial meningitis from *Haemophilus influenzae, Streptococcus pneumoniae,* or *Neisseria meningitides* may cause a subarachnoid inflammatory reaction that can lead to vessel occlusion and aneurysmal formation

b) Tuberculous meningitis is characterized by thick exudate causing panarteritis of basal arteries, particularly the MCA and lenticluostriate branches leading to cerebral infarction

c) Meningovascular syphilis is characterized by endarteritis obliterans of the medium sized meningeal arteries and leads to ischemic lesions. Infarction from thrombosis of small penetrating arteries due to perivascular infiltrates is also common

3) Viral Infections

a) VZV

   (i) Typically 2-6 weeks after initial vesicular zoster eruption, patients can develop arteriopathy

   (ii) More common after herpes zoster ophthalmicus than other segmental herpes zoster and often vasculopathy occurs on the side of the skin lesion

   (iii) Virus reaches arterial wall by direct neural passage along the trigeminal nerve and primarily affects large cerebral arteries

b) HIV

   (i) increased risk of ischemic and hemorrhagic stroke due to secondary causes related to complications associated with HIV/AIDS , a prothrombotic state, and HIV associated vasculopathy

   (ii) vasculopathy may be small vessel leading to microinfarcts or medium/large vessel characterized by occlusion, fusiform aneurysmal formation or stenosis

4) Fungal infections

a) CNS fungal infections may occlude small subarachnoid blood vessels or lead to formation of mycotic aneurysms
b) Of the most common fungal infections, stroke is most likely to occur with angioinvasive Aspergillus
c) Rhinocerebral mucormycosis, especially in diabetics, may extend into the cavernous sinus and lead to carotid artery thrombosis
d) Parasitic infections
e) Neurocysticercosis is the most common parasitic infection of the CNS. Inflammatory response leads to leptomeningeal thickening, occlusion of small perforator vessels and lacunar strokes
f) American trypanosomiasis (Chagas' disease) is widespread throughout Latin America with approximately 10 million individuals infected. Rarely causes direct CNS infection however cardiomyopathy is common and leads to CNS embolism in 19% of those patients

Hereditary and Genetic Conditions

Small Vessel Hereditary Conditions

1) Several hereditary conditions affecting small blood vessels of the brain have been identified: CADASIL (Cerebral Autosomal Dominant Arteriopathy with Subcortical Infarcts and Leukoencephalopathy); CARASIL (Cerebral Autosomal Recessive Arteriopathy with Subcortical Infarcts and Leukoencephalopathy); RVCL (Retinal Vasculopathy with Cerebral Leukodystrophy) and Fabry disease
2) CADASIL (Cerebral Autosomal Dominant Arteriopathy with Subcortical Infarcts and Leukoencephalopathy)
   a) AD disorder characterized by mutation in *Notch 3* gene which is expressed in vascular smooth muscle cells. Causes accumulation of granular osmiophilic material (GOM) in these cells and in capillaries
   b) Mean age of onset is 45 years and typically leads to death within 10 to 25 years of onset

    c) Symptoms include
        (i) TIA or ischemic stroke- Initial presentation in up to 70% of cases
        (ii) Migraine with aura (often atypical and prolonged)
        (iii) Mood disorders
        (iv) Cognitive decline and dementia beginning in 5th decade
    d) MRI findings may include lacunar infarctions, confluent symmetric leukoariosis, and hyperintensities at the temporal poles
    e) Electron microscopy can detect GOM in muscle or skin biopsies but definitive diagnosis is made with genetic analysis for *Notch3* mutation

3) CARASIL (Cerebral Autosomal Recessive Arteriopathy with Subcortical Infarcts and Leukoencephalopathy)
    a) small vessel disease described in Japanese and Chinese patients with vascular degeneration in the absence of GOM
    b) autosomal recessive disorder associated with HTRA 1 gene mutations
        (i) leads to increased signaling of TGF-β, upregulation of extracellular matrix proteins and subsequent vascular fibrosis-onset in young adulthood with average clinical course < 10 years
    c) common symptoms include ischemic stroke (in 2/3 of cases), alopecia, bone lesions, severe intervertebral disc disease, progressive mental and motor deterioration and dementia

4) RVCL (Retinal Vasculopathy with Cerebral Leukodystrophy)-
    a) small vessel vasculopathy with fibrinoid necrosis of vessel walls in the brain, retina and kidneys
    b) caused by mutations in gene *TREX1* which leads to accumulation of the TREX1 enzyme triggering abnormal immune responses
    c) Three previous distinct diseases now considered phenotypic variants of RVCL; HERNS (Hereditary Endotheliopathy with Retinopathy, Nephropathy and Stroke), HVR (Hereditary Vascular Retinopathy) and CRV (Cerebroretinal Vasculopathy)

d) onset usually in 3rd or 4th decade with progressive visual loss, stroke, dementia, migraines, nephropathy and psychiatric disease

e) radiologic findings include contrast-enhancing, space-occupying tumor-like lesions in the frontoparietal region related to areas of infarct with blood brain barrier breakdown, edema and astrocytic gliosis

f) progresses to neurovegetative state and death typically within 10 yrs of diagnosis

5) Fabry Disease

a) X linked disorder caused by deficiency in α-galactosidase A

b) symptoms begin in 1st or 2nd decade with neuropathic pain, angiokeratomas, hypohidrosis and corneal opacities

c) neurologic, cardiac and renal disease follow in early adulthood

d) men typically more severely affected than heterozygous women whose symptoms present at later age

e) deposition of glycosphingolipid leads to development of intracranial artery dolichoectasia and progressive occlusion of small arteries and arterioles

f) after cerebral ischemia, approximately 50% will die within 8 years. Majority of mortality linked to recurrent stroke or renal failure

g) Enzyme replacement therapy clears endovascular deposits and should begin as soon as clinical signs are present

Heritable connective tissue disorders

1) Ehlers-Danlos

a) group of >10 connective tissue diseases that involve a genetic defect in collagen and connective-tissue synthesis

b) Type IV EDS

(i) most individuals with cerebrovascular complications have Type IV

(ii) Autosomal dominant abnormal production of type III procollagen which is the major type found in blood vessels

(iii) complications include arterial dissections, intracranial aneurysms and carotid-cavernous fistulae

2) Marfan's Syndrome
   a) autosomal dominant connective disorder which results from mutations in the fibrillin-1 (*FBN1*) gene on chromosome 15
   b) symptoms result from defect in fibrillin which serves as a substrate for elastin in the skin, aorta, and all three layers of the arterial wall
   c) cerebrovascular events occur in the setting of dissection or aneurysm of the aorta, internal carotid or vertebral arteries
3) Pseudoxanthoma elasitcum (PXE)
   a) inherited connective tissue disorder that causes fragmentation of elastic fibers predominantly in the skin, eyes and blood vessels
   b) cutaneous manifestations begin with small yellow papules that resemble xanthomas that can coalesce and progress to a lax, wrinkled, cobblestone appearance
   c) 85% of patients have angiod streaks on their retina
   d) vascular involvement can lead to GI hemorrhage, cardiac disease and cerebrovascular disease including intracranial aneurysms with SAH and occlusive cervicocranial disease
   e) both autosomal dominant and autosomal recessive forms exist with common genetic defect in the ABCC6 gene
4) Osteogenesis Imperfecta (OI)
   a) disorder of congenital bone fragility caused by mutations in the genes encoding type I procollagen
   b) Cerebrovascular complications are rare, but can present with aneurysms, dissections, fistulas, and stenosis of cerebral vessels

Mitochondrial Disorders

1) Multisystemic progressive degenerative disorders resulting from mutations in mitochondrial DNA
2) Respiratory chain protein dysfunction primarily affects tissue with high metabolic demand (e.g. brain and muscle)
3) MELAS (Mitochondrial myopathy, encephalopathy, lactic acidosis, and stroke-like episodes)
   a) clinical presentation reflects name of disorder in addition to seizures, exercise intolerance, sensorineural hearing

loss, migraines, diabetes, short stature and cognitive decline

   b) fever and infections causing increased metabolic demand have been implicated as possible triggers for stroke-like episodes

   c) most common defect, present in 80% of patients, is a point mutation in the transfer RNA for leucine but at least 30 different point mutations are known

   d) MRI demonstrates ischemic appearing lesions not confined to vascular territories that may resolve with time, subcortical white matter lesions and generalized tissue loss

   e) CSF typically has elevated lactate and muscle biopsy may show ragged red fibers

   f) false negative tissue diagnosis possible due to heteroplasmy

   g) most patients die by the fourth decade of medical complications

4) Kearns-Sayre syndrome and MERRF (Myoclonic Epilepsy with Ragged Red Fibers)

   a) Stroke like episodes have also been reported due to similar mitochondrial dysfunction

Hematologic / Prothrombotic States

1) Quantitative and qualitative abnormalities of cellular constituents and clotting factors

2) Red Blood Cells

   a) Polycythemia-increases blood viscosity, decreases CBF, increases risk thrombosis

   b) Sickle cell anemia- occlusive disease of small penetrating vessels and large vessel arteriopathy

3) Platelets

   a) Thrombobytosis- either essential or myeloproliferative with counts typically >1million associated with stroke

   b) Sticky platelet syndrome (SPS)- autosomal dominant platelet disorder associated with arterial and venous thromboembolic events and characterized by hyperaggregability of platelets

Table 1. Genetic and acquired disorders that alter coagulation cascade

MTHFR (Methyltetrahydrofolate reductase) gene mutation
Factor V Leiden mutation
Prothrombin gene mutation
Antithrombin III deficiency
Protein C deficiency
Protein S deficiency
Activated Protein C resistance
Antiphospholipid antibodies
Lupus anticoagulant
Anticardiolipin antibodies
Anti-beta 2 GPI antibodies
Anti-phosphatidylserine antibodies

4) White Blood Cells
   a) Leukemia- extremely elevated WBC counts can lead to micro-infarcts
   b) Intravascular Lymphoma- causes multifocal vascular occlusions
5) Hyperviscosity- Waldenstrom's macroglobulinemia, multiple myeloma, and chylomicra have all been associated with stroke
6) Clotting factor abnormalities/Hypercoagulability

Table 2. Other Prothrombotic states

Cancer
Trousseau's syndrome seen with pancreatic, ovarian, prostate and lung adenocarcinoma
Certain chemotherapeutic agents
Marantic endocartiditis
Pregnancy
Oral contraceptive use and hormone therapy
Increased levels of factor V, VII, and VIII occurs in inflammatory conditions
Inflammatory bowel disease
Disseminated intravascular coagulation (DIC)
Thrombotic Thrombocytopenic Purpura (TTP)
Heparin Induced Thrombocytopenia (HIT) with thrombosis
Polycystic Kidney Disease
Scorpion stings
Falciparum Malaria

Cryoglobulinemia
Macroglobulinemia
Nephrotic syndrome
Postoperative or post-traumatic state
Exogenous administration of clotting factors

Disorders of the Arterial Wall

1) Moyamoya disease and syndrome- progressive stenosis of the intracranial carotid arteries and their proximal branches. Leads to compensatory development of abnormally dilated collateral vessels that resemble a "puff of smoke"
   a) Pathophysiology.
      (i) Moyamoya disease is idiopathic. Characterized by thickening of intimal and medial layers and fragmentation of the internal elastic lamina.
      (ii) Moyamoya syndrome has many associated risk factors including but not limited to; sickle cell disease, Neurofibromatosis type 1, cranial irradiation, Down's syndrome, advanced atherosclerosis and hypercoagulable states
         1) most are chronic states that lead to ischemia with subsequent proliferation of small vessels in the proximal branches of the MCA
   b) Epidemiology
      (i) two peaks; children <14 and adults between 25 and 49
      (ii) Female to male ratio 1.8:1
      (iii) Incidence is 10x higher in Japan than Europe
   c) Treatment
      (i) Given the progressive nature of the disease, revascularization (direct or indirect) is the treatment of choice. In moyamoya syndrome, management is also directed at the underlying etiology
         1) Direct revascularization performed with anastomosis of ECA branches to a cortical artery
            a) immediate effects but more challenging in the pediatric population with extremely small vasculature

      2) Indirect revascularization (ie. EDAMS, encephaloduroarteriomyosynangiosis) involves placement of vascularized tissue supplied by the ECA in direct contact with the cortex

        a) takes months to form collaterals however has favorable long term effect

2) Cervico-cephalic Arterial Dissections

  a) Pathophysiology

    (i) Tear in the intima causes stenosis and occlusion while a tear between the media and adventitia typically leads to pseudoaneurysm formation

    (ii) May occur spontaneously or from trauma

    (iii) Traumatic dissections occur with c-spine fracture & blunt or penetrating neck injury, as well as instances that lead to forceful exertion or rotation of the neck including sports, chiropractic manipulation, intubation and delivery

    (iv) Spontaneous dissections are either idiopathic or linked to a connective tissue disorder; Marfan's Syndrome, Ehlers-Danlos, Osteogenesis Imperfecta, Pseudoxanthoma elasticum, Polycystic Kidney Disease, Fibromuscular Dysplasia, Erdheim-Gsell segmental cystic medionecrosis

  b) Epidemiology

    (i) Cause 2.5% of all strokes but up to 20% of strokes in the young.

    (ii) Incidence has been reported <3/100,000 although likely number is higher as more cases are being diagnosed with increased awareness and more accurate non-invasive neuroimaging

  c) Diagnosis

    (i) Symptoms can be related to arterial occlusion, embolism from intramural clot or local compression from expanding pseudoaneurysm

    (ii) Besides ischemic stroke or SAH (reported in intracranial vertebral artery dissection), local signs and symptoms include headache, face & neck pain, Horner's Syndrome, pulsatile tinnitus, lower cranial nerve palsies

    (iii) MRI and MRA may demonstrate luminal compromise as well as intramural hematoma with T1 fat suppressed images
  d) Treatment
    (i) Anticoagulation or antiplatelet agents are both reasonable as there is no randomized controlled trial comparing the two
    (ii) In the US, the general consensus for dissections that have led to stroke is to anticoagulate until the vessel heals or for 3-6 months
 3) Fibromuscular Dysplasia- proliferation of smooth muscle cells in arterial walls causing constricting bands and characteristic string of beads appearance on imaging.
  a) commonly found in middle aged women in both extracranial and intracranial arteries with predilection for ICA's and renal arteries
  b) Often asymptomatic but may lead to dissection or ischemic stroke

References

[1] *Vasculitis of the nervous system.* Younger DS Curr Opin Neurol. 2004;17:317-36.

[2] *Vasculitis in the central nervous system.* Calabrese LH, Duna GF, Lie JT Arthritis Rheum. 1997;40:1189-201.

[3] *Cerebral autosomal recessive arteriopathy with subcortical infarcts and leukoencephalopathy.* Yanagawa et. al Neurology. 2002; 58 817-820.

[4] *Summary of the proceedings of the First International Workshop on CADASIL.* MG Bousser and E Tournier-Lasserve Stroke 1994;25;704-707.

[5] *[CADASIL and CARASIL]* López JI, Vilanova JR. Neurologia. 2009;2:125-30.

[6] *A new cause of hereditary small vessel disease: Angiopathy of retina and brain.* Martin Dichgans, Neurology 2003;60:8–9.

[7] *C-terminal truncations in human 3'-5' DNA exonuclease TREX1 cause autosomal dominant retinal vasculopathy with cerebral leukodystrophy.* Richards, Anna et. al. Nature Genetics. 200;39:1068-1070.

[8]   *Hematologic disorders and ischemic stroke. A selective review.* RG Hart and MC Kanter Stroke 1990;21;1111-1121.

[9]   *Hereditary endotheliopathy with retinopathy, nephropathy, and stroke (HERNS)* J. Jen, et. al Neurology 1997;49:1322-1330.

[10]   *Genetics of Ischemic stroke.* Dichgans M. Lancet Neurology 2007;6:149-161.

[11]   *MRI findings in Susac's syndrome.* Susac JO et. al Neurology. 2003;61:1783-7.

[12]   *Cerebrovascular complications of Fabry's disease.* Mitsias P, Levine SR Ann Neurol. 1996;40:8-17.

[13]   *Pathogenesis and treatment of sickle cell disease.* Bunn HF N Engl J Med. 1997;337:762-9.

[14]   *Sticky platelet syndrome.* Mammen EF. Semin Thromb Hemost. 1999;25:361-5.

[15]   *Varicella zoster virus vasculopathies: diverse clinical manifestations, laboratory features, pathogenesis, and treatment.* Gilden D, Cohrs RJ, Mahalingam R, Nagel MA Lancet Neurol. 2009;8:731-40.

[16]   *Neurological symptoms in type A aortic dissections.* Gaul C, Dietrich W, Friedrich I, Sirch J, Erbguth FJ Stroke. 2007;38:292-7.

[17]   *Bechet's syndrome: a report of 41 patients with emphasis on neurological manifestations.* Farah S, et. al J Neurol Neurosurg Psychiatry. 1998;64:382-4.

[18]   *Sarcoidosis presenting as brainstem ischemic stroke.* Navi BB, DeAngelis LM Neurology. 2009;72:1021-1022.

[19]   *Moyamoya Disease and Moyamoya Syndrome* R. Michael Scott, M.D., and Edward R. Smith, M.D. N Engl J Med 2009;360:1226-37.

Textbooks

[1]   *Adams and Victor's Principles of Neurology.* Eigth Edition, Ropper and Brown.

[2]   *Stroke Practical Management.* Third Edition, Warlow et. Al.

[3]   *Stroke: Pathophysiology, Diagnosis, and Management.* Fourth Edition, Mohr et. Al. Uncommon Causes of Stroke Second Edition. Louis R. Caplan, Julien Bogousslavsky.

In: Handbook of Stroke and Neurocritical Care   ISBN: 978-61324-786-0
Editor: Vivien H. Lee   © 2012 Nova Science Publishers, Inc.

Chapter VIII

Ischemic Stroke – Acute Therapy (IV)

Shawna Cutting and Shyam Prabhakaran
Department of Neurological Sciences,
Section of Stroke and Neurocritical care,
Rush University Medical Center, Chicago, IL, USA

Introduction

1) Background
   a) IV tPA is one of three treatments, besides aspirin and stroke unit care, shown to have benefit in randomized clinical trials for ischemic stroke patients
   b) It was approved by the United States Food and Drug Administration due in large part to the convincing study by the National Institute of Neurological Disorders and Stroke (NINDS) in 1996, showing improved clinical outcome at three months among those patients who received IV tPA.[1]
   c) ECASS-III extended the treatment window to 4.5 hours for select populations.

    d) Despite strong evidence of the benefit of treatment with IV tPA, less than 10% of ischemic stroke victims receive this therapy, even though up to 25% arrive within 3 hours.[2]

    e) Summary of relevant research studies on acute ischemic stroke (see table)

2) National Institute of Health Stroke Scale (NIHSS)

    a) Designed as a research tool designed to help evaluate stroke severity.

    b) 11 part assessment of language, motor, and sensory functioning; allows the medical professional to quickly identify neurologic deficits and determine eligibility for acute treatment with IV tPA.

    c) Emergency physicians, neurologists, nurses, hospitalists, clinical research raters and medical students can be certified in administering this scale.

    d) This scale should be administered as soon as a patient is suspected of having an acute stroke. A brief history may be taken before administering the scale. This should focus on time of symptom onset, nature of symptoms, and presence of any possible factors that would complicate or contraindicate treatment or suggest an alternative non-cerebrovascular diagnosis.

NIHSS Standard Images

1) Patients should be asked to describe the scene, name the objects, and read the sentences.

2) In addition, the patient should be asked to repeat:

- Mama
- Tip-top
- Fifty-fifty
- Thanks
- Huckleberry
- Baseball Player

(Year published)	Type of study	Patients	Findings
NINDS (1995)	Randomized double blind placebo controlled two part trial looking at benefit of IV tPA in patients treated within 3 hours of symptom onset First part investigated whether tPA had clinical activity evidenced by improvement of 4 points on NIHSS score or resolution of symptoms Second part used global test statistic to assess clinical outcomes at three months according to Barthel index, modified Rankin scale, Glasgow outcome scale, and NIHSS score	624 patients Ischemic stroke with clearly defined time of onset. Measurable deficit on NIHSS Baseline CT that showed no evidence of intracranial hemorrhage Exclusion criteria match those listed later in chapter	Part one: No significant difference between the tPA group and placebo. Improved clinical outcome on all four outcome measures at 3 months in IV tPA group Part two: Long-term clinical benefit for tPA confirmed: global odds ratio for favorable outcome 1.7 Symptomatic intracranial hemorrhage higher incidence in tPA group (6.4% vs 0.6%) Mortality not statistically different between two groups at 90 days
ECASS-I (1995)	Randomized, prospective, multi-center, double-blind, placebo-controlled trial looking at IV tPA (1.1 mg/kg) up to 6 hours after symptom onset. Primary endpoint modified Rankin scale and Barthel Index at 90 days Secondary endpoint Combined Barthel Index and Rankin scale; Scandinavian Stroke Scale (SSS) at 90 days; 30-day mortality Tertiary endpoint early neurologic recovery on SSS; duration of in-hospital stay.	620 patients Acute ischemic stroke Moderate to severe neurologic deficit No major early infarct changes on initial CT Scandinavian stroke scale used	No difference in primary endpoints in the intention to treat analysis; target population analysis showed a significant difference (p=0.035) in the Rankin scale score in favor of IV tPA treated patients. Combined Barthel Index and Rankin Scale favored IV tPA treated patients (P < .001). SSS at 90 days significantly better in IV tPA treated patients in the target population (P = .03). In-hospital stay shorter in the IV tPA treatment arm; no difference in the mortality rate at 30 days or overall incidence of intracerebral hemorrhages. Occurrence of large parenchymal hemorrhages was more frequent in the IV tPA treated patients.

Inset (Continued)

Trial (Year published)	Type of study	Patients	Findings
ECASS-II (1998)	Randomized, prospective, double-blind, placebo-controlled trial looking at IV tPA (0.9 mg/kg) within 6 hours of stroke onset Primary endpoint modified Rankin scale at 90 days, divided into favorable (0-1) and unfavorable (2-6) outcome Secondary endpoints change from baseline to day 30 on NIH stroke scale; combined Barthel Index and modified Rankin scale Tertiary endpoints Barthel Index at 90 days; SSS at 90 days; duration of hospital stay; quality of life at 90 days	800 patients Clinical diagnosis of moderate to severe stroke No or only early minor signs of infarction on initial CT Swelling <33% of MCA territory Scandinavian stroke scale and NIH stroke scale used	No difference in modified Rankin scale at 90 days; when divided into dependence (3-6) vs independence (0-2) statistically significant difference noted. Other endpoints with no difference except median change in NIH stroke scale more in IV tPA group More deaths in first 7 days due to intracerebral hemorrhage in IV tPA group; higher rate of intraparenchymal hemorrhage in IV tPA group
ATLANTIS (1999)	Placebo-controlled, double-blind, randomized study looking at administration of IV tPA between 3 and 5 hours after symptom onset Primary outcome NIHSS <=1 Secondary outcome Barthel Index, modified Rankin scale, and Glasgow Outcome Scale at 30 and 90 days.	613 patients Ischemic stroke with clearly defined time of onset. Measurable deficit on NIHSS Baseline CT that showed no evidence of intracranial hemorrhage	No significant difference between placebo and treatment group in primary or secondary outcome measures Symptomatic intracerebral hemorrhage in 7.0% (p<0.001) of treatment group Mortality at 90 days 6.9% in placebo group and 11% in tPA group (p= 0.09)
AbESTT (2005)	Phase two randomized double blind placebo controlled study looking at administration of abciximab within 6 hours of symptom onset Primary safety endpoint ICH, either fatal or symptomatic	401 patients Acute ischemic stroke Clearly defined time of onset less than 6 hours prior to drug administration	Average time to randomization 4 h 30 m Average time to treatment after randomization 31-32 m Nonsignificant shift in favorable outcomes if treated with abciximab

published)			
ESTAT (2006)	Randomized, double-blind, placebo-controlled trial looking at ancrod infusion (purified pit viper venom) started within 6 hours of symptom onset Primary endpoint Barthel index at least equal to prestroke value Secondary endpoint Scandinavian Stroke Scale, modified Rankin scale, death rates at 3 and 12 months	1222 patients Scandinavian stroke scale <40 (lower numbers indicate more severe deficits) No CT evidence of developing infarction or hemorrhage	85% of patients treated between 3h and 6h Functional outcome no different between treatment and placebo Symptomatic hemorrhage in 7% (p=0.007)
DIAS-2 (2008)	Randomized, double-blind, placebo-controlled study looking at desmoteplase given at either 90μ/kg or 125 μ /kg between 3 and 9 hours after symptom onset; Primary endpoint Clinical improvement at day 90 measured by NIHSS, Barthel Index and modified Rankin scale, and infarct volume (as measured by MRI). Secondary endpoint Change from baseline infarct volume at day 30 (measured by MRI or perfusion CT).	193 patients NIHSS from 4 up to 24 Distinct penumbra (at least 20%) involving MCA, ACA, or PCA as identified by perfusion CT, perfusion imaging on MR or DWI imaging on MRI	Median NIHSS 9 Average time to treatment 388-402 minutes in three subgroups No statistically significant difference in clinical outcome with desmoteplase Symptomatic hemorrhage in 4% of desmoteplase groups Asymptomatic hemorrhage in 35% of lower dose, 33% of higher dose, and 33% of placebo
ECASS-III (2008)	Randomized double blind placebo controlled study looking at IV tPA up to 4.5 hours after symptom onset Primary endpoint disability at 90 days; favorable vs unfavorable outcome divided between modified Rankin 0-1 vs 2-6 Secondary endpoint global outcome analysis using Barthel index, modified Rankin scale, Glasgow outcome scale, and NIHSS	821 patients Acute ischemic stroke Clearly defined time of onset 3 to 4.5 hours prior to drug administration Age 18-80 Symptoms present for at least 30 min with no significant improvement prior to treatment Expanded exclusion criteria	Average time to tPA 3 h 59 m More patients in tPA group with favorable outcome at 90 days (odds ratio 1.3) Increased incidence of any intracranial hemorrhage (27% vs 17.6%) and symptomatic intracranial hemorrhage (2.4 vs 0.2%) in tPA group No difference in mortality between two groups.

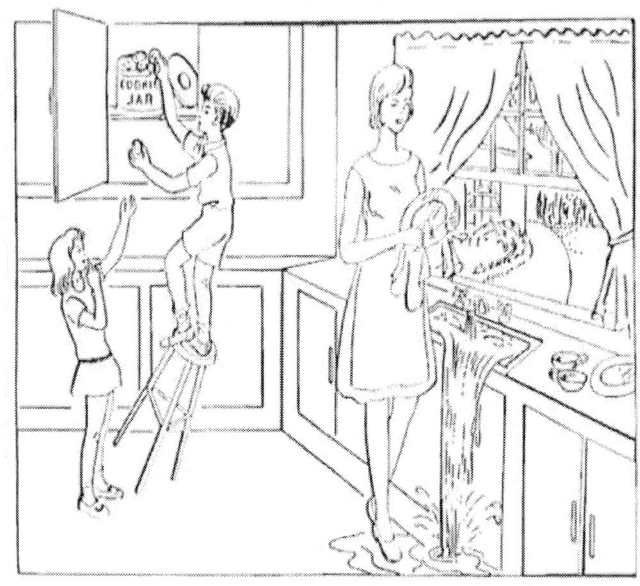

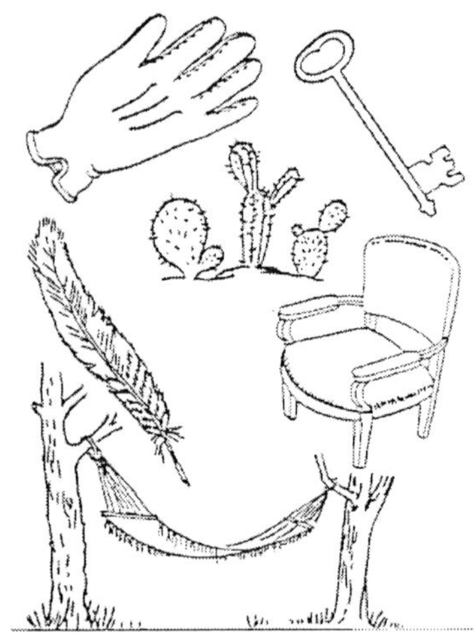

You know how.

Down to earth.

I got home from work.

Near the table in the dining room.

They heard him speak on the radio last night.

Scoring of NIHSS in Special Populations

1) Non-English speaking
   a) All attempts should be made to obtain proper translation through an on-site or phone interpreter.

    b)   If unable to obtain translation through professional means, a family member may be used.

    c)   Spanish translation is included in on-site materials at many larger hospitals. A Spanish cross-cultural adaptation of the NIHSS has been developed [3], but is not currently approved for use.

2) Comatose

    a)   The comatose patient will automatically receive an NIHSS of at least 15.

    b)   Coma does not exclude a patient from receiving IV tPA, but additional care will be needed in determining who may give consent for treatment, the exact time of onset of symptoms, and risk of treatment complications.

3) Patients with prior stroke or known pre-existing deficits

    a)   Patients with a prior stroke should be scored for both chronic and acute deficits.

    b)   An estimated NIHSS of baseline deficits can be determined if other family members are available to provide collateral history or if the patient can do so themselves.

    c)   Both the current NIHSS and the estimated baseline NIHSS should be used by the physician in determining eligibility for IV tPA.

4) Other deficits (broken limb, immobilization/joint fusion, amputees)

    a)   Patients should not receive points on the standard scale for immobility at the shoulder or hip or if they are absent a limb. Strictly speaking, they should be scored as a '9'. Practically speaking, this piece of information will likely not be useful in determining eligibility for IV tPA.

5) Blind patients

    a)   Blind patients will automatically score 3 points for visual field deficits.

    b)   Language can be assessed by placing objects in the patient's hands, having them repeat, and asking them to spontaneously produce speech.

    c)   Visual extinction should not be scored.

6) Illiterate patients

    a)   Patients who are not able to read the sentences should be asked to repeat them instead.

7) Under 18 years of age
  a) These patients should be scored the same as those over 18 years of age.
  b) Patients who cannot read should be asked to repeat phrases and sentences as directed above.
  c) Consent for IV tPA should be given by the guardian of the child. Assent must be obtained from the patient (for discussion of consent and assent, see below).

Common Mistakes when Scoring and Performing the NIHSS

1) Checking the sensory exam using light touch and not pinprick
2) Scoring for ataxia when cerebellar exam is not out of proportion to weakness
3) Scoring for extinction/neglect when cannot be determined due to primary sensory loss or other reason.
4) Improperly identifying the time of onset
  a) This is the time that the patient was last known normal, which is not always the time the patient notices the symptoms.
  b) In cases where a person has evolving symptoms (i.e. blurred vision, then hemiparesis), the time of onset should be documented as time of first symptom.
     - Examples
       - Patient went to bed at 10 pm, awoke at 6 am with left sided weakness → Time of onset is 10 pm.
       - Patient was talking to family at 5 pm, at 6 pm family heard a thump from the bedroom; they went in and found the patient on the floor → Time of onset is 5 pm.
       - Patient was talking on phone at 3 pm, when person on phone noticed the patient suddenly started slurring their speech. The patient last saw a co-worker at 2:30 pm → Time of onset is 3 pm.

Interpreting the NIHSS

1) Studies have shown that with an NIHSS score greater than 10 there was a 96% positive predictive value of large artery occlusion [4]
   a) However, there is no minimum NIHSS score used to select a group of patients that would benefit from angiographic imaging/intervention [5]
2) Specific items within the NIHSS have been found to be predictors of central occlusion confirmed by angiography, as shown in the table below (from Fischer et al, 2005) [4]:

NIHSS at baseline & odds ratio for large vessel occlusion (ICA, M1, M2, basilar artery)

NIHSS items	Odds ratio vessel occlusion	P value using univariate model	Odds ratio for Vessel occlusion	P value using multivariate model
LOC	3.3	0.001		
LOC alertness	3.0	0.001		
LOC questions	2.7	0.002	4.0	<0.001
LOC commands	2.7	0.005		
Gaze	4.6	<0.001	2.9	<0.001
Visual fields	2.8	0.021		
Facial palsy	2.1	0.129		
Motor arm	4.5	0.002		
Motor leg	5.2	<0.001	4.2	0.001
Ataxia	0.4	0.1		
Sensation	2.5	0.005		
Language	1.7	0.079		
Dysarthria	1.3	0.4		
Neglect	3.5	0.002	3.2	0.013

LOC=level of consciousness.

3) Left hemisphere lesions tend to have higher NIHSS than right hemisphere lesions that are equal in size due to the incongruous weight that aphasia carries on scoring [6]
4) Initial NIHSS is the major predictor of hospital disposition among patients who receive IV tPA; for every 5 point increase on the scale, relative risk of discharge to nursing home or rehabilitation facility increased dramatically, as seen in the table below (from Schlegel et al, 2004): [7]

Predictor	Rehabilitation Center	Skilled Nursing Facility
Age per year	1.01	*1.09
Male	0.76	0.57
White race	0.78	*0.50
Initial NIHSS		
<=5	Referent	Referent
6-10 vs <=5	1.78	2.31
11-15 vs <=5	*2.66	*5.05
16-20 vs <=5	*5.31	*16.30
>20 vs <=5	*8.36	*27.40

*= statistically significant, all p<0.05.

Initial Studies

Imaging (in the order they would be considered in most Hospitals)*

1) CT brain without contrast (AKA 'plain brain' or 'CT without'); 3-5 minutes
   a) The most rapid imaging technique available at most hospitals.
   b) In patients eligible for IV tPA, it should show no acute effects of brain ischemia but may show early ischemic changes (EIC) such as loss of gray-white differentiation, blurring of the lentiform nucleus, and sulcal effacement.
      (i) Presence of these signs is not a contraindication for IV tPA.
      (ii) Early ischemic changes correlate with more severe strokes; they are not independently associated with any increased risk of adverse outcome [8].
      (iii) Presence of hypodensity in > 1/3 of the MCA territory was an exclusion criterion in the ECASS trials due to concern of increased hemorrhagic risk and the possibility of erroneous time estimation.
      (iv) However, in the NINDS tPA trial, retrospective analysis did not reveal any association with EIC and clinical outcomes [9].

---

* For further information on imaging, please refer to chapter 17 (Neuroimaging)

(1) In instances where CT changes are obvious (i.e. > 1/3 MCA hypodensity) despite reported time of onset < 3 hours, the clinician should carefully re-question the patient and/or family to ensure the accuracy of the time of onset.

c) CT can, however, reliably exclude intraparenchymal hemorrhage, subarachnoid hemorrhage, subdural hematoma, epidural hematoma, or other mass that can explain acute focal symptoms.

d) Large artery thrombus can be inferred by the following signs:

   (i) hyperdense middle cerebral artery (a horizontal line just above the circle of Willis or a dot in or near the sylvian fissure) – for an example of this please see chapter 17 on Neuroimaging

   (ii) hyperdense basilar (a dot at the top of the basilar just below the circle of Willis);

   (iii) presence of these signs is not a contraindication for IV tPA.

2) CT angiography/CT perfusion (AKA 'CT angio' or 'CT A and P'); 10-20 minutes

   a) Includes a CT brain without contrast as its first sequence.

   b) Angiography and perfusion images should always be ordered simultaneously.

   c) CT angiogram provides direct visualization of the major intracranial and extracranial vessels

   d) CTA is indicated when:

      (i) The patient arrives to the ER in a timely manner in the above situations and the delay in obtaining the extra sequences will not delay tPA administration significantly.

      (ii) There is suspicion for large artery occlusion.

         1) A NIHSS score > 10 has been strongly correlated with acute proximal large arterial occlusions; other studies have shown high NIHSS scores can be seen in both cardioembolic and large artery atherothrombotic stroke etiologies [4] [10]

      (iii) Likelihood of response to IV tPA alone is poor and endovascular treatment options are being considered.

  e) CT perfusion gives information about cerebral blood flow, mean transit time, and cerebral blood volume.

    (i) Perfusion images can help identify tissue with decreased blood flow that could potentially be salvaged (the penumbra).

    (ii) Can be considered in select patients with unknown onset ischemic stroke as a means to direct treatment strategies.

      1) For example, a patient who wakes up with stroke symptoms (last known normal at 10 pm the previous evening) may have large areas of penumbra (salvageable tissue) and might benefit from revascularization therapies

      2) Though single-arm registry and phase two trials suggest some benefit in this perfusion-based selection of patients [11], [12], it should be noted that to date, randomized clinical trials using penumbra-based treatment decisions have failed to show benefit [13] and await further clinical trials [14], [15].

  f) Consider dye allergies, impaired renal function, radiation dosage, and implications for later studies (including intra-arterial intervention).

3) MRI brain/ MR angiography; 30 minutes

  a) Provides the most detailed information about acute changes in patients with suspected stroke.

  b) Ischemia appears on DWI within minutes of onset.

  c) Small or posterior fossa infarctions better visualized than CT; avoids exposure to ionizing radiation.

  d) Gadolinium contrast is not required for visualization of intracranial vessels using time-of-flight imaging.

    (i) However, TOF-MRA has poor resolution for small or distal arteries, over-estimates degree of stenosis, and is prone to movement artifacts.

  e) Perfusion images with gadolinium contrast can also be obtained if desired and can help determine the penumbra using a bolus-tracking method similar to CT perfusion. However, this adds approximately 20 minutes in the scanner.

f) Use of this study is largely limited by cost, time, and potential for contraindications in large subsets of the stroke population (i.e. implanted metallic hardware such as pacemakers, claustrophobia, and obesity).

Serum Studies

1) Coagulation tests (prothrombin time/international normalization ratio (PT/INR) and activated partial thromboplastin time (aPTT)).
2) Complete blood count (CBC) including platelet count.
   a) However, the most recent AHA/AHA guidelines recommend not delaying tPA administration while waiting for the results of coagulation or platelet tests unless a bleeding disorder is suspected.
   b) Several reports have confirmed that less than 0.5% of patients have an unsuspected coagulopathy (0.3% with unsuspected thrombocytopenia [16]). One study found, with 100% sensitivity and 94% specificity, that if the answers to these three questions were "no" that the PT/INR and aPTT values would be within normal range [17]:
      (i) Does the patient take warfarin?
      (ii) Has the patient been using heparin or low molecular weight heparin?
      (iii) Is the patient on hemodialysis?
   c) Administering tPA prior to obtaining coagulation results are known is safe and not associated with increased risk of hemorrhage [18].
3) Comprehensive metabolic panel (CMP or SMA-10).
   a) The serum glucose level is critical to assess for possible mimic presentations due to hypo- or hyperglycemia, which should be corrected and neurologic examination repeated, before administering tPA.
   b) In addition, hyperglycemia has been shown to worsen outcomes following ischemic stroke and increase the risk of symptomatic hemorrhage following tP [19].
4) Pregnancy test.

Other Studies may be Indicated, Including

5) Arterial blood gas (when concerned for hypoxia)
6) Urine toxicology screen and blood alcohol level

Additional Non-Neurologic Imaging Studies

1) Chest x-ray.
2) If fracture is suspected, portable films may be of use to exclude trauma as a source of weakness.

Inclusion Criteria (based on the Criteria used in the NINDS tPA Trial)

1) Suspected ischemic stroke of clearly defined onset less than three hours
2) Measurable deficit on the NIHSS
3) A CT of the brain that shows no evidence of hemorrhage

For use of IV tPA up to 4.5 hours in ECASS-3 [20], the following additional criteria are:

1) Age 18 to 80 years
2) Stroke symptoms present for at least 30 minutes with no significant improvement before treatment

Exclusion Criteria for 3 Hour Window

1) Pregnancy
   a) Considered pregnancy category C (uncertain safety).
   b) No large or controlled studies have been done to evaluate its use in pregnancy.
   c) Both mother and fetus are thought to be at increased risk of hemorrhage.
   d) Main concerns relate to premature labor, placental abruption, and fetal demise.

e)   Several papers have reported on the use of IV and intra-arterial thrombolysis during pregnancy (either intentional or inadvertent):

(i)   One paper reviewing the literature in 2007 discovered that 30 pregnant patients had been reported in the literature having received tPA during pregnancy for one of several thrombotic causes; 6 of these patients received iv tPA. Complication rates were similar to nonpregnant patients with no apparent impact on fetal outcome [21].

(ii)   A review of off-label use of thrombolysis for acute stroke found that one of 11 pregnant patients treated with either intra-arterial or intra-venous thrombolysis developed symptomatic intracranial hemorrhage; of the 11 fetuses, 6 died (one due to maternal demise, three due to elective abortion, two due to miscarriages) [6].

(iii)   Another review of the literature found 8 patients treated with IV tPA, urokinase, or intra-arterial TPA; 3 of those were treated with IV tPA and one of the 3 died from complications of angioplasty. All three of these fetuses died in this series (two from termination of pregnancy, one when the mother died) [22].

2)   Persistent hypertension

a)   SBP>185 or DBP>110 mg Hg despite antihypertensive therapy is thought to be a risk factor for hemorrhagic transformation.

b)   Studies have shown that a higher baseline systolic blood pressure is associated with parenchymal hemorrhage after IV tPA [23].

c)   Given that the rate of increased hemorrhage is increased in patients given IV tPA after 3 hours (when compared to those given IV tPA prior to 3 hours), caution should be taken when considering IV tPA in patients with elevated blood pressure who are within the 4.5 hour window but not the 3 hour window.

(i)   A protocol for staged blood pressuring lowering prior to tPA has been recommended (see table). A retrospective study did find that aggressive BP lowering using intravenous drips is safe and not associated with elevated risk of hemorrhage [24]

3) Rapidly resolving or mild deficits
   a) At least two studies suggest that patients with mild or rapidly resolving deficits had a larger risk for poor outcome or a larger stroke syndrome than initially thought.
   b) In both studies, over 25% of those patients who presented within 3 hours but were felt to have resolving symptoms died prior to discharge or had severe disability at time of discharge [25], [26].
   c) In order to truly be certain this is a resolving deficit, it must resolve 'monotonically and dramatically.'[27].
   d) If symptoms fluctuate, IV tPA should still be considered and given [28]
   e) A small study also found that tPA administration in those with mild or resolving deficits is safe with no increased risk of hemorrhage [29]

4) Seizure at onset
   a) The goal of excluding patients who have seizure at onset is to eliminate the possibility of a post-ictal paralysis being confused with hemiparesis due to an ischemic event.
   b) That being said, some patients will have focal seizures with stroke onset (<5%).
   c) Benefits may outweigh the risks if an ischemic event is suspected.
   d) CT angiography and perfusion or MRI may be of particular use in this situation in defining true ischemic events by presence of vascular occlusions, hypoperfusion, or restricted diffusion in the appropriate locations (i.e. matching clinical syndrome).

5) Ischemic stroke or serious head trauma within prior 3 months
   a) Intended to prevent unnecessary risk of hemorrhage into abnormal tissue
   b) This also excludes those patients who do not have a new ischemic event or new occlusion but simply 'unmask' prior deficits due to metabolic abnormalities, infection, or sedation [30].
   c) Some amount of clinical judgement is needed, as some patients may still benefit from IV tPA with relatively little increased risk.

       (i) A prior small lacunar infarct or TIA would not have the same risk of hemorrhage as a prior large hemispheric infarct.

       (ii) Collateral history will be of great importance in these patients, as the clinician will want to know date and severity of prior stroke, whether it was seen on imaging and was it CT or MRI, and if symptoms resolved completely or only partially.

       (iii) In most instances, the size of the prior stroke can be estimated from the baseline CT scan.

6) Prior or current intracerebral hemorrhage

   a) This is an absolute exclusion criterion.

   b) However, if a patient has a prior stroke of unknown etiology, the CT scan should be reviewed to determine if that stroke precludes IV tPA use. If CT is unable to visualize any prior stroke, the validity of the reported history should be questioned.

7) Gastrointestinal or Genitourinary hemorrhage within 21 days

   a) Discussion with the patient's gastroenterologist, urologist, or obstetrician/ gynecologist is recommended as he or she may feel the risk of bleeding is much lower than a neurologist would assume it to be. Alternatively, should bleeding occur, it may be readily more treatable than the outcome following ischemic stroke without tPA treatment.

       (i) Likewise, mild bleeding (i.e. from hemorrhoids) may be minor compared to the effects of a devastating stroke.

       (ii) Women with active, heavy menstruation have been safely and effectively treated with IV tPA; urgent uterine artery embolization or ligation can be performed to halt uncontrolled bleeding without difficulty, and transfusions may be required [31].

8) Arterial puncture at a non-compressible site within 7 days; Major surgery within the last 14 days

   a) Compressible sites include groin, wrist, forearm, neck; it is also possible to compress the subclavian artery in some patients. Thus, this should be a rarely cited exclusion criterion

b) Discussion with the surgeon who performed the surgery is recommended; again, the morbidity of a major stroke may outweigh the risks of rebleeding at the operative site.

c) No data exists regarding recent lumbar puncture, the clinician should take into account whether the procedure was a difficult one and explain that risk is unknown to person consenting for IV tPA.

9) Elevated aPTT>1.5 normal; Elevated INR>1.7; current anticoagulant use

a) The initial intention of this criterion was to exclude patients actively being anticoagulated (with oral anticoagulants or IV heparin).

b) The final package insert for tPA after FDA approval allowed for patient inclusion as long as the INR was below 1.7.

   (i) A recent retrospective paper evaluated a small subset of warfarin-treated patients with INR < 1.7 who were treated with IV tPA and found an 10-fold elevated risk of symptomatic ICH (30.8 vs. 3.2%, $P = 0.004$). Hence, the safety of tPA in warfarin-treated patients remain uncertain [32].

c) Presence of active anticoagulation is an absolute contraindication for patients within the 4.5 hour time window.

d) If patients received heparin (i.e. hemodialysis), aPTT should be checked and < 1.5x normal prior to administering tPA.

10) Platelet count <100,000

a) No data exists which suggests increased risk for patients with thrombocytopenia.

b) One study asserts that unsuspected thrombocytopenia accounts for 0.3% of all stroke patients presenting for evaluation. Stated another way, if every person with thrombocytopenia treated with IV tPA had a fatal hemorrhage (as opposed to an excellent outcome), then 3 out of 1000 treated with IV tPA would be harmed by it [33].

c) The treating physician should thus take platelet count into consideration, but may in the absence of other contraindications decide to proceed with IV tPA.

11) Glucose<50 or >400 mg/dl
    a) Normoglycemia is essential prior to giving IV tPA and should be maintained following its administration:
       (i) In those patients with altered mental status contributing to the NIHSS, correction of glucose can sometimes reverse many deficits (some of which may simply be unmasking of prior stroke).
       (ii) Patients with persistent hyperglycemia are at increased risk of parenchymal hemorrhage; one study found an odds ratio of 6.64 towards parenchymal hemorrhage following ischemic stroke in those patient with hyperglycemia at onset and 24 hours later [34].

Hour Window

1) ECASS-3 investigated the use of IV tPA in patients presenting between 3 and 4.5 hours post symptom onset.
2) They found that patients had significantly better clinical outcomes compared to placebo, despite the increased risk of symptomatic intracranial hemorrhage.
3) To limit the risk of intracranial hemorrhage attributable to IV tPA, the following additional exclusions were proposed:

   a) Oral anticoagulants regardless of INR
   b) Heparin use within the prior 48 hours with a PTT exceeding the upper limit of normal range
   c) NIHSS>25
   d) CT findings of >1/3 MCA territory infarct
   e) Both a history of stroke AND diabetes

Common Misconceptions about IV tPA

1) tPA will harm patients without stroke (i.e. stroke mimics)
   a) One recent study found no occurrence of symptomatic ICH among patients who received IV tPA but were later determined not to have ischemic stroke by MRI. [35]
2) tPA does not really work or risks outweigh benefits

a) Some studies have suggested that the outcomes in treatment and placebo limbs are similar [36], or that patients treated with tPA failed to improve more rapidly in the acute phase than placebo treated patients (questioning the benefit of the intervention) [37]. However, the multiple international studies, meta-analyses, and community and post-marketing studies have replicated the NINDS results [38].

3) As long as tPA is given by the end of the time window, you have met the standard of care.

a) There is a clear relationship between efficacy and time to treatment of tPA [39]. Thus, the earlier the treatment is given, the more likely the patient will have a good outcome (modified Rankin score 0-1).

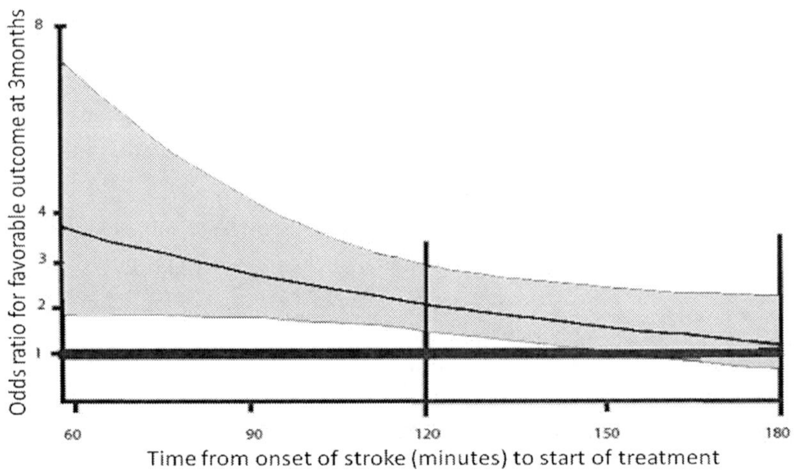

Graph showing odds ratio for favorable outcome at three months if given tPA (from Marler et al, 2000).

4) The narrow time window make implementation of tPA protocols not feasible due to limited time to examine patient, obtain consent, and perform necessary tests.

a) An expedited stroke protocol eliminating delays due to waiting for coagulation tests, chest xray, written (not verbal) consent and official read of CT scan is feasible and appears safe [40].

    b)   Goal time from ER triage to tPA administration is less than 60 minutes.

5)   tPA can only be given if assessed by a neurologist trained in vascular fellowship

    a)   In the original NINDS trial, 30 of the 40 participating sites were community hospitals; many of the patients were assessed and treated by either emergency room physicians or community neurologists [41].

    b)   Many teaching hospitals allow neurology residents to be the evaluating and treating physician.

6)   tPA does not work in large vessel occlusions or not all stroke subtypes respond to tPA

    a)   Though the rate of recanalization is higher with smaller clot burden (distal branch occlusions > proximal stem occlusion), the rate of recanalization is substantial and treatment of large artery subtypes of AIS is associated with better outcomes than placebo[1,11].

    b)   In the NINDS subgroup analyses, all ischemic stroke subtypes showed statistically significant benefit from tPA versus placebo. Therefore, withholding tPA based on suspected stroke subtype is not recommended[11].

    c)   One study found that patients with diabetes and extracranial carotid occlusions will infrequently recanalize [42]; patients with both MCA and ICA occlusions may benefit from more aggressive treatment [43].

So you've decided to give IV tPA...

Consent

1)   In order to give informed consent for IV tPA, the patient must demonstrate two things: the ability to make a voluntary choice and evidence of decisional competence.

2)   This must be assessed by the physician administering the IV tPA.

3)   Patients who will not likely be able to give consent have one or more of the following:

    a)   Impaired level of consciousness

    b)   Wernicke's aphasia
    c)   Frontal lobe dysfunction
    d)   Known mental retardation or developmental delay
    e)   Age <18 years

4) In patients who cannot give consent, all attempts must be made to contact the durable power of attorney or health care proxy if one exists

5) Consent may be obtained over the phone and should be documented as such.

6) If the patient does not have a durable power of attorney or health care proxy, the next of kin (or parent) may be able to give consent.

7) In situations where no party with decision making capacity can be reached, the following statement may apply: As an approved therapy endorsed by evidence based guidelines, IV rtPA may be emergently administered under US regulations by implied consent.[14.]

8) Many studies have shown that better understanding of the proposed intervention/medical decision point occurs when the information given to the patient is highly structured, uses brief summaries of the overall topic and of the key points, incorporates visual aids, and uses straightforward consent forms [44].

Elements to include when Seeking informed Consent

1) Overview of the clinical situation in laymen's terms
    a)   What you think is going on (hopefully it's a stroke if you are thinking about tPA!)
    b)   What a stroke is (blocking artery to the brain, cutting off blood flow)
    c)   Lack of blood to one part of the brain explains symptoms
    d)   Restoring blood flow in a timely manner will improve symptoms and lead to less disability

2) Proposed treatment, again in laymen's terms
    a)   FDA approved treatment for acute stroke
    b)   Intravenous medication given over one hour

      c)   Breaks up clots in arteries
3)   Benefits
      a)   Restore blood flow
      b)   Reverse weakness/numbness/altered speech/clumsiness
      c)   Improve outcome – 30% more likely (from NINDS trial) to have minimal or no disability by 3 months after the stroke
4)   Risks
      a)   Increased risk of major bleeding into the brain (6% symptomatic ICH in NINDS, 7% symptomatic ICH in ECASS-3)
      b)   Risk of systemic bleeding
      c)   No benefit

TPA for Cerebral Ischemia within 3 Hours of Onset-Changes in Outcome Due to Treatment

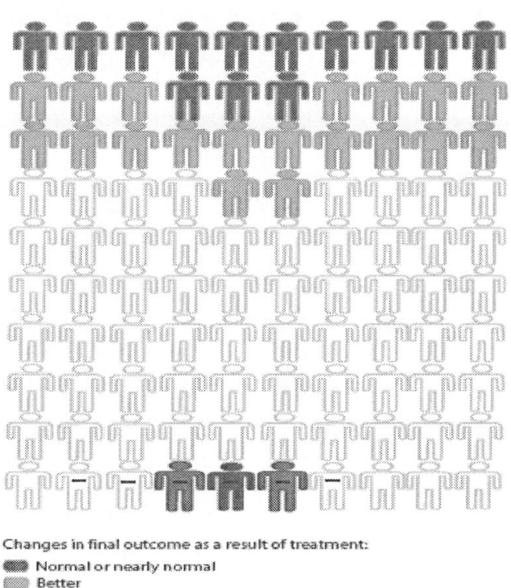

(Prepared by UCLA for the American Heart Association website) [45].

Legal Pitfalls

1) The most important thing you can do to protect yourself is to document (legibly) the discussions, decisions, and people involved.
2) Discussions documented should include the major points of the informed consent you gave.
3) Always note if other physicians were involved, the names of the family member/power of attorney/healthcare proxy involved in the decision, and the specific time of arrival, assessment, etc as closely as possible.
4) If the decision to give or not give IV tPA is made, a succinct explanation why with specific reasons should be documented.
5) Although the perception exists that giving IV tPA exposes treating healthcare professionals to risk of legal action, reviews of the litigation suggest that liability is mostly associated with failure to provide tPA (negligence) and for tPA-related adverse events [46], [47], [48].

Dosing/Rate

1) IV tPA should be given as a one time dose of 0.9 mg/kg, with a maximum dose of 90 mg.
2) The first 10% should be given as a bolus (IV push over 1 minute). The remaining amount should be given over one hour.
3) Dosing Errors
   a) Overdose of tPA happens due to inaccurate estimation of weight [49], poor communication and medication dosing errors (dosing of tPA for STEMI is higher than for ischemic stroke), and giving more the maximal allowable dose (90mg).
      (i) It is well-documented that medical professionals are not adept at estimating patient weight, with a mean absolute error of 9 to 10 kg; in contrast, patient self-estimates of actual weight were generally off by about 3 kg [50].

(ii) Data from the cardiology literature suggests an increased odd ratio for intracranial hemorrhage when doses of tPA greater than 1.5 mg/kg were given [51].

(iii) All attempts should be made to obtain an actual weight or a patient's estimate of their weight to prevent dosing error. Dose should be confirmed before initiation of administration.

Monitoring

1) During infusion of IV tPA
   a) Vital signs including blood pressure and neurologic exams should be checked every 15 minutes for the first two hours after starting the infusion.
   b) Treatment of blood pressure should be as follows:

If blood pressure is:	You can give	Or consider
>140 diastolic	nicardipine gtt	Labetalol gtt nitroprusside gtt
>230 systolic or 121-140 diastolic	20 mg IV labetalol push (repeat q10 min, max 150 mg)	labetalol gtt
180-230 systolic or 105-120 diastolic	10 mg IV labetalol push (repeat q10 min, max 150)	labetalol gtt

   c) If there is any sign of neurologic deterioration during administration of IV tPA, or the patient develops headache, nausea, vomiting, or acute hypertension, then hemorrhage should be suspected and the physician should do the following:
   (i) Stop infusion of IV tPA
   (ii) Obtain a stat head CT
   (iii) Recheck PT, PTT; check fibrinogen
   (iv) If a type and cross has not been done already obtain one now
   (v) Place 6-8 units of cryoprecipitate (containing factor VIII) and 6-8 units of platelets on hold and administer if hemorrhage seen on CT
   (vi) If hemorrhage present on CT, consult neurosurgery +/- hematology

2) After infusion of IV tPA
   a) Blood pressure should be checked every 15 minutes for the first 2 hours, then every 30 minutes for 6 hours, and then every hour until 24 hours after tPA treatment.
   b) Neurological checks should be done at the same time as blood pressure checks.
   c) The patient should be observed in an intensive care unit for the first 24 hours.
   d) Cardiac telemetry should be placed on the patient.
   e) Bleeding precautions should be followed, and the patient should be regularly assessed for any signs of bleeding.
   f) The patient should be kept on bed rest (to prevent unnecessary risks from falls).
   g) No antithrombotic agents should be given for the first 24 hours including subcutaneous heparin, aspirin, clopidogrel, dipyridamole, warfarin, or NSAIDs.
   h) No additional arterial or central lines should be placed within the first 24 hours unless for another emergency (i.e. hemodynamically unstable).
   i) Foley catheters should not be inserted for the first 24 hours
   j) With any sign of neurologic deterioration the physician should follow the same protocol outlined during the infusion.

Use of tPA in Special Populations

1) Pediatric ischemic stroke
   a) Stroke in patients less than 18 years old is typically related to an transient arteriopathy that may be post-infectious (particularly related to upper respiratory infection) or inflammatory in nature [52]. Other common causes include hypercoagulability, congenital heart disorders, or cervical artery dissection.
   b) Most pediatric patients with ischemic stroke do not receive thrombolysis (a review of all children with ischemic stroke admitted within a three year period in the US revealed 1.6% received either intra-arterial or intra-venous tPA) [53].

a) This review found that children treated with tPA tended to have longer hospital stays and worse outcomes, although some have criticized this review due to incomplete information about stroke severity at presentation, time to treatment, and other important factors.

c) A published review of the literature found 6 reported cases of ischemic stroke treated with IV tPA and 10 treated with IA tPA; all of the cases treated with IV tPA received treatment within three hours of symptom onset and none had intracranial hemorrhage [54].

d) A multicenter observational cohort study expanded the number of cases treated with IV tPA to 9 and found that 2/9 experienced asymptomatic intracranial hemorrhage. Deviation from adult protocol occurred in 4/9 patients [55].

2) Stroke in the very old

a) Analysis of those patients within the original NINDS cohort with age greater than 80 showed that 3 month functional outcome was not associated with administration of tPA [56].

b) A small study of patients greater than 90 showed no mortality benefit for IV tPA, but also no increased risk of symptomatic hemorrhage was observed in these patients.

c) Given the overall poor functional outcome octagenarians with ischemic stroke, IV tPA should not be withheld in eligible patients.

When good Intentions aren't enough (Protocol Violations and Impact on Outcome)

1) Protocol violations occur in anywhere from 14-27% of patients [57],[46.]

2) Increased rate of hemorrhage, both symptomatic and asymptomatic, were seen in patients who received tPA outside the protocol proposed by the NINDS trial [58].

3) Stroke centers certification has emphasized the use of protocols and safety procedures to ensure safe and effective utilization of tPA with many examples of quality improvement [59], [60].

Risk of Spontaneous Intracerebral Hemorrhage

1) Pooled analysis of four prospective observational studies did not show any increased risk of symptomatic intracranial hemorrhage following IV tPA for subgroups thought to be at increased risk (those over 70, with an NIHSS greater than 20, with diabetes, with congestive heart failure, or of Hispanic origin) [61].
2) Other factors influencing hemorrhage risk include hyperglycemia, lower platelet counts, higher pre-treatment blood pressure, protocol violations, and early infarct changes or edema on brain imaging [62], [63].
3) Patients treated with antiplatelet medication at baseline may be at increased risk as well though the studies are conflicting [48],[64], [65].Warfarin use, even in the presence of an INR less than 1.7, may increase the risk of symptomatic intracerebral hemorrhage following IV tPA [33].

Drip and Ship/Telemedicine

1) Telephone, video consultation that results in IV tPA administration in a community emergency room can overcome hesitancy of ER physicians and allows for more patients who are eligible for tPA to receive it.
2) If the community hospital does not have stroke unit care or capabilities to care for stroke patients following tPA, treated patients may be transferred to a stroke center for further monitoring. In these "drip and ship" patients, studies suggest no statistical difference in outcomes compared to those who were treated with tPA at stroke centers [66], [67].
3) Starting IV tPA at a community hospital and transferring the patient for further intervention for large artery occlusions appears to be safe [68]. Transfer processes including phone

numbers, ambulance arrangements, and medical record transfer must be efficient.
4) Telemedicine using live video for examination and review of imaging has been shown to superior to telephone consultation in thrombolysis-eligible patients [69].

Future Directions in Research: Neuroprotective Therapy

1) Normothermia
   a) Normothermia has been shown to correlate with good outcome after stroke [70], [71].
   b) Temperatures below 36.5° C (97.7° F) using anti-pyretics and fever source control are recommended by the American Heart Association [72].
2) Hypothermia
   a) Used in cardiac arrest, in infants with hypoxic-ischemic events, and shown to improve neurologic outcomes.
   b) Reduces glucose metabolism, inflammation, and free radical formation.
   c) In animal models, its neuroprotective effect approaches that of prompt thrombolysis [73].
   d) No conclusive data exists about neuroprotective effects of hypothermia on outcome following ischemic stroke.
3) Statins
   a) Animal models suggest that administration of HMG-CoA reductase inhibitors (statins) given within the first hours of ischemic stroke reduces neuronal injury and infarct size.
   b) One study found that the window for IV tPA could be extended to 6 hours in rats when they were given atorvastatin prior to thrombolysis [74].
   c) Statins may also enhance the neuroprotective effects of hypothermia [75].
   d) Phase I clinical trials are investigating potential for high-dose statin therapy following acute stroke.
4) Albumin
   a) Albumin has been observed to reduce total infarct volume in animal models [76].

b) Albumin has been shown to decrease swelling, improve blood flow, improve microvascular flow within the ischemic cortex, and supply free fatty acids [77].

c) The ALIAS pilot trial suggested that patients who receive high-dose albumin along with IV tPA are more likely to achieve a good outcome [78].

d) A randomized clinical trial (ALIAS-2) is currently underway.

References

[1] The National Institute of Neurological Disorders and Stroke rt-PA Stroke Study Group. *Tisue plasminogen activator for acute ischemic stroke.* N Engl J Med 1995; 333:1581-7.

[2] Reeves MJ, Arora S, Broderick JP et al. *Acute stroke care in the US: results from 4 pilot prototypes of the Paul Coverdell National Acute Stroke Registry.* Stroke 2005; 36: 1232-1240.

[3] Dominguez R, Vila JF, Augustovski F et al. *Spanish Cross-Cultural Adaptation and Validation of the National Instities of Health Stroke Scale.* Mayo Clinic Proc. 2006; 81 (4): 476-480.

[4] Fischer U et al. *NIHSS score and Arteriographic Findings in Acute Ischemic Stroke.* Stroke 2005; 36:2121-2125.

[5] Maas M et al. *National Institutes of Health Stroke Scale Score Is Poorly Predictive of Proximal Occlusion in Acute Cerebral Ischemia.*

[6] Fink JN et al. *Is the association of National Institutes of Health Stroke Scale scores and acute MRI stroke volume equal for patients with right- and left- hemisphere ischemic stroke?* Stroke 2002; 33: 954-958.

[7] Schlegel DJ, Tanne D, Demchuk AM, Levine SR, Kasner SE. *Prediction of hospital disposition after thrombolysis for acute ischemic stroke using the National Institutes of Health Stroke Scale.* Arch Neurol. 2004;61:1061-1064.

[8] Patel SC et al. *Lack of Clinical Significance of Early Ischemic Changes on Computed Tomography in Acute Stroke.* JAMA 2001; 286: 2830-2838.

[9] Generalized Efficacy of tPA for acute stroke. *Subgroup analysis of the NINDS t-PA Stroke Trial.* Stroke 1997 Nov; 28 (11):2119-25.

[10] Hsia AW, Sachdev HS, Tomlinson J et al. *Efficacy of IV tissue plasminogen activator in acute stroke: Does stroke subtype really matter?* Neurology 2003; 61: 71-75.

[11]   Puetz V, Dzialowski I, Hill MD et al. *Malignant profile detected by CT angiographic information predicts poor prognosis despite thrombolysis within three hours from symptom onset.* Cerebrovasc Dis 2010; 29 (6): 584-91.

[12]   Noguiera RG, Liebeskind D, Gupta R et al. DWI/PWI and CTP *Assessment in the Triage of Wake-Up and Late Presenting Strokes Undergoing Neurointervention: The DAWN Trial.* Poster presented at International Stroke Conference, February 2009.

[13]   Hacke W, Furlan AJ, Al-Rawi Y et al. *Intravenous desmoteplase in patients with acute ischaemic stroke selected by MRI perfusion— diffusion weighted imaging or perfusion CT (DIAS-2): a prospective, randomised, double-blind, placebo-controlled study.* Lancet Neurol 2009 Feb; 8 (2): 141-150.

[14]   Davis SM, Donnan GA, Parsons MW et al. *Effects of alteplase beyond 3 h after stroke in the Echoplanar Imaging Thrombolytic Evaluation Trial (EPITHET): a placebo-controlled randomised trial.* Lancet Neurol 2008 Apr;7(4):299-309.

[15]   Kidwell CS et al. *MR and Recanalization of Stroke Clots Using Embolectomy (MR-Rescue).* Ongoing clinical trial, NCT00094588.

[16]   Cucchiara et al. *Usefulness of Checking Platelet Count before Thrombolysis in Acute Ischemic Stroke.* Stroke 2007; 38: 1639-1640.

[17]   Gottesman RF et al. *Predicting abnormal coagulation in ischemic stroke: Reducing delay in rt-PA use.* Neurology 2006; 67: 1665-1667.

[18]   Rost NS et al. *Unsuspected coagulopathy rarely prevents IV thrombolysis in acute ischemic stroke.* Neurology 2009; 73: 1957-1962.

[19]   Alvarez-Sabin J et al. *Effects of Admission Hyperglycemia on Stroke Outcome in Reperfused Tissue Plasminogen Activator-Treated Patients.* Stroke 2003; 34: 1235-1240.

[20]   Hacke W, Kast M, Bluhmki E et al. *Thrombolysis with Alteplase 3 to 4.5 Hours after Acute Ischemic Stroke.* N Engl J Med 2008; 359:1317-29.

[21]   De Keyser J et al. *Intravenous Alteplase for Stroke: Beyond the Guidelines and in Particular Clinical Situations.* Stroke 2007; 38: 2612-2618.

[22]   Murugappan A, Coplin WM, Al-Sadat AN et al. *Thrombolytic therapy of acute ischemic stroke during pregnancy.* Neurology 2006; 66: 768-770.

[23] Larrue V, von Kummer R, Muller A, and Bluhmki E. *Risk Factors for Severe Hemorrhagic Transformation in Ischemic Stroke Patients Treated With Recombinant Tissue Plasminogen Activator*: A Secondary Analysis of the European-Australasian Acute Stroke Study (ECASS II). Stroke 2001: 32: 438-441.

[24] Martin-Schild S et al. *Aggressive Blood Pressure-Lowering Treatment Before Intravenous Tissue Plasminogen Activator Therapy in Acute Ischemic Stroke.* Arch Neurol 2008; 65 (9):1174-1178.

[25] Barber PA, Zhang J, Demchuck A, et al. *Why are stroke patients excluded from TPA therapy?* Neurology 2001; 56: 1015-1020.

[26] Smith EE, Abdullah Ar, Petkovska I, et al. *Poor outcomes in patients who do not receive intravenous tissue plasminogen activator because of mild or improving ischemic stroke.* Stroke 2005,; 36: 2497-2499.

[27] Al-Khoury L and Lyden PD. *Intravenous Thrombolysis.* Insert book reference here.

[28] Ozdemir O et al. *Thrombolysis in Patients With Marked Clinical Fluctuations in Neurologic Status Due to Cerebral Ischemia.* Arch Neurol 2008; 65 (8): 1041-1043.

[29] Baumann CR et al. *Good Outcomes in Ischemic Stroke Patients Treated With Intravenous Thrombolysis Despite Regressing Neurological Symptoms.* Stroke 2006; 37: 1332-1333.

[30] Thal GD et al. *Exacerbation or Unmasking of Focal Neurologic Deficit by Sedatives.* Anesthesiology 1996; 85 (1): 21-25.

[31] Wein TH, Hickenbottom SL, Morgenstern LB et al. *Safety of Tissue Plasminogen Activator for Acute Stroke in Menstruating Women.* Stroke 2002; 33: 2506-2508.

[32] Prabhakaran S, Rivolta J, Vieira JR et al. *Symptomatic Intracerebral Hemorrhage Among Eligible Warfarin-Treated Patients Receiving Intravenous Tissue Plasminogen Activator for Acute Ischemic Stroke.* Arch Neurol 2010; 67 (5): E1-E5.

[33] Cucchiara BL, Jackson B, Weiner M, et al. *Usefulness of checking platelet count before thrombolysis in acute ischemic stroke.* Stroke 2007; 39: 1639-1640/

[34] Kaste M, Yong M. *Dynamic of Hyperglycemia as a Predictor of Stroke Outcome in the ECASS-II Trial.* Stroke 2008; 39: 2749-2755.

[35] Chernyshev O et al. *Safety of tPA in stroke mimics and neuroimaging-negative cerebral ischemia.* Neurology 2010; 74: 1-6.

[36] Hoffman JR, Schriger DL et al. *A Graphic Reanalysis of the NINDS trial.* Ann Emerg Med 2009 Sep; 54 (3): 329-336.

[37] Del Zoppo GJ. *Acute stroke: on the threshold of a therapy?* N Engl J Med 1995; 333: 1632-1633

[38] Albers GW et al. *Intravenous tissue-type plasminogen activator for treatment of acute stroke: the Standard Treatment with Alteplase to Reverse Stroke (STARS) study.* JAMA 2000 Mar; 283 (9): 1145-1150.

[39] Marler JR, Tilley BC, Lu M et al. **Early stroke treatment associated with better outcome: The NINDS rt-PA Stroke Study.** Neurology, Dec **2000**; 55: 1649 - 1655.

[40] Sattin JA et al. *An expedited Code Stroke Protocol is Feasible and Safe.* Stroke 2006; 37: 2935-2939.

[41] Haley EC et al. *Myths regarding the NINDS rt-PA Stroke Trial: Setting the Record Straight.* Ann Emerg Med 1997 Nov; 30 (5): 676-82.

[42] Zangerle A, Kiechl S, Spiegel M et al. *Recanalization after thrombolysis in stroke patients: predictors and prognostic implications.* Neurology 2007; 68 (1): 39-44.

[43] Linfante I, Llinas RH, Selim M et al. *Clinical and Vascular Outcome in Internal Carotid Artery Versus Middle Cerebral Artery Occlusions After Intravenous Tissue Plasminogen Activator.* Stroke 2002; 33: 2066-2071.

[44] White-Bateman SR, Schumaker HC, Sacco RL, Applebaum PS. *Consent for Intravenous Thrombolysis in Acute Stroke.* Arch Neurol 2007; 64:785-792.

[45] *http://www.americanheart.org/downloadable/heart/1269388918946U CLA%20tPA%20benefits%20and%20risks%20decision%20figure%20 matching.pdf.*   From http://www.americanheart.org/presenter.jhtml?identifier=3068375

[46] Liang B, Zivin J. *Empirical Characteristics of Litigation Involving Tissue Plasminogen Activator and Ischemic Stroke.* Ann Emerg Med 2008; 52 (2): 160-164.

[47] Liang B, Lew R, Zivin JA. *Review of Tissue Plasminogen Activator, Ischemic Stroke, and Potential Legal Issues.* Arch Neurol. 2008;65(11):1429-1433

[48] Weintraub M. *Thrombolysis (Tissue Plasminogen Activator) in Stroke: a medicolegal quagmire.* Stroke 2006; 37: 1917-1922.

[49] Messe SR et al. *Dosing errors may impact the risk of rt-PA for stroke: the Multicenter rt-PA Acute Stroke Survey.* J Stroke Cerebrovasc Dis 2004 Jan-Feb; 13 (1): 35-40.

[50] Anglemeyer BL et al. *The accuracy of visual estimation of body weight in the ED.* Am J Emerg Med. 2004; 22: 526-529.

[51] Cannon C. *Thrombolysis Medication Errors: Benefits of Bolus Thrombolytic Agents.* Am J Cardiol 2000; 85: 17C-22C.

[52] Amlie-Lefond C et al. *Predictors of Cerebral Arteriopathy in Children with Arterial Ischemic Stroke.* Circulation 2009; 119: 1417-1423.

[53] Janjua N et al. *Thrombolysis for Acute Ischemic Stroke in Children: Data from the Nationwide Inpatient Sample.* Stroke 2007; 38: 1850-1854.

[54] Arnold M et al. *Thrombolysis in Childhood Stroke: Report of 2 cases and Review of the Literature.* Stroke 2009; 40: 801-807.

[55] Amlie-Lefond C et al. *Use of alteplase in childhood arterial ischaemic stroke: a multicenter, observational, cohort study.* Lancet Neurol 2009; 8: 530-536.

[56] Longstreth WT et al. *Intravenous tissue plasminogen activator and stroke in the elderly.* Am J Emerg Med 2010; 28: 359-363.

[57] Nadeau et al. tPA *Use for Stroke in the Registry of the Canadian Stroke Network.* Can J Neurol Sci 2005 Nov; 32 (4) 433-439.

[58] Lopez-Yunez, Bruno A, Williams LS, Yilmaz E, Zurru C, Biller J. *Protocol violations in Community-Based rTPA Stroke Treatment Are Associated with Symptomatic Intracerebral Hemorrhage.* Stroke 2001; 32:12-16.

[59] Katzan IL, Furlan AJ, Lloyd LE et al. *Use of tissue type plasminogen activator for acute ischemic stroke: the Cleveland area experience.* JAMA 2000; 283 (9): 1151-8.

[60] Katzan IL, Hammer MD, Furlan AJ et al. *Quality improvement and tissue-type plasminogen activator for acute ischemic stroke: a Cleveland update.* Stroke 2003; 34 (3): 799-800.

[61] Sylaja et al. *Safety outcomes of Alteplase among acute ischemic stroke patients with special characteristics.* Neurocrit Care 2007 6: 181-185.

[62] Tanne D, Kasner SE, Demchuk AM, et al. *Markers of increased risk of intracerebral hemorrhage after intravenous recombinant tissue plasminogen activator therapy for acute ischemic stroke in clinical practice: The multicenter rt-PA stroke survey.* Circulation. 2002;105:1679-1685.

[63] The NINDS t-PA Stroke Study Group. *Intracerebral hemorrhage after intravenous t-PA therapy for ischemic stroke.* Stroke. 1997;28:2109-2118.

[64] Bravo Y, Marti-Fabregas J, Cocho D, et al. *Influence of antiplatelet pre-treatment on the risk of symptomatic intracranial haemorrhage after intravenous thrombolysis.* Cerebrovasc Dis. 2008;26:126-133.

[65] Uyttenboogaart M, Koch MW, Koopman K, Vroomen PC, De Keyser J, Luijckx GJ. *Safety of antiplatelet therapy prior to intravenous thrombolysis in acute ischemic stroke.* Arch Neurol. 2008;65:607-611.

[66] Martin-Schild S et al. *Is the Drip and Ship Approach to Delivering Thrombolysis For Acute Ischemic Stroke Safe?* J Emerg Med.

[67] Pervez MA et al. *Remote Supervision of IV-tPA for Acute Ischemic Stroke by Telemedicine or Telephone Before Transfer to a Regional Stroke Center is Feasible and Safe.* Stroke 2010; 41; e18-24.

[68] Pfefferkorn T et al. *Drip, Ship, and Retrieve: Cooperative Recanalization Therapy in Acute Basilar Artery Occlusion.* Stroke 2010; 41: 722-726.

[69] Meyer BC, Raman R, Hemmen T, Obler R, Zivin JA, Rao R, Thomas RG, Lyden PD. *Efficacy of site-independent telemedicine in the STRokE DOC trial: a randomised, blinded, prospective study.* Lancet Neurol. 2008 Sep;7(9):787-95.

[70] Wang Y, Lim LL, et al. *Influence of admission body temperature on stroke mortality.* Stroke. 2000;31:404–409.

[71] Hajat C, Hajat S, Sharma P. *Effects of poststroke pyrexia on stroke outcome: a meta-analysis of studies in patients.* Stroke. 2000;31:410–414.

[72] Adams HP Jr, Adams RJ, et al. *Guidelines for the early management of patients with ischemic stroke: a scientific statement from the Stroke Council of the American Stroke Association.* Stroke. 2003;34:1056 – 1083.

[73] Schaller B, Graf R. *Hypothermia and Stroke: The pathophysiological background.* Pathophysiology 2003; 10 (3): 7-35.

[74] Zhang L, Chopp M et al. *Atorvastatin extends the therapeutic window for tPA to 6h after the onset of embolic stroke in rats.* J Cerebral Blood Flow Metabolism 2009 Nov; 29 (11): 1816-24.

[75] Lee SH, Kim YH et al. *Atorvastatin enhances hypothermia-induced neuroprotection after stroke.* J Neurol Sci 2008 Dec 15; 275 (1-2): 64-8.

[76] Belayev L, Liu Y et al. *Human Albumin Therapy of Acute Ischemic Stroke : Marked Neuroprotective Efficacy at Moderate Doses and With a Broad Therapeutic Window.* Stroke 2001: 32; 553-560.

[77] Ginsberg MD. *Neuroprotection for Ischemic Stroke: Past, Present, and Future.* Neuropharmacology 2008 Sept; 55 (3): 363-389.

[78] Palesch YY, Hill MD et al. *The ALIAS Pilot Trial: a dose-escalation and safety study of albumin therapy for acute ischemic stroke--II: neurologic outcome and efficacy analysis.* Stroke. 2006 Aug;37 (8):2107-14.

In: Handbook of Stroke and Neurocritical Care   ISBN: 978-61324-786-0
Editor: V. H. Lee   © 2012 Nova Science Publishers, Inc.

Chapter IX

Ischemic Stroke Acute Treatment Intraarterial Therapy

Michael Chen
Department of Neurological Sciences,
Section of Stroke and Neurocritical care,
Rush University Medical Center, Chicago, IL, USA

I.   Introduction

   a) Between 30-50% of stroke survivors fail to regain functional independence. [1]

   b) Smith evaluated brain CT angiography in 72 consecutive ischemic stroke patients and found that intracranial large vessel occlusion, involving either the vertebral, basilar, middle cerebral artery or carotid terminus, independently predicted a poor neurologic outcome at hospital discharge. [2] (Figures 1 & 2)

   c) Most of the 70 billion dollars spent annually in the US on stroke care is for the severely disabled, who likely have large vessel occlusions.

   d) The only FDA-approved therapy for acute ischemic stroke, namely intravenous thrombolysis, has been shown to lead to only modest recanalization rates for large vessel occlusions. [3]

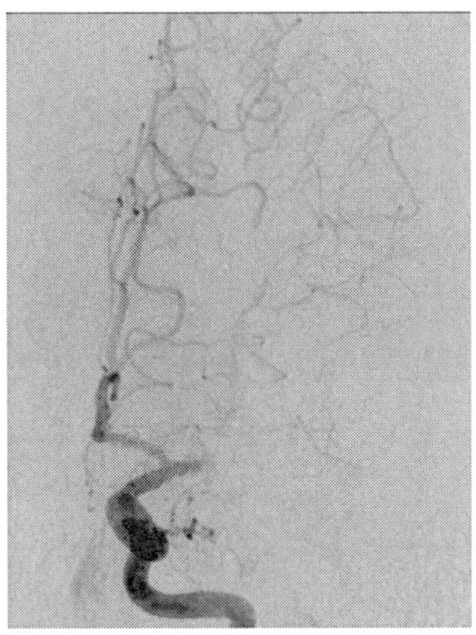

Figure 1. Left TIMI 0 M1 segment of MCA occlusion with pial collateral flow from the ipsilateral anterior cerebral artery branches.

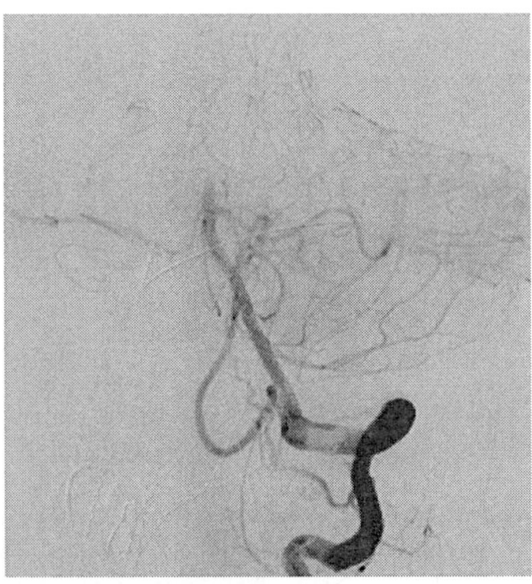

Figure 2. Mid-basilar TIMI 0 occlusion.

e)   The Prolyse in Acute Cerebral Thromboembolism (PROACT II) study represents the best study to date that studies intraarterial stroke thrombolysis with primary clinical outcome measures which showed significantly improved clinical outcomes and recanalization rates among the treatment group. [4]

f)   Although not approved by the FDA for the treatment of acute ischemic stroke, various physician organizations have made qualified endorsements for intraarterial stroke therapy with the belief that, "treating a suitable patient under appropriate clinical circumstances by means of intraarterial thrombolysis is a responsible medical decision even in the absence of strict scientific guidelines." [5]

II.   Practical considerations

a)   Evaluation and decision making must be done quickly
   (i)   Clinical diagnosis of acute ischemic stroke must be made
   (ii) Time of symptom onset should be established

b)   Patient selection is of fundamental importance

c)   Thrombolysis must be instituted quickly

d)   Logistical considerations for intraarterial therapy often significant
   (i)   Alert the angiography team of nurses, technicians, anesthesia staff as soon as possible such that room and devices can be prepared.
   (ii) The diagnostic cerebral angiogram can be performed while the anesthesia team is being mobilized
   (iii) Devices and thrombolytic medications should be obtained and prepared early.

III.   Informed consent (Table 2)

a)   Consent often obtained from family members or surrogates.

b)   Despite the desperate and traumatic situation, an efficient and effective discussion on stroke mechanism and treatment expectations is necessary.

c)   15% of patients with a large vessel occlusion, without intraarterial thrombolysis, may have a favorable functional outcome. [2]

    d) Risks of the procedure primarily concern symptomatic intracerebral hemorrhage, and consistently average around 10%. [4,6,7]

    e) Recanalization rates consistently average around 75%. [6,7]

    f) Rate of favorable clinical outcome after intraarterial thrombolysis consistently average around 30%. [6,7]

Table 2. Comparison of significant thrombolysis trials

Trial	Median NIHSS	Re-canalization rate (%)	Mortality rate (%)	Symptomatic ICH (%)	mRS <=2
IV-tPA [15] (n=333)	14	N/A	17	6	39%
PROACT II [4] (n=180) Control/ Treatment	17/17	18/66	27/25	2/10	25%/40%
Multi-Merci [6] (n=164)	19	69	34	9.8	36%
Penumbra [7] (n=125)	21	82	33	11	25%

IV.   Patient selection

    a) Time

        (i) Albeit important, a disproportionate emphasis is often given to duration of stroke symptoms in patient selection for intraarterial thrombolysis.

        (ii) The Desmoteplase in Acute Stroke Trial (DIAS) found favorable clinical outcomes with intravenous thrombolysis given from 3-9 hours if MR physiologic imaging suggested a viable ischemic penumbra. [8]

    b) Literature

        (i) PROACT II Exclusion criteria [4]

            1) NIHSS >30

            2) Coma

            3) Rapidly improving neurologic signs

            4) Stroke within previous 6 weeks

            5) Seizures at onset of presenting stroke

            6) Clinical presentation suggestive of subarachnoid hemorrhage

7) Previous intracranial hemorrhage, neoplasm or subarachnoid hemorrhage
8) Septic embolism
9) Suspected lacunar stroke
10) Surgery, biopsy of a parenchymal organ, trauma with internal injuries, or lumbar puncture within 30 days
11) Head trauma within 90 days
12) Active or recent hemorrhage within 30 days
13) Bleeding diathesis, INR >1.7, PTT > 1.5 times normal or platelet count less than $100 \times 10^9 \, L^{-1}$
14) Contrast agent sensitivity
15) Uncontrolled hypertension SBP >180mmHg or DBP >100mmHg on three occasions requiring IV medications
16) CT evidence of hemorrhage, tumor except small meningiomas, significant mass effect, hypodense parenchymal lesion or cerebral sulci effacement in more than 1/3 MCA vascular territory
17) Angiographic evidence for arterial dissection or stenosis precluding safe passage of microcatheter.

c) Physiology based imaging [9]

   (i) Critical questions:

      1) Absence of hemorrhage?

      2) Presence of intravascular thrombus amenable to thrombolysis?

      3) Does the visualized volume of irreversibly damaged brain significantly underrepresent the severity of new neurologic deficits?

   (ii) CT perfusion facilitates patient selection via: 1) excluding patients likely to hemorrhage and including those most likely to benefit, 2) extending the time window beyond 3 hours for intravenous thrombolytics and beyond 6 hours for intraarterial thrombolytics, including those who woke up with symptoms, 3) assist at times with disposition.

   (iii) Practically, CT perfusion is fast, available, safe and affordable. Typically it adds an additional 10 minutes to a standard noncontrast head CT and does not interfere with intravenous thrombolytics.

     (iv) CT perfusion interpretation scenarios

         1) CBV and CBF match

            a) No treatment indicated

         2) Large CBV, larger CBF

            a) Possible treatment based on time, size, etc.

            b) Consider no treatment if CBV changes >100cc.

         3) Small CBV, larger CBF

            a) Ideal intraarterial thrombolytic candidate

            b) Consider no treatment if time after ictus prolonged.

V.   Technique

   a) Patient preparation

     (i) Foley catheter in place

     (ii) Continuous arterial blood pressure monitoring

     (iii) Pharmacologic agents: t-PA, heparin, verapamil and protamine should be available.

   b) Anesthesia

     (i) In general, most anterior circulation strokes can be done without general anesthesia but may require careful titration of sedatives with the help from the anesthesia team. [10]

     (ii) Posterior circulation occlusions may be better treated under general anesthesia because of the alterations in level of consciousness which affects the ability to maintain airway. Intubation in the emergency room may save time.

   c) Access phase

     (i) A 6 or 8 F sheath is placed in the femoral artery.

     (ii) Focused cerebral angiogram used to determine:

         (1) Location of occlusion

            a) For M2 branch occlusions, evaluating areas of attenuated capillary blush and stagnant anterograde filling may help in localizing the occluded vessel.

         2) Vascular access to the occlusion and presence of tandem stenosis or occlusion.

        3) Degree of collateral supply to the affected territory

        4) Define the proximal and distal face of the clot if possible

    (iii) Hydrophilic exchange wire for guide catheter to be placed as distal as possible.

d) Technical approach: Based on the clinical exam, time, angiographic pictures and prior treatment with intravenous thrombolytics, the decision on whether to pursue further thrombolysis via pharmacologic, mechanical or some combination is made.

VI. Intraarterial approaches

a) Pharmacologic thrombolysis

    (i) Navigable microcatheter over a soft tipped microguidewire .

    (ii) J-shaped microguidewire tip.

    (iii) Being careful of perforators, the wire is gently advanced past the occlusive lesion.

    (iv) Microcatheter tip is advanced beyond occlusive lesion, which is generally at the next branch point.

    (v) Microcatheter angiography performed to confirm intravascular location

    (vi) The microcatheter is then withdrawn into the occlusive lesion and the thrombolytic agent, diluted, is injected slowly over several minutes.

        1) This author uses alteplase (t-PA) primarily because of its availability in 2mg doses diluted in 20cc of heparinized saline up to a maximum of 20mg.

b) Mechanical embolectomy

    (i) The Merci® Retrieval system (Concentric Medical, Mountain View, CA) was the first FDA-approved treatment option for embolectomy in cerebral arteries.

    (ii) Prospective, multi-center single arm study with 177 patients demonstrated 68% recanalization rate, symptomatic hemorrhage rate of 9.8%, with 36% of patients achieving functional independence. [6]

        1) The devices consist of a nitinol, helical shaped wire with suture threads bound to the wire to improve thrombus engagement.

2) After femoral artery access, an 8F sheath is inserted, sutured to the skin, and perfused with heparinized saline for the entirety of the procedure.

3) 2000 units of intravenous heparin may or may not be administered.

4) An 8F balloon guide catheter is advanced, usually over an exchange wire, into the carotid or vertebral artery that is occluded.

5) The microcatheter is advanced over a wire with the support of an intermediate sized distal access catheter (4-5F) past the occlusive lesion.

6) The microguidewire is withdrawn and contrast is gently injected into the microcatheter to confirm intravascular positioning.

7) The retriever device is advanced through the microcatheter and out of the distal end of the microcatheter, forming the helical loops

8) The deployed device is then withdrawn until the helical loops appear to conform to the clot.

9) The distal access catheter is advanced up to provide additional support prior to embolectomy.

10) Anterograde flow is arrested with inflation of the balloon on the guide catheter using a 3cc syringe and 50% contrast.

11) The rotating hemostatic valves on the guide catheter, distal access catheter and microcatheter are tightened.

12) A 60cc syringe is attached to the hub of the guide catheter and gentle aspiration performed.

13) The retrieval device is withdrawn, with the goal of maintaining the shape of the helical loops all the way down to the guide catheter.

14) If the loops stretch significantly, the retriever may 'slide through' the clot without removing it, so the retriever and microcatheter should then be repositioned and the clot pulled with slow steady tension.

c) Endovascular thromboaspiration

(i) The Penumbra Stroke System (Penumbra, Alameda, CA) was FDA approved in 2008 and is the most widely used thromboaspiration device in the US.

(ii) Prospective multi-center single arm study with 125 patients demonstrated an 82% recanalization rate, a 11% symptomatic hemorrhage rate, and only 25% of patients achieving at 90 days, functional independence. [7]

1) The device consists of a thrombus debulking and aspiration reperfusion reperfusion catheter along with a separator device that prevents obstruction of the catheter via fragmentation. [7]

2) After femoral artery access, an 6F sheath is inserted, sutured to the skin, and perfused with heparinized saline for the entirety of the procedure.

3) 2000 units of intravenous heparin may or may not be administered.

4) A 6F guide catheter is advanced into the carotid or vertebral artery that is occluded.

5) The reperfusion catheter is advanced over a wire within the occlusive lesion.

6) The microguidewire is withdrawn and contrast is gently injected into the reperfusion catheter to confirm intravascular positioning.

7) Intraarterial pharmacologic thrombolytics may be administered at this time.

8) The reperfusion is then connected to the aspiration tubing and the separator is then advanced within the reperfusion catheter.

9) Thromboaspiration is performed by activating the suction while advancing and withdrawing the separator in a to and fro motion for several minutes within the vicinity of the occlusive lesion.

10) Control guide catheter angiographic images can be obtained to evaluate the progress.

d) Thrombus entrapment
  (i) Analogous to recanalization of acute coronary occlusions, intracranial stent placement provides for rapid recanalization by entrapping the thrombus between the stent and vessel wall.
    1) The SOLITAIRE FR with Intention for Thrombectomy (SWIFT) study aims to compare this closed cell, stent attached to a wire with the Merci retrieval device with outcomes measures evaluating both clinical outcomes and angiographic recanalization rates. [11]
    2) The Stent-Assisted Recanalization in Acute Ischemic Stroke (SARIS) trial is studying the use primary self-expanding stent placement, including the Enteprise (Codman, Miami Lakes, FL) and Wingspan (Boston Scientific, Fremont, CA). [12]
e) Intraprocedural evaluation
  (i) Guide catheter angiography can be performed intermittently to evaluate for changes, either recanalization or contrast extravasation.
  (ii) When to stop:
    1) Vessel recanalization (Table 1) (Figure 3)
    2) Maximum dose of thrombolytic reached
    3) Signs of intracerebral hemorrhage
    4) Suspect established cerebral infarct using combination of prior physiologic imaging, time and other factors.

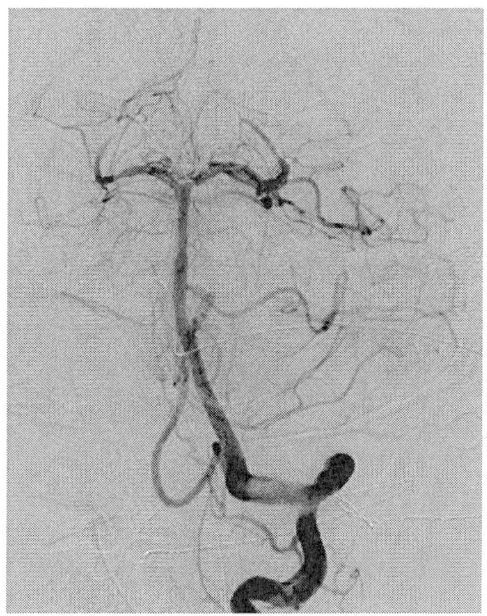

Figure 3. Recanalized TIMI 3 flow in basilar artery after mechanical intraarterial thrombolysis.

Table 1. Thrombolysis in myocardial infarction (TIMI) scale

Grade	Definition
0	No flow
1	Some penetration past the site of occlusion but no flow distal to occlusion
2	Distal perfusion but delayed filling of distal vessels
3	Distal perfusion with adequate perfusion of distal vessels

VII.   Post procedure care
- a) Noncontrast head CT should be obtained to evaluate for hemorrhage
  - (i) Artifact from extravasated contrast should be differentiated from hemorrhage.
- b) Patient should be admitted to neurointensive care unit for observation and blood pressure control
- c) Groin check protocol
- d) Secondary stroke prevention
- e) Rehabilitation or nursing care

VIII.   Complications:
  a) Intracerebral hemorrhage
    (i) Signs of intracerebral hemorrhage
       1) Severe headache
       2) New or worsening neurologic deficit
       3) Abrupt elevation in blood pressure or pulse
       4) Angiographic evidence for mass effect
    (ii) Needs to be differentiated from hemorrhagic transformation, which is limited, under hemostatic control, and attributable to ischemic vasculopathy.[13]
    (iii) Thrombolytic-related intracerebral hemorrhage, or parenchymal hematoma is related to loss of hemostatic control, often associated with greater mass effect.
    (iv) Established cerebral infarct is likely the most important predictor of thrombolytic-related intracerebral hemorrhage
       1) ASPECTS score of 7 or less raises hemorrhage risk.[14]
  b) Management of intracerebral hemorrhage
    (i) Asymptomatic small hemorrhage (<30cc)
       1) Reverse heparin if previously given
       2) Consider FFP and platelet transfusion
       3) Strict blood pressure contol
    (ii) Symptomatic significant hemorrhage (>30cc)
       1) Reverse heparin if previously given
       2) Consider FFP and platelet transfusion
       3) Strict blood pressure contol
       4) Consider intubation
       5) Consider mannitol 50g IV
       6) Ventriculostomy if hydrocephalus present
       7) Consider craniotomy for clot evacuation
  c) Femoral artery hemorrhage
    (i) Signs
       1) Obvious bleeding or enlarging subcutaneous hematoma
       2) Severe pain at puncture site
       3) Hypotension, bradycardia, anemia
    (ii) Management
       1) Manual compression

2) Reverse heparin if previously given
3) Consider FFP and platelet transfusion
4) Abdominal and pelvic CT scan to evaluate for hemorrhage
5) Volume expansion and PRBC transfusion if necessary.
6) Consider vascular surgery consultation

References

[1] Lloyd-Jones D, Adams RJ, Brown TM, Carnethon M, Dai S, De Simone G, Ferguson TB, Ford E, Furie K, Gillespie C, Go A, Greenlund K, Haase N, Hailpern S, Ho PM, Howard V, Kissela B, Kittner S, Lackland D, Lisabeth L, Marelli A, McDermott MM, Meigs J, Mozaffarian D, Mussolino M, Nichol G, Roger VL, Rosamond W, Sacco R, Sorlie P, Stafford R, Thom T, Wasserthiel-Smoller S, Wong ND, Wylie-Rosett J. *Executive summary: heart disease and stroke statistics--2010 update: a report from the American Heart Association.* Circulation 2010 Feb 23;121(7):948-54.

[2] Smith WS, Tsao JW, Billings ME, Johnston SC, Hemphill JC, 3rd, Bonovich DC, Dillon WP. *Prognostic significance of angiographically confirmed large vessel intracranial occlusion in patients presenting with acute brain ischemia.* Neurocrit Care 2006;4(1):14-7.

[3] Saqqur M, Uchino K, Demchuk AM, Molina CA, Garami Z, Calleja S, Akhtar N, Orouk FO, Salam A, Shuaib A, Alexandrov AV. *Site of arterial occlusion identified by transcranial Doppler predicts the response to intravenous thrombolysis for stroke.* Stroke 2007 Mar;38(3):948-54.

[4] Furlan A, Higashida R, Wechsler L, Gent M, Rowley H, Kase C, Pessin M, Ahuja A, Callahan F, Clark WM, Silver F, Rivera F. *Intra-arterial prourokinase for acute ischemic stroke. The PROACT II study: a randomized controlled trial. Prolyse in Acute Cerebral Thromboembolism.* JAMA 1999 Dec 1;282(21):2003-11.

[5] Intraarterial thrombolysis: ready for prime time? *Executive Committee of the ASITN. American Society of Interventional and Therapeutic Neuroradiology.* AJNR Am J Neuroradiol 2001 Jan;22(1):55-8.

[6]   Smith WS, Sung G, Saver J, Budzik R, Duckwiler G, Liebeskind DS, Lutsep HL, Rymer MM, Higashida RT, Starkman S, Gobin YP, Frei D, Grobelny T, Hellinger F, Huddle D, Kidwell C, Koroshetz W, Marks M, Nesbit G, Silverman IE. *Mechanical thrombectomy for acute ischemic stroke: final results of the Multi MERCI trial.* Stroke 2008 Apr;39(4):1205-12.

[7]   *The penumbra pivotal stroke trial: safety and effectiveness of a new generation of mechanical devices for clot removal in intracranial large vessel occlusive disease.* Stroke 2009 Aug;40(8):2761-8.

[8]   Hacke W, Albers G, Al-Rawi Y, Bogousslavsky J, Davalos A, Eliasziw M, Fischer M, Furlan A, Kaste M, Lees KR, Soehngen M, Warach S. *The Desmoteplase in Acute Ischemic Stroke Trial (DIAS): a phase II MRI-based 9-hour window acute stroke thrombolysis trial with intravenous desmoteplase.* Stroke 2005 Jan;36(1):66-73.

[9]   Shetty SK, Lev MH. *CT perfusion in acute stroke.* Neuroimaging Clin N Am 2005 Aug;15(3):481-501, ix.

[10]   Abou-Chebl A, Lin R, Hussain MS, Jovin TG, Levy EI, Liebeskind DS, Yoo AJ, Hsu DP, Rymer MM, Tayal AH, Zaidat OO, Natarajan SK, Nogueira RG, Nanda A, Tian M, Hao Q, Kalia JS, Nguyen TN, Chen M, Gupta R. *Conscious sedation versus general anesthesia during endovascular therapy for acute anterior circulation stroke: preliminary results from a retrospective, multicenter study.* Stroke 2010 Jun;41(6):1175-9.

[11]   Castano C, Dorado L, Guerrero C, Millan M, Gomis M, Perez de la Ossa N, Castellanos M, Garcia MR, Domenech S, Davalos A. *Mechanical thrombectomy with the Solitaire AB device in large artery occlusions of the anterior circulation: a pilot study.* Stroke 2010 Aug;41(8):1836-40.

[12]   Levy EI, Siddiqui AH, Crumlish A, Snyder KV, Hauck EF, Fiorella DJ, Hopkins LN, Mocco J. *First Food and Drug Administration-approved prospective trial of primary intracranial stenting for acute stroke: SARIS (stent-assisted recanalization in acute ischemic stroke).* Stroke 2009 Nov;40(11):3552-6.

[13]   Trouillas P, von Kummer R. *Classification and pathogenesis of cerebral hemorrhages after thrombolysis in ischemic stroke.* Stroke 2006 Feb;37(2):556-61.

[14] Singer OC, Kurre W, Humpich MC, Lorenz MW, Kastrup A, Liebeskind DS, Thomalla G, Fiehler J, Berkefeld J, Neumann-Haefelin T. *Risk assessment of symptomatic intracerebral hemorrhage after thrombolysis using DWI-ASPECTS.* Stroke 2009 Aug;40(8):2743-8.

[15] *"Tissue plasminogen activator for acute ischemic stroke. "The National Institute of Neurological Disorders and Stroke rt-PA Stroke Study Group."* N Engl J Med (1995). 333(24): 1581-1587.

In: Handbook of Stroke and Neurocritical Care   ISBN: 978-61324-786-0
Editor: V. H. Lee   © 2012 Nova Science Publishers, Inc.

Chapter X

Ischemic Stroke in Hospital Management

Neil Rosenberg and Shyam Prabhakaran
Department of Neurological Sciences,
Section of Stroke and Neurocritical care,
Rush University Medical Center, Chicago, IL, USA

Key Points

1) Aspirin safely prevents recurrent stroke and reduces mortality.
2) In general, anticoagulation is not beneficial in acute stroke.
3) Blood pressures up to 220/120 mmHg should be tolerated immediately after stroke, unless thrombolysis is used. Hypotension should be avoided.
4) Organized stroke units improve outcomes after stroke.
5) Measuring cardiac enzymes, obtaining echocardiograms and cardiac telemetry may help detect comorbid cardiac disease.
6) Fever may worsen outcomes in stroke.
7) Elevate the head of the bed, use frequent oral suctioning, and screen for dysphagia in order to help prevent pneumonia.
8) Remove urinary catheters when possible.
9) Turn immobile stroke patients frequently.
10) DVT prophylaxis should be used for stroke patients.

11) Start feeding patients as soon as possible.

12) Control blood glucose with a target of 140-180 mg/dL.

Non-Thrombolytic Treatment

1) Based on large trials, aspirin at doses between 160-300 mg started within 48 hours of onset and continued for at least 2 weeks is associated with approximately 10 fewer recurrent strokes or deaths per 1000 patients treated[1,2]. The risk of recurrent stroke was 2.8% vs. 3.9% in favor of aspirin with no increase in intracerebral hemorrhage (0.9 vs. 0.8%).

2) Combination antiplatelet therapy (aspirin plus clopidogrel) has not been extensively studied in acute stroke patients[3].

3) Full dose anticoagulation for acute ischemic stroke has not been shown to be beneficial. In a meta-analysis, anticoagulation with heparin or heparinoids reduced recurrent ischemic stroke at the cost of increasing intracranial hemorrhages [4,5].

4) Heparin given subcutaneously at a dose of 5000 units started during first 48 hours and twice daily also resulted in a small but significant reduction in ischemic stroke].

5) Bridging with heparinoids is generally not recommended in patients who require long-term full anticoagulation with warfarin (i.e. atrial fibrillation). In the Heparin Aspirin Embolic Stroke Trial, there was no significant difference in early recurrent stroke risk in those receiving the low-molecular weight heparinoid, dalteparin, compared to aspirin prior to warfarin therapy for atrial fibrillation].

6) Clinical case-by-case exceptions may be made for the following:
    a) Presence of intra-cardiac or intra-vascular thrombus in the presence of a small cerebral infarct or TIA
    b) Cerebral venous thrombosis. Small trials suggest heparinoids are beneficial in this disease, even in the presence of intracerebral hemorrhage.
    c) Large-artery stenosis subtype. Subgroup analysis from the TOAST trial suggested more favorable outcomes among those treated with danaparoid[7].

7) The value of induced hypothermia after ischemic stroke remains unproven (see "Ongoing Trials")[8].

Blood Pressure Management in Ischemic Stroke Patients

1) Most ischemic stroke patients have some degree of hypertension at presentation, with systolic blood pressures above 150-160 mmHg[9,10]. This often reflects a history of hypertension (diagnosed or undiagnosed), but pain, nausea, increased sympathetic tone, and elevated intracranial pressure may also contribute.

2) Blood pressure derangements at presentation bear a U-shaped relationship to prognosis. Both hypotension and extreme hypertension have been associated with poor outcomes[9].

3) Even in the absence of treatment, elevated baseline blood pressures tend to decline somewhat over 24 hours to 1 week[11,12].

4) In acute stroke patients not receiving thrombolytic therapy, only systolic blood pressures > 220 mmHg or diastolic pressures > 120 mmHg should be treated with medications, with a goal of lowering blood pressure by about 15% in 24 hours, according to expert consensus]. In theory, this strategy of "permissive hypertension" may maximize perfusion of the stroke penumbra. However, this has not been demonstrated in large, prospective trials. Previous studies have variously associated blood pressure reduction over 24 hours with better functional outcomes[10,14], no benefit[15], and infarct growth and poor outcome[11,16].

5) Patients with other indications for blood pressure control (e.g., myocardial infarction or aortic dissection) should receive antihypertensive medications[13].

6) Following thrombolysis or thrombectomy, blood pressure should be maintained below 180/105 mmHg for at least 24 hours after treatment[13]. Elevated blood pressures are associated with an increased risk of hemorrhagic transformation after thrombolysis[15]. Table 1 outlines a sample approach to treating hypertension.

7) In stable patients previously diagnosed with hypertension, antihypertensive medications should be gradually restarted approximately 24 hours after onset [13]. In one randomized trial, ischemic stroke patients who continued antihypertensive medications had an 8% absolute risk reduction in death or

dependence at 2 weeks compared to those who stopped their medications [17].

Table 1. Suggested algorithm for blood pressure management after reperfusion therapy [13]

Monitor blood pressure every 15 minutes during treatment and then for another 2 hours, then every 30 minutes for 6 hours, and then every hour for 16 hours
Blood pressure level Systolic 180 to 230 mm Hg or diastolic 105 to 120 mm Hg
Labetalol 10 mg IV over 1 to 2 minutes, may repeat every 10 to 20 minutes, maximum dose of 300 mg; Or Labetalol 10 mg IV followed by an infusion at 2 to 8 mg/min
Systolic >230 mm Hg or diastolic 121 to 140 mm Hg
Labetalol 10 mg IV over 1 to 2 minutes, may repeat every 10 to 20 minutes, maximum dose of 300 mg; or Labetalol 10 mg IV followed by an infusion at 2 to 8 mg/min; or Nicardipine infusion, 5 mg/h, titrate up to desired effect by increasing 2.5 mg/h every 5 minutes to maximum of 15 mg/h
If blood pressure not controlled, consider sodium nitroprusside

8) While long-term management should focus on achieving normotension in order to reduce recurrent stroke risk (see Chapter 11, "Vascular Risk Factor Modification"), the optimal time to begin treatment is not known. In many series, antihypertensive treatment during the first 1-7 days after stroke onset does not appear to affect long-term outcomes[10,11]. Another trial randomizing patients to candesartan immediately or after 7 days showed no difference in 3-month functional outcomes[18].

9) In patients not previously on antihypertensives, we suggest gradually controlling blood pressure beginning 3 to 7 days after stroke onset. Some degree of blood pressure control is often necessary for procedures (e.g., placement of feeding tubes) and

prior to transferring patients (e.g., to rehabilitation or skilled nursing facilities).

10) There is no preferred antihypertensive agent in stroke prevention though there is more data on use of ACE inhibitors and ARBs; however, the choice of medication should be dictated by a patient's comorbidities (e.g., ACE inhibitors in diabetics, or beta-blockers in atrial fibrillation).

11) Hypotension should be avoided. When detected, an underlying cause should be sought and treated. Interventions should focus on correcting hypovolemia and optimizing cardiac output.

12) Induced hypertension (with vasopressors) is not recommended for unselected stroke patients[13]. The safety of such a strategy has not been demonstrated in large trials. However, permissive and perhaps induced hypertension may benefit some patients. If vasopressors and volume expanders are used, patients must be monitored carefully for side effects, including myocardial ischemia and congestive heart failure.

Stroke Units

1) Stroke units are typically dedicated wards with care coordinated between specialized medical, nursing and therapy staff. In contrast to general medical wards, these units organize processes and create pathways that improve outcomes and potentially decrease medical complications after stroke.

2) Stroke units reduce the odds of death or dependence at 1 year by 21% when compared to less organized services, such as general medical wards[19]. They also reduce hospital length of stay by 2 to 6 days.

3) The mechanism by which stroke units improve outcomes remains speculative but may include better diagnostic procedures, earlier attention to medical complications, better nursing care, and/or more effective rehabilitation].

4) Primary Stroke Center designation requires the presence of a stroke unit[21].

Prevention and Detection of Medical Complications

1) Most medical complications occur within in first few weeks of stroke onset and those with severe, disabling strokes are most susceptible[22].
2) Medical complications prolong hospital stays, worsen functional outcomes, and increase the risk of death following stroke.
3) Prevention is possible in many cases, and early detection and treatment can reduce the morbidity and mortality associated with these complications.

Cardiac Complications

1) Risk factors for cardiac complications
   a) Cardiac conditions tend to be comorbid with stroke. Furthermore, acute stroke may predispose patients to cardiac abnormalities, which tend to occur early after stroke onset.
   b) Those with known coronary artery disease, peripheral artery disease, diabetes, and those with more severe strokes may be more prone[23].
   c) Large artery ischemic stroke patients may harbor the greatest risk of having concomitant coronary artery disease].
   d) In general, there is little consensus regarding how screening for cardiac comorbidities ought to proceed.
2) MI and cardiomyopathy
   a) In various studies, the incidence of myocardial infarction following stroke is 0.5-6%. Patients with large-artery strokes may be at higher risk.
   b) Cardiac troponins may also be elevated due to autonomic dysregulation (e.g., with infarctions involving the right insula) or as a stress response following ischemic stroke]. Although no clear troponin cutoff value exists, symmetric T-wave inversions on EKG may help to identify this disorder.

c) Congestive heart failure may occur with volume overload, acute myocardial infarction, or from neurogenic causes. Careful attention should be paid to patients' volume status.

d) Although long associated with subarachnoid hemorrhage, "stunned myocardium," or takotsubo cardiomyopathy, may occur in 1-2% of patients within 24 hours of an ischemic stroke]. The syndrome is typically marked by ST segment elevation on EKG and apical ballooning on echocardiogram. Most patients recover cardiac function over time and require only supportive care.

e) We suggest that ischemic stroke patients be initially screened for abnormal cardiac biomarkers and with echocardiography.

3) Cardiac arrhythmias

a) The detection of arrhythmias responsible for stroke, particularly atrial fibrillation, plays an important role in reducing the risk of recurrent stroke.

b) Other arrhythmias may occur following stroke, with an incidence of 2-8%[27].

c) Risk factors for developing arrhythmias may include baseline QTc prolongation and involvement of the right insula[28].

d) Patients with acute stroke should be monitored with cardiac telemetry for at least 24-48 hours [29]. In some cases, Holter monitoring may increase the sensitivity for detecting arrhythmias.

Fevers and Infections

1) Fever

a) Fever has been associated with increased mortality and worse outcomes in a number of neurological conditions, including ischemic stroke and hemorrhagic stroke.

b) At present, little evidence supports the use of acetaminophen or other active fever treatments in stroke, including active cooling to normothermia, though they may ameliorate the negative effects on fever on the injured brain].

2) Pneumonia
   a) In various series, the incidence of pneumonia following ischemic stroke is 4-22%[31] and occurs in the first several days following stroke.
   b) Risk factors include old age, speech impairment, cognitive impairment, disabling stroke, dysphagia, severe facial palsy, brainstem] stroke, and multifocal infarct[32]. Other factors may include mechanical ventilation, decreased level of consciousness, and poor or weakened cough from pharyngeal or expiratory muscle weakness.
   c) Pneumonia increases the odds of death after stroke threefold[33]. Furthermore, persistent, or even transient but severe, hypoxemia may worsen neurologic outcomes following stroke.
   d) The most common cause is aspiration], which can cause both an infectious pneumonia (pharyngeal flora aspiration) and a chemical pneumonitis (gastric contents aspiration).
   e) Aspiration pneumonia is associated with desaturation, consolidation on x-rays (may lag behind clinical exam), and requires antimicrobial therapy. Aspiration pneumonitis is typically self-limited without antimicrobial therapy.
   f) Prevention strategies include dysphagia screening in all stroke patients, semi-upright positioning, frequent oral suctioning and good oral hygiene in those at risk.
   g) Monitoring of pulse oximetry with goal oxygen saturation > 92% is generally recommended[13].
3) Urinary tract infections (UTI)
   a) UTIs occur in 6-31% of stroke patients, with risk factors including old age, indwelling urinary catheters, severe stroke and female gender(27).
   b) Its impact on outcomes is unclear, although related fevers may worsen neurologic recovery.
   c) UTI risk may be reduced by removing/avoiding catheters in cognitively intact, voiding patients. Antibiotic-impregnated catheters may also be of value.
4) Decubitus ulcers
   a) Ulcers are common due to immobility and urinary and fecal incontinence, and they may become sources of infection.

    b)   The sacrum and buttocks are common sites that require regular examination in bed-ridden patients.

    c)   Prevention entails early mobilization and frequent turning (every 2 hours), use of air mattresses and padded heel supports [29].

Hematologic Complications

Deep Venous Thrombosis (DVT) and Pulmonary Embolism (PE)

1) DVT is quite common, varying from 0.2-4% in some retrospective series and in up to 40% of patients undergoing routine screening[27].

2) Risk factors include old age, immobility, and dehydration.

3) Untreated, DVT can lead to pulmonary embolism in up to 15% of patients. PE is a major cause of death and occurs most commonly between 2-4 weeks following stroke.

4) DVTs can be diagnosed using lower extremity Doppler or MRI of the pelvis and lower extremities. PEs are generally diagnosed using helical CT angiography of the chest.

5) Routine screening for DVTs in the absence of symptoms is not generally recommended. Evaluation for DVT may be useful in patients with lower extremity swelling or low-grade, unexplained fevers.

6) Mechanical or pharmacological DVT prophylaxis should be used in non-ambulatory stroke patients within 2 days of hospitalization].

7) Pneumatic compression devices may be used for mechanical DVT prophylaxis. Compression stocking are no longer considered safe given the risks of skin necrosis and lack of evidence in reduction of DVT, PE, or mortality].

8) Enoxaparin 40mg subcutaneously, given daily, is superior to unfractionated heparin 5000 units subcutaneously, given twice daily, as shown in a recent randomized trial. The incidence of DVT was 10% vs. 18%, respectively ($p = 0.0001$). Although the incidence was low, major extracranial bleeding occurred more frequently with enoxaparin (1% vs. 0%, p=0.015)[35].

9) Although few data are available, most experts agree that anticoagulation (e.g., for DVTs) may be started after 2-4 weeks following an ischemic stroke, depending on its size.

GI Bleeding

1) The prevalence of GI bleeding is 1.5-3% in acute stroke studies[27].
2) Risk factors include severe stroke, history of peptic ulcer disease, cancer, sepsis, renal failure, abnormal LFTs, anticoagulation, feeding through NG tube (but not PEG).
3) GI bleeding can lead to recurrent strokes, MI, and venous thromboembolism owing to anti-thrombotic medication cessation.
4) Proton-pump inhibitors, H-2 blockers, and sucralfate may all help to prevent GI bleeding though the first two classes are associated with increased risks of pneumonia [36].

GI Complications

Dysphagia

1) Strokes may cause dysphagia by causing weakness, sensory loss, alterations of consciousness or attention, or apraxia [31]. Since cortical input is often asymmetric in healthy individuals, even unilateral hemispheric strokes can cause dysphagia [37].
2) Dysphagia occurs in 29 to 78% of non-obtunded, hospitalized stroke patients [38].
3) Patients with dysphagia have a 2- to 5-fold higher risk of developing pneumonia within days to months of stroke, and frank aspiration increases this risk [38].
4) Dysphagia improves in up to 79% of stroke patients during the first month and, rarely, develops in a delayed fashion [39].
5) All stroke patients should be screened for dysphagia within the first 24 hours of admission [29].
6) Several bedside screening tests are available for initial patient assessment [40,41]. A sample is shown in Table 2.

Table 2. Acute Stroke Dysphagia Screen [40]

If any of the following questions are answered with a yes, stop and refer to speech pathology.
1) Is the Glasgow Coma Scale score < 13? 2) Is there facial asymmetry/weakness?

<table>
<tr><td>

3)   Is there tongue asymmetry/weakness?

4)   Is there palatal asymmetry/weakness?

If all findings for the first four questions are NO, proceed to the 3 oz. water test.

Administer 3 oz. of water for sequential drinks, note any throat clearing, cough or change in vocal quality immediately after and 1 minute following the swallow. If clearing, coughing, or change in vocal quality is noted, refer to speech therapy.

5)   Are there signs of aspiration during the 3 oz. water test?

If all of the answers to the above questions are NO, then start the patient on a regular diet.

</td></tr>
</table>

7) If dysphagia is suspected on a screening test or based on other clinical grounds, patients should be made strict NPO. Alternate nutritional routes should be initiated (e.g., nasogastric tubes) until formal evaluation can be performed.

8) Patients with suspected dysphagia should be referred to speech pathologists. The gold standard for diagnosing dysphagia is videofluoroscopic swallow studies.

Nutrition

1) Undernutrition is common in stroke patients and may increase mortality [42].

2) Timing and route/method of nutrition initiation in stroke patients was assessed in the FOOD trial [43]. Early nasogastric tube feeding was associated with a small decrease in risk of death at 6 months compared to delayed feeding (avoid feeding for 7 days) but did not improve functional outcomes. Early percutaneous gastrostomy tube placement was associated increased risk of death or dependency at 6 months compared to early NG tube feeding.

3) It is recommended that nutrition be started as soon as possible and that early nasogastric tube feeding is preferred over early PEG placement.

Hyperglycemia and Hypoglycemia

1) Hyperglycemia is common after stroke, with a prevalence exceeding 60% in some series[44]. This may represent a stress response, diabetes/impaired glucose tolerance, or a combination of the two.

2) Initial hyperglycemia is associated with increased long-term mortality and decreased functional independence].

3) Bloood glucose should be controlled during inpatient hospitalization, with target levels of approximately 140-180 mg/dL.

   a) A number of prospective studies have evaluated the safety and feasilibility of aggressive hyperglycemia treatment strategies, e.g., with continuous infusions and blood glucose goals <110-130 mg/dL, versus "sliding scales" or goals of <200 or 300 mg/dL [47-49].

   b) Aggressive strategies more effectively lower blood glucose. They do this at the expense of causing hypoglycemia in 15-35% of aggressively treated patients, compared to 0-4% in routine care.

   c) In these small series assessing stroke patients, hypoglycemia did not appear to have long-term adverse consequences. However, in much larger observational studies, hypoglycemia is strongly associated with poor outcome [45], and in critically ill adults, more aggressive strategies are associated with increased mortality].

   d) Based on these data, "tight" glucose control should be avoided. Ongoing studies may further clarify the optimum glucose goal in stroke patients.

4) Stroke patients should probably be screened with a hemoglobin A1c. Recent guidelines establish two values greater than or equal to 6.5% as diagnostic for diabetes. Moreover, previously undiagnosed diabetes may be present in more than 20% of ischemic stroke patients [44].

Surgical Treatment of Ischemic Stroke

1) Decompressive Hemicraniectomy for Malignant cerebral ischemia
   a) Space-occupying 'malignant' middle cerebral artery territory (MCA) infarction accounts for over 10% of supratentorial ischemic strokes. Patients with malignant MCA infarction show clinical worsening as manifested by progressive deterioration in their level of conciousness due to increasing cerebral edema early in the course of their hospitalization (most frequently within the first 1-2 days after the onset of stroke symptoms). If this cascade of worsening cerebral edema is left unchecked, cerebral herniation and death will occur in over 80% of patients. [52, 53]
   b) Risk factors for malignant cerebral infarction include: NIHSS >20 in infarction of the dominant hemisphere or >15 in the non-dominant hemisphere, infarction of ½ to 2/3 of the territory of the MCA or >145 cm^3 of the MCA territory, infarction of the ipsilateral ACA or PCA territory.
   c) Aggressive neurocritical care with standard measures to control ICP (head of bed elevation to 30-45 degrees, early intubation for compromised airway reflexes or hypoventilation, adequate sedation to prevent agitation and ventilator dyssynchrony, aggressive fever control, etc) as well as hyperosmolar therapy with mannitol or hypertonic saline are advocated as medical measures to prevent and manage malignant cerebral edema, yet these measures have not been proven to decrease mortality or improve outcome in malignant cerebral infarction.
   d) In the past decade, 3 small prospective randomized trials compared standard medical management to early decompressive hemicraniectomy [54, 55, 56].
      (i) HAMLET study (Hemicraniectomy After Middle cerebral artery infarction with Life-threatening Edema Trial)
      (ii) DECIMAL (DEcompressive Craniectomy In MALignant middle cerebral artery infarction)

        (iii) DESTINY (DEcompressive Surgery for the Treatment of malignant INfarction of the middle cerebral artery)

        (iv) Recruitment was stopped early in DECIMAL and DESTINY. In HAMLET, surgical decompression had no effect on the primary outcome measure of functional outcome.

e) Metaanalysis of 3 trials (HAMLET, DECIMAL, DESTINY) [57]

        (i) included 93 patients aged 18-60 years old randomized to decomrpessive hemicraniectomy vs conversative therapy

        (ii) randomized within 48 hours of onset of symptoms

        (iii) 51patients were randomized to decompressive hemicraniectomy and 42 to conservative treatment.

        (iv) Outcome measures were the score on the mRS at 1 year, dichotomized into 0 to 4 and 5+6 as well as 0 to 3 and 4 to 6 and the case fatality at 1 year. A total of 93 patients were included, of whom 51 were randomized to decompressive surgery and 42 to conservative treatment.

        (v) Results demonstrated that after decompressive surgery, more patients had an mRS ≤ 4 (75% vs 24%; P <0.0001), with a pooled absolute risk reduction (ARR) of 51% (95% CI, 34%–69%). In addition, more patients had an mRS ≤ 3 (43% vs 21%; $P =$ 0.014), with a pooled ARR of 23% (95% CI, 5%–41%). The case fatality rate in the surgical group was 78% versus 29% in the conservative treatment group ($P < 0.0001$), indicating a pooled ARR of 50% (95% CI, 33%–67%).

        (vi) The resulting numbers needed to treat are 2 for survival with an mRS ≤ 4, 4 for survival with an mRS ≤ 3, and 2 for survival irrespective of outcome

        (vii) Conclusion: in patients with malignant MCA infarction, decompressive surgery undertaken within 48 h of stroke onset reduces mortality and increases the number of patients with a favourable functional outcome.

2) Cerebellar Infarction
    a) The surgical management of cerebellar infarction lacks prospective controlled trials to guide management and thus remains based upon expert opinion and local practice.
    b) Most physicians would advocate posterior fossa decompression in a patient with multiple terriotory infarction with effacement of the fourth ventricle and/or obstructive hydrocephalus
    c) placing an extraventicular drain carries the risk for upward herniation of the posterior fossa contents.

Box Ongoing and Upcoming Clinical Trials

- TARDIS: Triple Antiplatelets for Reducing Dependency after Ischemic Stroke (ISRCTN47823388). A multi-center, open-label trial assessing the efficacy, safety, and tolerability of adding clopidogrel to aspirin and dipyridamole in patients at high risk of recurrent stroke.
- COMPRESS: COMbination of Clopidogrel and Aspirin for Prevention of Early REcurrence in Acute Atherothrombotic Stroke (NCT00814268). A randomized, double-blind study to assess if aspirin+clopidogrel versus aspirin alone prevents recurrent stroke, mortality and improves outcomes.
- VENTURE: Valsartan Efficacy on Modest Blood Pressure Reduction in Acute Ischemic Stroke (NCT00874601). A randomized, open-label trial to assess the effect of blood pressure reduction on 90-day functional outcomes.
- CHIL: The Cerebral Hypothermia in Ischemic lesion Trial (ACTRN12609000690257). A randomized, controlled trial evaluating the effect of systemic and local mild hypothermia on infarct growth, penumbral salvage, and 90-day functional outcomes.
- ICTuS2/3: The Intravascular Cooling in the Treatment of Stroke 2/3 (NCT01123161). A randomized trial comparing hypothermia vs. normothermia after t-PA, on 90-day outcomes.
- CLOTS-3: A RCT to Establish the Effectiveness of Intermittent Pneumatic Compression to Prevent Post Stroke DVT

(NCT00789542). A randomized trial of intermittent pneumatic compression in preventing DVTs.

- ATTRACT: Acute Venous Thrombosis: Thrombus Removal With Adjunctive Catheter-Directed Thrombolysis (NCT00790335). A randomized trial to determine if rt-PA delivered into a symptomatic DVT prevents the post-thrombotic syndrome.
- INSULINFARCT: Efficacy and Safety of Continuous Intravenous Versus Usual Subcutaneous Insulin in Acute Ischemic Stroke (NCT00472381). A prospective, randomized trial comparing glucose control strategies in patients with stroke in the carotid artery territory.
- SHINE: Stroke Hyperglycemia Insulin Network Effort (Proposed). A prospective, randomized trial comparing insulin infusion with target glucose concentration 80mg/dl – 130 mg/dL or control sliding scale insulin with a target of 80mg/dL - 185 mg/dL in acute ischemic stroke patients treated within 12 hours of symptom onset.

References

[1] CAST: randomised placebo-controlled trial of early aspirin use in 20,000 patients with acute ischaemic stroke. *CAST (Chinese Acute Stroke Trial) Collaborative Group.* Lancet 1997;349:1641-9.

[2] The International Stroke Trial (IST): a randomised trial of aspirin, subcutaneous heparin, both, or neither among 19435 patients with acute ischaemic stroke. *International Stroke Trial Collaborative Group.* Lancet 1997;349:1569-81.

[3] Kennedy J, Hill MD, Ryckborst KJ, et al. *Fast assessment of stroke and transient ischaemic attack to prevent early recurrence (FASTER): a randomised controlled pilot trial.* Lancet Neurol 2007;6:961-9.

[4] Sandercock P, Gubitz G, Counsell C. *Anticoagulants for Acute Ischemic Stroke.* Stroke 2004;35:2916-7.

[5] Sandercock PA, Counsell C, Kamal AK. *Anticoagulants for acute ischaemic stroke.* Cochrane Database Syst Rev 2008;(4):CD000024.

[6] Berge E, Abdelnoor M, Nakstad PH, Sandset PM. *Low molecular-weight heparin versus aspirin in patients with acute ischaemic stroke and atrial fibrillation: a double-blind randomised study. HAEST Study Group. Heparin in Acute Embolic Stroke Trial.* Lancet 2000;355:1205-10.

[7]   Low molecular weight heparinoid, ORG 10172 (danaparoid), and outcome after acute ischemic stroke: a randomized controlled trial. *The Publications Committee for the Trial of ORG 10172 in Acute Stroke Treatment (TOAST) Investigators.* JAMA 1998;279:1265-72.

[8]   Lazzaro MA, Prabhakaran S. *Induced hypothermia in acute ischemic stroke.* Expert Opin Investig Drugs 2008;17:1161-74.

[9]   Leonardi-Bee J, Bath PM, Phillips SJ, Sandercock PA, IST Collaborative Group. *Blood pressure and clinical outcomes in the International Stroke Trial.* Stroke 2002;33:1315-20.

[10]   Sare GM, Ali M, Shuaib A, Bath PM, VISTA Collaboration. *Relationship between hyperacute blood pressure and outcome after ischemic stroke: data from the VISTA collaboration.* Stroke 2009;40:2098-103.

[11]   Oliveira-Filho J, Silva SC, Trabuco CC, Pedreira BB, Sousa EU, Bacellar A. *Detrimental effect of blood pressure reduction in the first 24 hours of acute stroke onset.* Neurology 2003;61:1047-51.

[12]   Potter J, Mistri A, Brodie F, et al. *Controlling hypertension and hypotension immediately post stroke (CHHIPS)--a randomised controlled trial.* Health Technol Assess 2009;13:iii, ix,xi, 1-73.

[13]   Adams HP,Jr, del Zoppo G, Alberts MJ, et al. *Guidelines for the early management of adults with ischemic stroke: a guideline from the American Heart Association/American Stroke Association Stroke Council, Clinical Cardiology Council, Cardiovascular Radiology and Intervention Council, and the Atherosclerotic Peripheral Vascular Disease and Quality of Care Outcomes in Research Interdisciplinary Working Groups: the American Academy of Neurology affirms the value of this guideline as an educational tool for neurologists.* Stroke 2007;38:1655-711.

[14]   Toyoda K, Fujimoto S, Kamouchi M, Iida M, Okada Y. *Acute blood pressure levels and neurological deterioration in different subtypes of ischemic stroke.* Stroke 2009;40:2585-8.

[15]   Yong M, Kaste M. *Association of characteristics of blood pressure profiles and stroke outcomes in the ECASS-II trial.* Stroke 2008;39:366-72.

[16]   Castillo J, Leira R, Garcia MM, Serena J, Blanco M, Davalos A. *Blood pressure decrease during the acute phase of ischemic stroke is associated with brain injury and poor stroke outcome.* Stroke 2004;35:520-6.

[17] Robinson TG, Potter JF, Ford GA, et al. *Effects of antihypertensive treatment after acute stroke in the Continue or Stop Post-Stroke Antihypertensives Collaborative Study (COSSACS): a prospective, randomised, open, blinded-endpoint trial.* Lancet Neurol 2010;9:767-75.

[18] Schrader J, Luders S, Kulschewski A, et al. T*he ACCESS Study: evaluation of Acute Candesartan Cilexetil Therapy in Stroke Survivors.* Stroke 2003;34:1699-703.

[19] Stroke Unit Trialists' Collaboration. *Organised inpatient (stroke unit) care for stroke.* Cochrane Database Syst Rev 2007;(4):CD000197.

[20] Kalra L, Evans A, Perez I, Knapp M, Swift C, Donaldson N. *A randomised controlled comparison of alternative strategies in stroke care.* Health Technol Assess 2005;9:iii,iv, 1-79.

[21] Alberts MJ, Hademenos G, Latchaw RE, et al. *Recommendations for the establishment of primary stroke centers. Brain Attack Coalition.* JAMA 2000;283:3102-9.

[22] Johnston KC, Li JY, Lyden PD, et al. *Medical and neurological complications of ischemic stroke: experience from the RANTTAS trial. RANTTAS Investigators.* Stroke 1998;29:447-53.

[23] Liao J, O'Donnell MJ, Silver FL, et al. *In-hospital myocardial infarction following acute ischaemic stroke: an observational study.* Eur J Neurol 2009;16:1035-40.

[24] Touze E, Varenne O, Calvet D, Mas JL. *Coronary risk stratification in patients with ischemic stroke or transient ischemic stroke attack.* Int J Stroke 2007;2:177-83.

[25] Ay H, Koroshetz WJ, Benner T, et al. *Neuroanatomic correlates of stroke-related myocardial injury.* Neurology 2006;66:1325-9.

[26] Yoshimura S, Toyoda K, Ohara T, et al. *Takotsubo cardiomyopathy in acute ischemic stroke.* Ann Neurol 2008;64:547-54.

[27] Kumar S, Selim MH, Caplan LR. *Medical complications after stroke.* Lancet Neurol 2010;9:105-18.

[28] Abboud H, Berroir S, Labreuche J, Orjuela K, Amarenco P, GENIC *Investigators. Insular involvement in brain infarction increases risk for cardiac arrhythmia and death.* Ann Neurol 2006;59:691-9.

[29] Summers D, Leonard A, Wentworth D, et al. *Comprehensive overview of nursing and interdisciplinary care of the acute ischemic stroke patient: a scientific statement from the American Heart Association.* Stroke 2009;40:2911-44.

[30] Kalafut MA, Llanes J, Kidwell C, Starkman S, Saver JL. *Can Prophylactic Acetaminophen Prevent Hyperthermia in Acute Stroke?: Results of the Normothermia and Stroke Outcome (NOTHOT) Pilot Clinical Trial.* Stroke 2000;32:381C.

[31] Kumar S. *Swallowing and dysphagia in neurological disorders.* Rev Neurol Dis 2010;7:19-27.

[32] Sellars C, Bowie L, Bagg J, et al. *Risk factors for chest infection in acute stroke: a prospective cohort study.* Stroke 2007;38:2284-91.

[33] Katzan IL, Cebul RD, Husak SH, Dawson NV, Baker DW. *The effect of pneumonia on mortality among patients hospitalized for acute stroke.* Neurology 2003;60:620-5.

[34] CLOTS Trials Collaboration, Dennis M, Sandercock PA, et al. *Effectiveness of thigh-length graduated compression stockings to reduce the risk of deep vein thrombosis after stroke (CLOTS trial 1): a multicentre, randomised controlled trial.* Lancet 2009;373:1958-65.

[35] Sherman DG, Albers GW, Bladin C, et al. *The efficacy and safety of enoxaparin versus unfractionated heparin for the prevention of venous thromboembolism after acute ischaemic stroke (PREVAIL Study): an open-label randomised comparison.* Lancet 2007;369:1347-55.

[36] Herzig SJ, Howell MD, Ngo LH, Marcantonio ER. *Acid-suppressive medication use and the risk for hospital-acquired pneumonia.* JAMA 2009;301:2120-8.

[37] Hamdy S, Aziz Q, Rothwell JC, et al. *Explaining oropharyngeal dysphagia after unilateral hemispheric stroke.* Lancet 1997;350:686-92.

[38] Martino R, Foley N, Bhogal S, Diamant N, Speechley M, Teasell R. *Dysphagia after stroke: incidence, diagnosis, and pulmonary complications.* Stroke 2005;36:2756-63.

[39] Smithard DG, O'Neill PA, England RE, et al. *The natural history of dysphagia following a stroke.* Dysphagia 1997;12:188-93.

[40] Edmiaston J, Connor LT, Loehr L, Nassief A. *Validation of a Dysphagia screening tool in acute stroke patients.* Am J Crit Care 2010;19:357-64.

[41] Trapl M, Enderle P, Nowotny M, et al. *Dysphagia bedside screening for acute-stroke patients: the Gugging Swallowing Screen.* Stroke 2007;38:2948-52.

[42] Davalos A, Ricart W, Gonzalez-Huix F, et al. *Effect of malnutrition after acute stroke on clinical outcome.* Stroke 1996;27:1028-32.

[43] Dennis MS, Lewis SC, Warlow C, *FOOD Trial Collaboration. Effect of timing and method of enteral tube feeding for dysphagic stroke patients (FOOD): a multicentre randomised controlled trial.* Lancet 2005;365:764-72.

[44] Gray CS, Scott JF, French JM, Alberti KG, O'Connell JE. *Prevalence and prediction of unrecognised diabetes mellitus and impaired glucose tolerance following acute stroke.* Age Ageing 2004;33:71-7.

[45] Ntaios G, Egli M, Faouzi M, Michel P. *J-Shaped Association Between Serum Glucose and Functional Outcome in Acute Ischemic Stroke.* Stroke 2010;.

[46] Ahmed N, Davalos A, Eriksson N, et al. *Association of admission blood glucose and outcome in patients treated with intravenous thrombolysis: results from the Safe Implementation of Treatments in Stroke International Stroke Thrombolysis Register (SITS-ISTR).* Arch Neurol 2010;67:1123-30.

[47] Johnston KC, Hall CE, Kissela BM, Bleck TP, Conaway MR, GRASP Investigators. *Glucose Regulation in Acute Stroke Patients (GRASP) trial: a randomized pilot trial.* Stroke 2009;40:3804-9.

[48] Bruno A, Kent TA, Coull BM, et al. *Treatment of hyperglycemia in ischemic stroke (THIS): a randomized pilot trial.* Stroke 2008;39:384-9.

[49] Gray CS, Hildreth AJ, Sandercock PA, et al. *Glucose-potassium-insulin infusions in the management of post-stroke hyperglycaemia: the UK Glucose Insulin in Stroke Trial (GIST-UK).* Lancet Neurol 2007;6:397-406.

[50] NICE-SUGAR Study Investigators, Finfer S, Chittock DR, et al. *Intensive versus conventional glucose control in critically ill patients.* N Engl J Med 2009;360:1283-97.

[51] International Expert Committee. *International Expert Committee report on the role of the A1C assay in the diagnosis of diabetes.* Diabetes Care 2009;32:1327-34.

[52] Hacke W, Schwab S, Horn M, Spranger M, De Georgia M, von Kummer R. *Malignant middle cerebral artery territory infarction: clinical course and prognostic signs.* Arch Neurol 1996; 53: 309–15.

[53] Berrouschot J, Sterker M, Bettin S, Koster J, Schneider D. *Mortality of space-occupying (malignant) middle cerebral artery infarction under conservative intensive care.* Intensive Care Med 1998; 24: 620–23.

[54] Hofmeijer J, Kappelle LJ, Algra A, Amelink GJ, van Gijn J, van der Worp HB; HAMLET investigators. *Surgical decompression for space-occupying cerebral infarction (the Hemicraniectomy After Middle Cerebral Artery infarction with Life-threatening Edema Trial [HAMLET]): a multicentre, open, randomised trial.* Lancet Neurol. 2009; 8: 326–333

[55] Vahedi K, Vicaut E, Mateo J, et al. *Sequential-design, multicenter, randomized, controlled trial of early decompressive craniectomy in malignant middle cerebral artery infarction (DECIMAL trial).* Stroke 2007; 38: 2506-2517.

[56] Jüttler E, Schwab S, Schmiedek P, et al. *Decompressive Surgery for the Treatment of Malignant Infarction of the Middle Cerebral Artery (DESTINY): a randomized, controlled trial.* Stroke 2007; 38: 2518-2525.

[57] Vahedi K, Hofmeijer J, Juettler E, et al. *Early decompressive surgery in malignant infarction of the middle cerebral artery: a pooled analysis of three randomised controlled trials.* Lancet Neurol 2007; 6: 215-222.

In: Handbook of Stroke and Neurocritical Care   ISBN: 978-61324-786-0
Editor: V. H. Lee   © 2012 Nova Science Publishers, Inc.

Chapter XI

Ischemic Stroke- Secondary Stroke Prevention

Vivien Lee
Department of Neurological Sciences,
Section of Stroke and Neurocritical care,
Rush University Medical Center, Chicago, IL, USA

Secondary stroke prevention in ischemic stroke typically involves a combination of anti-thrombotic medication and vascular risk factor modification.

Anti-Platelet Medications

1) Aspirin
   a) 2 large trials that showed a modest but significant benefit when treatment with aspirin was initiated within 48 hours of stroke.
   b) Chinese Acute Stroke Trial (CAST) [1]
      (i) 21,106 pts w/acute ischemic stroke w/in 48 hr of onset randomized to ASA 160 mg/d vs placebo

        (ii) Results- ASA group had significant reduction in early mortality (3.3% vs 3.9%, p=0.04) and recurrent ischemic strokes (1.6% vs 2.1%, p=0.01)

        (iii) at discharge, smaller proportion dead/dependent (30.5% vs 31.6%, p=0.08)

    c) The International Stroke Trial (IST) [2]

        (i) Unblinded trial, 19,435 pts (36 countries), Randomized w/in 48 hrs of onset to: ASA 300 QD, Heparin SQ (5000 BID or 12,500U BID), Both, or Nothing

        (ii) Tx started prior to CT in 1/3 of cases, PTT not followed

        (iii) Results- Data analyzed with 2 heparin groups combined

        (iv) Heparin group- no sig difference in 14 d mortality or 6 mo outcome

        (v) At 14 d, recurrent ischemic strokes significantly reduced (3.8% to 2.9%) but hemorr stroke significantly increased (0.4% to 1.2%) yielding no net benefit

        (vi) the higher dose (12,500U BID) assoc. with more bleeding, risk of death at 14 d

        (vii) ASA- no effect on death at 14 days, but improvement at 6 mo

        (viii) significantly fewer recurrent ischemic strokes (2.8% vs 3/9%)

        (ix) no excess of hemorrhagic stroke (0.9% vs 0.8%)

        (x) trend toward a reduction in death/dependence at 6 mos (61.2% vs 63.5%)

        (xi) pts who received both low-dose heparin and ASA had the lowest rate of stroke recurrence, or PE, and no significant increase in bleeding risk

        (xii) Interpretation- ASA and low-dose Heparin are good

    d) IST & CAST trials demonstrate ASA in tx of acute ischemic stroke is safe and produces a small but definite net benefit

        (i) For every 1000 acute strokes tx w/ASA

            1) ~ 9 deaths or stroke recurrence will be prevented in the 1st 4 wks

            2) ~ 13 fewer pts will be dead or dependent at 6 mo

      (ii)   Interpretation- Give ASA early

      (iii) Aspirin remains the only oral antiplatelet agent that has been evaluated for the treatment of acute ischemic stroke, and data on clopidogrel or combination aspirin and dipyridamole for treatment of acute ischemic stroke are not available.

2) Ticlopidine
   a)   Ticlopidine Aspirin Stroke Study Group (TASS) [3]
      (i)   3,069 pts enrolled w/in 3 mos of minor stroke or TIA
      (ii)   Ticlid 250 BID vs ASA 650 BID
      (iii) 21% Relative risk reduction for stroke w/ticlid at 3 yr
      (iv) 9% RRR in end pt (stroke/MI/Vasc death) at 3 yr
      (v)   0.9% w/severe neutropenia w/in 3 mo of tx
      (vi) Interpretation: Ticlid was more effect than ASA in preventing strokes, but risk of side effects greater

3) Clopdiogrel (Plavix)
   a)   CAPRIE [4]
      (i)   Randomized, blinded, multicenter trial
      (ii)   19,185 pts enrolled, Clopidogrel vs ASA
      (iii) Composite outcome of stroke/MI/vascular death
      (iv) Results: Clopidigrel had 5.32% annual risk of composite outcome vs 5.83% w/ASA
      (v)   RRR of 8.7% in favor of clopidogrel (p= 0.04)
      (vi) Clopidogrel is better than ASA for combined vascular endpoint with similar side effect (significance was driven by reduction in PAD patients)

4) Dipyridamole (Aggrenox)
   a)   ESPS-1 [5]
      (i)   1306 patients with TIA, RIND or stroke in one single center of Kuopio in Finland
          a)   aspirin 990 mg + dipyridamole 225 mg/day
          b)   Placebo
      (ii)   for 2 years or until an endpoint
      (iii) endpoints were stroke or death from any cause
      (iv) the combination of aspirin/dipyridamole superior to placebo in the prevention of stroke and transient ischemic attack (TIA)
   b)   ESPS-2 [6]
      (i)   Multicenter, randomized, blinded, placebo-controlled study

      (ii) Cerebrovascular trial (only pts w/stroke or TIA enrolled)

      (iii) 6,602 pts w/prior stroke/TIA, followed 2 years

      (iv) 4 tx groups:

         1) ASA 25 BID

         2) ER Dipyridamole 200 BID

         3) both

         4) none

      (v) Results: Stroke risk compared to placebo was reduced by

         1) 16% with ER DP alone

         2) 18% with ASA only

         3) 37% with both ASA + ER DP

c) ESPIRIT [7]

      (i) randomized controlled trial, open (but auditing was blinded)

         1) aspirin (30–325 mg QD) + (n=1363) dipyridamole (200 mg BID)

         2) aspirin (30–325 mg QD) (n=1376)

      (ii) within 6 months of a TIA or minor stroke

      (iii) primary outcome event was the composite of death from all vascular causes, stroke, myocardial infarction, or major bleeding complication, whichever happened first

      (iv) Mean follow-up was 3·5 years

      (v) Primary outcome events in 173 (13%) patients on aspirin + dipyridamole and in 216 (16%) on aspirin alone (absolute risk reduction 1% per year)

5) Dual anti-platelet medication MATCH [8]

a) Randomized, double-blinded, placebo-controlled trial

      (vi) Plavix 75mg

      (vii) ASA 75mg + Plavix

b) Followed 18 mos

c) Primary endpoint was composite stroke/MI/vascular death

d) Absolute risk reduction 1% (16.7 to 15.7%, a Non-significant difference

e) higher life threatening bleeding

f) Interpretation- No benefit to adding ASA to Plavix, more bleeding.

g) Dual anti-platelet medication use (aspirin plus clopidogrel) has been shown to have no benefit in secondary stroke prevention, and therefore is generally not recommended for ICAS. [9]

6) For secondary stroke prevention, aspirin, aggernox, or clopidogrel monothreapy are all acceptable options for initial anti-platelet medications.[10,11]

Anti-Coagulants

1) Heparinoids
   a) TOAST study (Trial of Org 10172 in Acute stroke treatment) [12]
      (i) a randomized blinded placebo controlled trial of IV infusion of a low molecular weight heparinoid (danaparoid, ORG 101732) versus placebo
      (ii) No benefit of heparinoid overall
          1) may be beneficial for large artery atherosclerosis (LAA) subtype(based upon subgroup analysis which revealed a benefit in favorable outcome at 3 months for patient with LAA)
2) Coumadin
   a) Warfarin-Aspirin Recurrent Stroke Study (WARS)[13]
      (i) multicenter, double-blind, randomized trial
          1) 2206 pt, ischemic stroke w/in past 30 d (warfarin (INR 1.4-2.8) vs
          2) ASA (325 QD)
          3) combined primary end point of recurrent ischemic stroke or death from any cause w/in 2 yr
          4) 17.8 % warfarin
          5) 16% ASA (P=0.25)
          6) rates of major hemorrhage were low
          7) 2.22 per 100 patient-yrs in warfarin group
          8) 1.49 per 100 patient-yrs in ASA group
          9) Over 2-yr period, no difference btw ASA and warfarin in prevention of recurrent ischemic stroke or death or in rate of major hemorrhage
          10) Warfarin offered no additional benefit over aspirin in preventing recurrent ischemic stroke

b) WASID (see Chapter 3). Aspirin should be used in preference to warfarin for patients with intracranial arterial stenosis

c) Atrial fibrillation (see Chapter 5)

Surgery- Carotid Stenosis- CEA (See Chapter 3)

Vascular Risk Factor Modification

Management of vascular risk factors should be done in all ischemic stroke patients for secondary prevention, per AHA guidelines. (Table 1)

Table 1. AHA/ASA Recommendations for secondary stroke prevention [10,14]

Risk factor	Recommendation	Level of Evidence
Modifiable Behavior Risk Factors		
Smoking	All ischemic stroke or TIA patients who have smoked in the past year should be strongly encouraged not to smoke. Avoid environmental smoke. Counseling, nicotine products, and oral smoking cessation medications have been found to be effective for smokers.	Class I, Level C Class IIa, Level C Class IIa, Level B
Icohol	Patients with prior ischemic stroke or TIA who are heavy drinkers should eliminate or reduce their consumption of alcohol. Light to moderate levels of ≤ 2 drinks per day for men and 1 drink per day for nonpregnant women may be considered.	Class I, Level A Class IIb, Level C
Obesity	Weight reduction may be considered for all overweight ischemic stroke or TIA patients to maintain the goal of a BMI of 18.5 to 24.9 kg/m2 and a waist circumference of <35 in for women and <40 in for men. Clinicians should encourage weight management through an appropriate balance of caloric intake, physical activity, and behavioral counseling.	Class IIb, Level C

Physical activity	For those with ischemic stroke or TIA who are capable of engaging in physical activity, at least 30 minutes of moderate-intensity physical exercise most days may be considered to reduce risk factors and comorbid conditions that increase the likelihood of recurrence of stroke. For those with disability after ischemic stroke, a supervised therapeutic exercise regimen is recommended.	Class IIb, Level C
Treatable Vascular Risk Factors		
Hypertension	Antihypertensive treatment is recommended for prevention of recurrent stroke and other vascular events in persons who have had an ischemic stroke and are beyond the hyperacute period. Because this benefit extends to persons with and without a history of hypertension, this recommendation should be considered for all ischemic stroke and TIA patients.	Class I, Level A Class IIa, Level B Class IIa, Level B
Risk factor	Recommendation	Level of Evidence
	An absolute target BP Level And reduction are uncertain and should be individualized, but benefit has been associated with an average reduction of ~10/5 mm Hg and normal BP levels have been defined as <120/80 by JNC-7. Several lifestyle modifications have been associated with BP reductions and should be included as part of a comprehensive approach antihypertensive therapy. Optimal drug regimen remains uncertain; however, available data support the use of diuretics and the combination of diuretics and an ACEI. Choice of specific drugs and targets should be individualized on the basis of reviewed data and consideration, as well as specific patient characteristics (eg, extracranial cerebrovascular occlusive disease, renal impairment, cardiac disease, and DM).	Class IIb, Level C Class I, Level A

Table 1. (Continued)

Diabetes	More rigorous control of blood pressure and lipids should be considered in patients with diabetes. Although all major classes of antihypertensives are suitable for the control of BP, most patients will require >1 agent. ACEIs and ARBs are more effective in reducing the progression of renal disease and are recommended as first-choice medications for patients with DM.	Class IIa, Level B Class I, Level A
	Glucose control is recommended to near-normoglycemic levels among diabetics with ischemic stroke or TIA to reduce microvascular complications.	Class I, Level A
	The goal for Hb A1c should be $\leq 7\%$.	Class IIa, Level B
Cholesterol	Ischemic stroke or TIA patients with elevated cholesterol, comorbid coronary artery disease, or evidence of an atherosclerotic origin should be managed according to NCEP III guidelines, which include lifestyle modification, dietary guidelines, and medication recommendations.	Class I, Level A
	Statin agents are recommended, and the target goal for cholesterol lowering for those with CHD or symptomatic atherosclerotic disease is an LDL-C level of < 100 mg/dL.	Class I, Level A
Risk factor	Recommendation	Level of Evidence
Recommendations for anti-platelet therapy		
	An LDL-C < 70 mg/dL is recommended for very high-risk persons with multiple risk factors.	
	On the basis of the SPARCL trial, administration of statin therapy with intensive lipid- lowering effects is recommended for patients with atherosclerotic ischemic stroke or TIA and without known CHD to reduce the risk of stroke and cardiovascular events.	Class I, Level B
	Ischemic stroke or TIA patients with low HDL cholesterol may be considered for treatment with niacin or gemfibrozil.	Class IIb, Level B
	For patients with noncardioembolic ischemic stroke or TIA, antiplatelet agents rather than oral anticoagulation are recommended to reduce the risk of recurrent stroke and other cardiovascular events.	Class I, Level A
	Aspirin (50 to 325 mg/d) monotherapy, the combination of aspirin and extended-release	Class I, Level A

	dipyridamole, and clopidogrel monotherapy are all acceptable options for initial therapy.	
	The combination of aspirin and extended-release dipyridamole is recommended over aspirin alone.	Class I, Level B
	Clopidogrel may be considered over aspirin alone on the basis of direct-comparison trials.	Class IIb, Level B
	For patients allergic to aspirin, clopidogrel is reasonable.	Class IIa, Level B
	The addition of aspirin to clopidogrel increases the risk of hemorrhage. Combination therapy of aspirin and clopidogrel is not routinely recommended for ischemic stroke or TIA patients unless they have a specific indication for this therapy.	

1) Modifiable predictors
   a) Hypertension
   b) Diabetes
   c) Hyperlipidemia
   d) Smoking
   e) Alcohol
   f) Obesity/physical inactivity

References

[1] CAST (Chinese Acute Stroke Trial) Collaborative Group. *CAST: randomized placebo-controlled trial of early aspirin use in 20,000 patients with acute ischaemic stroke.* Lancet. 1997;349:1641–1649.

[2] International Stroke Trial Collaborative Group. *The International Stroke Trial (IST): a randomised trial of aspirin, subcutaneous heparin, both, or neither among 19435 patients with acute ischaemic stroke.* Lancet. 1997;349:1569-1581.

[3] Hass W, Easton J, Adams H, et al., *Randomized trial comparing ticlopidine hydrochloride with aspirin for the prevention of stroke in high-risk patients. Ticlopidine Aspirin Stroke Study Group.* The New England Journal of Medicine. 1989;321:501–507.

[4] CAPRIE Steering Committee. *A randomized, blinded, trial of clopidogrel versus aspirin in patients at risk of ischaemic events.* Lancet 1996; 348:1329–1339.

[5] ESPS Group. *European Stroke Prevention Study.* Stroke. 1990;21:1122-30.

[6]   Diener HC, Cunha L, Forbes C, Sivenius J, Smets P, Lowenthal A. *European Stroke Prevention Study 2: dipyridamole and acetylsalicylic acid in the secondary prevention of stroke.* J Neurol Sci 1996; 143:1–13.

[7]   ESPRIT Study Group. *Aspirin plus dipyridamole versus aspirin alone after cerebral ischaemia of arterial origin (ESPRIT): randomised controlled trial.* Lancet 2006; 367:1665–1673.

[8]   MATCH investigators. *Aspirin and clopidogrel compared with clopidogrel alone after recent ischaemic stroke or transient ischaemic attack in high-risk patients (MATCH): randomised, double-blind, placebo-controlled trial.* Lancet 2004; 364: 331–37.

[9]   Diener HC, Bogousslavsky J, Brass LM, Cimminiello C, Csiba L, Kaste M, Leys D, Matias-Guiu J, Rupprecht HJ, on behalf of the MATCH investigators. *Aspirin and clopidogrel compared with clopidogrel alone after recent ischaemic stroke or transient ischaemic attack in high-risk patients (MATCH): randomised, double-blind, placebo-controlled trial.* Lancet 2004; 364: 331–37.

[10]   Sacco RL, Adams R, Albers G, Alberts MJ, Benavente O, Furie K, Goldstein LB, Gorelick P, Halperin J, Harbaugh R, Johnston SC, Katzan I, Kelly-Hayes M, Kenton EJ, Marks M, Schwamm LH, Tomsick T; *American Heart Association; American Stroke Association Council on Stroke; Council on Cardiovascular Radiology and Intervention; American Academy of Neurology. Guidelines for prevention of stroke in patients with ischemic stroke or transient ischemic attack: a statement for healthcare professionals from the American Heart Association/American Stroke Association Council on Stroke: co-sponsored by the Council on Cardiovascular Radiology and Intervention: the American Academy of Neurology affirms the value of this guideline.* Stroke. 2006;37:577-617.

[11]   Adams RJ, Albers G, Alberts MJ, Benavente O, Furie K, Goldstein LB, Gorelick P, Halperin J, Harbaugh R, Johnston SC, Katzan I, Kelly-Hayes M,. Kenton EJ, Marks M, Sacco RL and Schwamm LH. *Update to the AHA/ASA Recommendations for the Prevention of Stroke in Patients with Stroke and Transient Ischemic Attack.* Stroke. 2008;39;1647-1652.

[12]   *The Publications Committee for the Trial of ORG 10172 in Acute Stroke Treatment (TOAST) Investigators. Low molecular weight heparinoid, ORG 10172 (danaparoid), and outcome after acute ischemic stroke: a randomized controlled trial. JAMA.* 1998;279:1265-1272.

[13] Warfarin-Aspirin Recurrent Stroke Study Group. *A Comparison of Warfarin and Aspirin for the Prevention of Recurrent Ischemic Stroke..* N Engl J Med 2001;345:1444-51.).

[14] Adams RJ, Albers G, Alberts MJ, Benavente O, Furie K, Goldstein LB, Gorelick P, Halperin J, Harbaugh R, Johnston SC, Katzan I, Kelly-Hayes M,. Kenton EJ, Marks M, Sacco RL and Schwamm LH. *Update to the AHA/ASA Recommendations for the Prevention of Stroke in Patients With Stroke and Transient Ischemic Attack.* Stroke. 2008;39;1647-1652.

In: Handbook of Stroke and Neurocritical Care   ISBN: 978-61324-786-0
Editor: V. H. Lee   © 2012 Nova Science Publishers, Inc.

Chapter XII

Intracerebral Hemorrhage

Sayona John and Rajeev Garg
Department of Neurological Sciences,
Section of Stroke and Neurocritical care,
Rush University Medical Center, Chicago, IL, USA

Incidence

1) Intracerebral hemorrhage (ICH) is the second most common cause of stroke
2) accounts for between 8-15% of all strokes in high-income countries [1, 2]
3) estimated incidence of 10-25 per 100,000 populations. [3, 4]
4) ICH is more common in men than in women, particularly in those older than 55 years of age.

Etiology

1) Hypertension (primary): Hypertension is the most important risk factor for spontaneous ICH.
   a) Risk is increased in patients who are non compliant with antihypertensive medications, are 55 years of age or older, or are smokers.

    b)   Common locations for hypertensive ICH are the basal ganglia, thalamus, pons, cerebellum, and cerebral lobes (Figure 1).

    c)   Hemorrhage results from the rupture of small penetrating arteries that have been damaged by degenerative changes in the vessel wall from chronic hypertension.

2)   Cerebral Amyloid Angiopathy (CAA):

    a)   CAA is characterized by the deposition of β amyloid protein in the blood vessels of the cerebral cortex and leptomeninges. This deposition is a risk factor for ICH in persons >60 years of age.

    b)   The presence of ε2 and ε4 alleles of the apolipoprotein E gene is associated with a tripling of the risk of recurrent hemorrhages among survivors of lobar ICH related to amyloid angiopathy.

3)   Warfarin Relate Hemorrhage:

    a)   The risk of ICH in patients on long term anticoagulation is 8 to 11 times that of patients of similar age who are not on anticoagulation.

    b)   Advanced age (>70), hypertension, and concomitant use of aspirin doubles the rate of ICH. Most ICH occurs in the first year of anticoagulation use. Intensity of anticoagulation and leukoariosis increase the risk of warfarin associated ICH.

    c)   Hematoma size in this type of hemorrhage is associated with a high mortality (46% to 68%).

    d)   Hemorrhages show a characteristic blood-fluid level on non-contrast CT.

4)   Direct-Thrombin Inhibitors Related Hemorrhage:

    a)   With the recent FDA approval of the oral direct thrombin inhibitor Dabigatran for the secondary prevention of ischemic strokes in the setting of atrial fibrillation, patients taking this medication will represent a new sub-group of patients with intracerebral hemorrhage.

5)   Fibrinolytic Therapy:

    a)   Tissue-type plasminogen activator (t-PA) used in acute MI, pulmonary embolus, and ischemic strokes is associated with increased risk of intracerebral hemorrhage in the range of 1 to 6%. Hemorrhages occur in the lobar and deep location and are associated with a high mortality (45%).

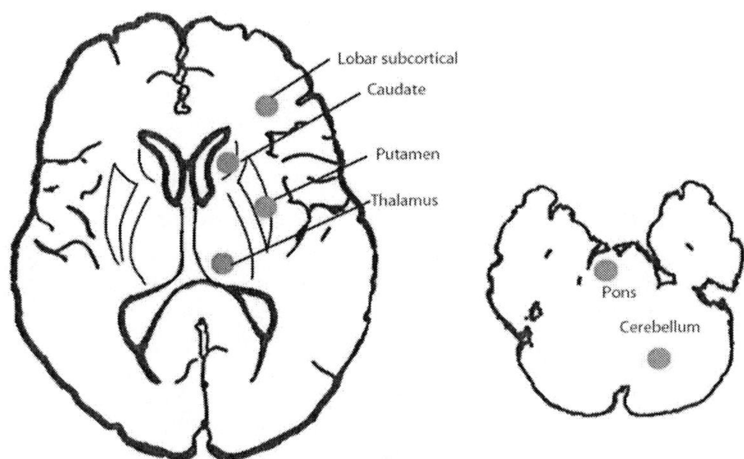

Figure 1. Hypertensive hemorrhage typical locations.

6) Coagulopathy: Impaired clotting function related to uremia, liver dysfunction, hemophilia, platelet dysfunction, or other abnormalities of coagulation, can lead to spontaneous ICH.

7) Excessive use of alcohol use: Excessive ethanol use increases the risk of ICH by impairing coagulation and directly affecting the integrity of blood vessels.

8) Vascular Malformations:

   a) Arteriovenous Malformations (AVM), Angiomas, and Cavernous Malformations have been implicated in cases of ICH. These lesions need to be considered in lobar hemorrhages occurring in persons who are younger with no history of hypertension. MRI is useful in the detection of these lesions.

   b) Cavernous angiomas are best seen on T2 weighted sequences as irregular lesions with a central core of mixed signal.

   c) AVMs are seen on MRI as dilated arteries with flow voids due to the fast flow. After a hemorrhage, the diagnosis of AVMs is best made with a CT angiogram or a conventional cerebral angiogram.

9) Sympathomimetic Drugs: Intravenous methamphetamine, pseudoephedrine, phenylpropanolamine, and cocaine have all been associated with intracerebral hemorrhage. The ICH is commonly lobar in location and is thought to be related to transient hypertension associated multifocal arterial changes due to vasospasm, or less commonly vasculitis.

10) Vasculitis: Granulomatous angitis is a rare cause for ICH. It is a primary cerebral vasculitis occurring in the absence of systemic involvement. Diagnosis is favored by the finding of lymphocytic pleocytosis in the CSF associated with elevated protein, and angiographic evidence of beading in medium and small sized intracranial arteries. Occasionally, a meningeal biopsy is needed to confirm the diagnosis.

11) Venous Sinus Thrombosis:
    a) Cerebral sinus thrombosis is a rare cause for ICH (incidence of 2-4 per million per year) affecting predominantly women in their middle ages.
    b) Risk factors include primary hypercoagulable states, local or systemic inflammatory disorders, and local infections (e.g. mastoiditis, otitis, or sinusitis).
    c) Magnetic resonance imaging, CT venography, and conventional angiography are all potential diagnostic imaging modalities to evaluate for this disease.

12) Primary Intracranial Tumors:
    a) Brain tumors are an uncommon cause of ICH. Majority of tumors are malignant, either primary or metastatic.
    b) Glioblastoma Multiforme (GBM) is the leading primary brain tumor causing ICH with hemorrhage location deep in the hemispheres, basal ganglia or corpus callosum.
    c) MRI with contrast can help differentiate tumors as the cause of hemorrhage.

13) Metastatic Tumors:
    a) Metastatic lesions to the brain from certain primary tumors have a tendency to bleed.
    b) These include melanoma, renal cell carcinoma, thyroid, and choriocarcinoma.
    c) Occasionally, non-small cell lung cancer of the brain will also have intratumoral hemorrhage.

Clinical Features

1) Abrupt onset of focal neurological symptoms with associated findings of headache, coma or decreased level of consciousness, systolic BP >220, and progression over minutes or hours all suggest ICH though none of these findings are specific.

   a) Patients with a large hematoma usually have a decreased level of consciousness as a result of increased intracranial pressure and the direct compression of the thalamic or brain-stem reticular activating system.

2) Supratentorial ICH involving the basal ganglia and thalamus result in a contralateral sensory-motor deficit of varying severity owing to the involvement of the internal capsule. Abnormalities indicating higher-level cortical dysfunction, including aphasia, neglect, gaze deviation, and hemianopia, may occur as a result of the disruption of connecting fibers in the subcortical white matter and functional suppression of overlying cortex.

3) In patients with an infratentorial ICH, signs of brainstem dysfunction include abnormalities of gaze, cranial-nerve palsies, and contralateral motor deficits. Ataxia, nystagmus, and dysmetria are prominent when the intracerebral hemorrhage involves the cerebellum.

4) Early deterioration is common in the first few hours after ICH onset

   a) 20% of patients experiencing a decrease in the Glasgow Coma Scale (GCS) score of ≥2 points between onset of symptoms and initial evaluation in the Emergency Room.

   b) An additional 15% of patients demonstrate a further ≥2 point decline in GCS within the first hour or presentation to a hospital. The high rate of neurological deterioration after ICH is in part related to active bleeding that may persist for hours after symptom onset.

   c) Worsening cerebral edema is also implicated in neurologic deterioration that occurs within 24 to 48 hours after the onset of hemorrhage.[5, 6]

Diagnosis

1) CT is very sensitive for identifying an acute hemorrhage and is considered the gold standard. Gradient echo and T2 susceptibility weighted MRI are as sensitive as CT for detection of acute blood and are more sensitive for identification of prior hemorrhage.[7, 8]

2) CT angiography (CTA) and contrast enhanced CT may identify patients at high risk of hematoma expansion based on the presence of contrast extravasation within the hematoma. The presence of contrast extravasation has been coined the "spot sign".[9, 10]

3) Abnormalities on angiography are seen in 49 percent of patients with lobar hemorrhage and 65 percent of patients with isolated intraventricular hemorrhage.

4) Patients who are 45 years of age or younger and have no history of hypertension should undergo conventional angiography as 48% of these patients have abnormalities on angiography.

Management

1) Initial management of patients with acute intracerebral hemorrhages should focus on the ABCs of emergency neurology. The following questions should be asked of every patient that is being evaluated:

2) Airway: Is the patient protecting and maintaining a patent airway?

3) Breathing: Is the patient oxygenating and ventilating appropriately?

4) Circulation: Is the patient hemodynamically stable?

5) Although these factors are likely to be managed by your emergency medicine or intensivist colleagues, patients with ICH can have rapidly progressive and/or fluctuating exams, which require frequent re-evaluations.

6) The main goal of treatment during the first 24 hours after an intracerebral hemorrhage is to limit hematoma expansion. Associated is the prevention of further neurologic injury that can occur with ICH, including seizures, elevated intracranial pressure, and herniation. Much of the data available on the treatment of acute ICH is based upon studies in hypertensive and warfarin related ICH. Thus, current treatments are largely focused on blood pressure control and reversal of coagulopathies, both of which are factors in hematoma expansion. In addition to management of the neurologic

injury, concurrent systemic problems such as neurogenic fever, respiratory failure, myocardial infarction, acute renal failure, deep venous thrombosis, and hyperglycemia need to evaluated and managed.

7) Blood pressure is often elevated during an acute intracerebral hemorrhage.

    a) This may be a systemic response to maintain cerebral perfusion pressure in the setting of rapidly increasing intracranial pressure. Conversely, the elevated blood pressure may be causal to the ICH.

    b) Blood pressure management during acute ICH has been a controversial subject and an area of active research.

    c) According to the 2010 American Stroke Association Guidelines[11], goal blood pressure should be based on tiered assessment of the patient's intracranial pressure.

        (i) Therefore, goal SBP/MAP in patients with elevated intracranial pressure (typically defined as an ICP > 20 cm H2O) should be reduced to maintain a cerebral perfusion pressure of at least 60 mm Hg.

        (ii) In patients with normal intracranial pressure, the SBP/MAP should be reduced modestly (absolute numbers not provided by the ASA) while following the patient's exam.

8) The INTERACT[12] and the ATACH [13] studies collectively showed that aggressive blood pressure reduction (irrespective of intracranial pressure status) was safe and effective in controlling hematoma expansion.

    a) INTERACT

        (i) patients were randomized to either blood pressure control of SBP < 140 or SBP < 180.

        (ii) The study showed a trend towards lower hematoma growth in the intensive blood pressure group. Although the study was not powered to assess this, no differences in outcomes were measured between the two groups.

    b) ATACH

        (i) a Phase I feasibility trial, blood pressure reduction to SBP of 110 to 140 mg Hg

           (ii) ATACH was considered safe and provided the basis for the larger ATACH II trial, which will evaluate the impact of blood pressure reduction on outcomes.

    c) In a recent study, however, MAP lowering > 40% was associated with the presence of diffusion weight imaging lesions on MRI in patients with ICH. [14]

9) Antithrombotic therapy may also be a factor in hematoma expansion.

    a) With regards to antiplatelet therapy, it remains unclear whether prior antiplatelet use leads to larger hematomas. It further remains unclear whether frozen platelets or desmopressin should be administered to patients who have taken antiplatelet therapy.

    b) The general recommendation for warfarin related hemorrhages is the prompt reversal of the coagulopathy.

           (i) Treatments include fresh frozen plasma, prothrombin complex concentrate, and recombinant Factor VIIa.

           (ii) Adjunctive therapy with vitamin K (preferably intravenous) can also help with reversal. Prothrombin complex concentrate is increasingly becoming the preferred reversal agent due to its rapidity of administration, and possibly quicker reversal of INR when compared to FFP.[12]

           (iii) Recombinant factor VIIa (Novo-seven) was successful in a phase II trial in limiting hematoma expansion, however, this did not affect clinical outcomes.[15]

    c) With dabigatran, no specific antidotes exist for its reversal. The short duration of action of the drug upon discontinuation may eliminate its anticoagulation effects. Current, data on hematoma expansion in dabigatran related ICH is limited.

10) Surgical evacuation of supratentorial spontaneous intracerebral hemorrhage was

    a) STICH trial [16] - results of the trial showed no difference in outcomes between those patients who underwent early surgery versus those treated by medical management alone, especially if the patient's bleed was > 1 cm from the cortex or the GCS < 8.

    b) Cerebellar Infarction and Hemorrhage

1) The surgical management of cerebellar infarction lacks prospective controlled trials to guide management and thus remains based upon expert opinion and local practice.
2) Most physicians would advocate posterior fossa decompression in a patient with multiple terriotory infarction with effacement of the fourth ventricle and/or obstructive hydrocephalus
3) placing an extraventicular drain carries the risk for upward herniation of the posterior fossa contents.
4) surgical management of primary cerebellar hemorrhage also lacks prospective controlled trials but there is a greater consensus amongst surgeons that a hemorrhage of 3cm or larger in maximal diameter who are deteriorating neurologically or who have brainstem compression and/or hydrocephalus from ventricular obstruction

11) With regard to hemorrhages with mass effect, although no randomized controlled trials have been done, it is generally accepted that these patient have emergent evacuation to relieve the elevated intracranial pressure.[12]

12) CH related to venous sinus thrombosis.
   a) Although there is risk for hematoma expansion, several studies have suggested that patients treated either with unfractionated heparin or low-molecular weighted heparin to prevent clot progression have improved outcomes. [17]
   b) Failure of clot resolution or further intracerebral hemorrhage may be an indication for endovascular therapy.[18]

13) Besides management of the hemorrhage, several other neurologic and systemic complications can occur with this neurologic injury.
   a) Seizures have been reported in 2.7 to 17% of patients with acute ICH, with most occurring at ictus. Data on whether prophylactic anti-convulsant therapy reduces this incidence is unclear. There is data to suggest that the use of prophylactic anti-convulsant therapy, specifically phenytoin, may lead to worse neurologic outcomes.[19]
   b) Fever is a common complication in patients with ICH, especially with basal ganglionic bleeds or extensive intraventricular hemorrhage. Although fever has been

associated with worse outcomes in patients, whether induced normothermia can alter this course is unclear. [12]

14) Timing of safe re-introduction of antiplatelet or anticoagulant therapy during and after ICH remains unknown.

Outcomes

1) Only 20% of patients with ICH are expected to be functional at 6 months [20]

2) between 25-48% of patients are dead between 21 days and 1 month.[21]

3) Within the United States, long-term mortality has been estimated at > 50% at 1 year.[22]

4) Despite advances in the field of stroke and neurocritical care, the 30-day mortality has not changed significantly over the past 20 years.[4]

5) Morbidity and mortality in this type of brain injury is strongly predicted by the ICH score, which is a weighted composite of various clinical factor, including Glascow Coma Scale, age, location of hemorrhage, ICH volume, and presence of intraventricular blood. [23, 24] Broderick et al._found that the mortality rate at one month was best predicted by determining the initial score on the Glasgow Coma Scale and the initial volume of the hematoma.[25]

6) ICH volume growth has been described to occur up to 20 hours after ICH ictus with hematoma expansion and final volume each being associated with poor outcomes [5]

7) Most patients with intracerebral hemorrhage who die do so during the initial acute hospitalization. This is mostly due to withdrawal of life support due to physician biases regarding patient prognosis. These same biases are in place during the development of the aforementioned prognostic indicators, and therefore may lead to a self-fulfilling prophecy in predicting outcomes [26, 27]

Research

1) Many questions still remain regarding the diagnosis, management, and outcomes in patients with ICH. Safety and efficacy of blood pressure reduction in reducing hematoma growth is being evaluated in the large multi-center ATACH II trial.

2) Minimally invasive surgical evacuation of blood products in the cerebral cortex and ventricles is being examined in MISTIE and CLEAR IVH, respectively. If blood break down products induce inflammation in the brain, early removal via endoscopic or catheter based approaches may prevent the associated reactive cerebral edema.

3) Early identification of various types of vasculopathy and structural vascular malformations are being evaluated to develop treatments and prevent hemorrhages. Better models to predict outcomes in these patients to help them and their families make decisions are being developed.

References

[1] Feigin VL, L.C., Bennett DA, Barker-Collo SL, and Parag V, *Worldwide stroke incidence and early case fatality reported in 56 population-based studies: a systematic review.* Lancet Neurology, 2009. 8: p. 355-69.

[2] Broderick JP, B.T., Tomsick T, Miller R, Huster G., *Intracerebral hemorrhage more than twice as common as subarachnoid hemorrhage.* Journal of Neurosugery, 1993. 78: p. 188-19.

[3] Qureshi AI, Mendelow AD, Hanley DF. *Intracerebral haemorrhage.* Lancet. 2009; 373:1632-1644.

[4] van Asch CJ, Luitse MJ, Rinkel GJ, van der Tweel I, Algra A, Klijn CJ. *Incidence, case fatality, and functional outcome of intracerebral haemorrhage over time, according to age, sex, and ethnic origin: A systematic review and meta-analysis.* Lancet Neurol. 2010;9:167-176.

[5] Brott T, Broderick J, Kothari R, Barsan W, Tomsick T, Sauerbeck L, Spilker J, Duldner J, Khoury J. *Early hemorrhage growth in patients with intracerebral hemorrhage.* Stroke. 1997;28(1):1-5.

[6]   Davis SM, Broderick J, Hennerici M, Brun NC, Diringer MN, Mayer SA, Begtrup K, Steiner T; *Recombinant Activated Factor VII Intracerebral Hemorrhage Trial Investigators. Hematoma growth is a determinant of mortality and poor outcome after intracerebral hemorrhage.* Neurology. 2006;66:1175–1181.

[7]   Goldstein LB, Simel DL. *Is this patient having a stroke?.* JAMA. 2005 May 18;19:2391-402.

[8]   Chalela JA, Kidwell CS, Nentwich LM, Luby M, Butman JA, Demchuk AM, Hill MD, Patronas N, Latour L, Warach S. *Magnetic resonance imaging and computed tomography in emergency assessment of patients with suspected acute stroke: a prospective comparison.* Lancet. 2007; 369:293–298.

[9]   Goldstein JN, Fazen LE, Snider R, Schwab K, Greenberg SM, Smith EE, Lev MH, Rosand J. *Contrast extravasation on CT angiography predicts hematoma expansion in intracerebral hemorrhage.* Neurology. 2007;68:889–894.

[10]   Kim J, Smith A, Hemphill JC 3rd, Smith WS, Lu Y, Dillon WP, Wintermark M. *Contrast extravasation on CT predicts mortality in primary intracerebral hemorrhage.* AJNR Am J Neuroradiol. 2008;29:520–525.

[11]   Morgenstern LB, Hemphill III JC, Anderson C, Becker K, Broderick JP, Connolly Jr. ES, Greenberg SM, Huang JN, MacDonald RL, Messe SR, Mitchell PH, Selim M, Tamargo RJ.*Stroke* 2010;41:2108-2129.

[12]   Anderson, C., et al., *Intensive blood pressure reduction in acute cerebral haemorrhage trial (INTERACT): a randomised pilot trial.* Lancet Neurol, 2008. 7(5): p. 391-399.

[13]   ATACH Investigators, Qureshi A., *Antihypertensive treatment of acute cerebral hemorrhage.* Critical Care Medicine, 2010;38(2): p. 637-48.

[14]   Prabhakaran S, G.R., Ouyang B, John S, Temes RE, Mohammad Y, Lee VH, Bleck TP, *Acute brain infarcts after spontaneous intracerebral hemorrhage: a diffusion-weighted imaging study.* Stroke, 2010. 41: p. 89-94.

[15]   Mayer SA, Brun NC, Begtrup K, Broderick J, Davis S, Diringer MN, Skolnick BE, Steiner T, FAST *Investigators.* New England Journal of Medicine,2008;358(20):2174-6.

[16] Mendelow AD, Gregson BA, Fernandes HM, Murray GD, Teasdale GM, Hope DT, Karimi A, Shaw MD, Barer DH. *Early surgery versus initial conservative treatment in patients with spontaneous supratentorial intracerebral haematomas in the international surgical trial in intracerebral haemorrhage (STICH): A randomised trial.* Lancet. 2005;365:387-397.

[17] Einhaupl K, Stam J, Boursser MG, De Brujin SFTM, Ferro JM, Martinelli I, Masuhr F. *EFNS guideline on the treatment of cerebral venous and sinus thrombosis in adult patients.* European Journal of Neurology. 2010 Oct;17(10):1229-1235.

[18] Medel R, Monteith SJ, Crowley W, Dumont AS. *A review of therapeutic strategies for the management of cerebral venous thrombosis.* Neurosurgery Focus. 2009;27(5):1-9.

[19] Naidech AM, Garg RK, Liebling S, Levasseur K, Macken MP, Schuele SU, Batjer HH. *Anticonvulsant use and outcomes after intracerebral hemorrhage.* Stroke. 2009 Dec; 40(12):39810-5.

[20] Counsell C, B.S., Dennis M, Sandercock P, Bamford J, Burn J, and Warlow C., *Primary intracerebral hemorrhage in the Oxfordshire Community Stroke Project, 2: prognosis.* Cerebrovascular Diseases, 1995. 5: p. 26-34.

[21] Feigin VL, L.C., Bennett DA, Barker-Collo SL, and Parag V, *Worldwide stroke incidence and early case fatality reported in 56 population-based studies: a systematic review.* Lancet Neurology, 2009. 8: p. 355-69.

[22] Flaherty ML, H.M., Sekar P, Kissela B, Kleindorfer D, Moomaw CJ, Sauerbeck L, Schneider A, Broderick JP, Woo D, *Long-term mortality after intracerebral hemorrhage.* Neurology, 2006. 66(8): p. 1182-6.

[23] Hemphill, J., et al., *The ICH Score: a simple, reliable grading scale for intracerebral hemorrhage.* Stroke, 2001. 32: p. 891-897.

[24] Hemphill III JC, F.M., and Neill Jr. TA, *Prospective validation of the ICH score for 12-month functional outcome.* Neurology, 2009. 73: p. 1088-1094.

[25] Broderick JP, Brott TG, Duldner JE, Tomsick T, Huster G. *Volume of intracerebral hemorrhage. A powerful and easy to use predictor of 30 day mortality.* Stroke. 1993;24(7):987-93.

[26] Naidech AM, Bernstein RA, Bassin SL, Garg RK, Liebling S, Bendock BR, Batjer HH, Bleck TP. *How patients die after intracerebral hemorrhage.* Neurocritical Care. 2009;11:45-49.

[27] Zurasky JA, Aiyagari V, Zazulia AR, Shackelford A, Diringer MN. *Early mortality following spontaneous intracerebral hemorrhage.* Neurology. 2005;64:725-727.

In: Handbook of Stroke and Neurocritical Care   ISBN: 978-61324-786-0
Editor: V. H. Lee   © 2012 Nova Science Publishers, Inc.

Chapter XIII

Subarachnoid Hemorrhage

Richard Temes
Department of Neurological Sciences,
Section of Stroke and Neurocritical care,
Rush University Medical Center,
Chicago, IL, USA

Epidemiology

Traumatic head injury is the most common cause of SAH. Among spontaneous SAH, the majority of cases are the result of cerebral aneurysms. Arteriovenous malformations and intracranial dissection contribute up to 15% of spontaneous SAH.

Angiographic negative subarachnoid hemorrhage comprises 10-15% of cases, with perimesencephalic hemorrhage being the more common presentation. The annual incidence of aneurysmal subarachnoid hemorrhage (aSAH) exceeds 30,000 persons and occurs with a median age of 59[1]. It is estimated that 20% of all hemorrhages occur between the ages of 15 to 45 years [2].

There appears to be a female preponderance with females having up to a four-fold increase in risk in some studies [3].

Risk Factors

Increasing age, female gender and black race have all been implicated as non-modifiable risk factors for aSAH. Similar to other forms of cerebrovascular disease, traditional modifiable risk factors include cigarette smoking, heavy alcohol consumption, oral contraceptives, and hyperlipidemia. Although rare, certain heritable connective tissue diseases such as Ehler's-Danlos Syndrome type IV and pseudoxanthoma elasticum have been associated with aSAH. Autosomal dominant polycystic disease is associated with the formation of intracranial aneurysms and subsequent rupture.

Table 1. Risk Factors for aSAH

Clinical History
Onset of headache: abrupt, maximal at onset
Severity of headache: "worst of life", severe
Qualitative characteristics: first headache of this intensity, unique/different
Associated signs and symptoms
Loss of consciousness
Diplopia
Seizure
Focal neurological signs

Epidemiologic factors
Cigarette smoking
Hypertension
Alcohol consumption
Personal or family history
Polycystic kidney disease
Heritable connective tissue diseases
Ehlers-Danlos syndrome (type IV)
Pseudoxanthoma elasticum
Fibromuscular dysplasia
Other
Sickle cell anemia
Alpha$_1$ antitrypsin deficiency

Physical findings
Retinal or subhyaloid hemorrhage
Nuchal rigidity
Focal or generalized neurological signs

Diagnosis of Asah

Clinical Features

The predominant feature of aSAH is the presence of a sudden, severe headache. Accompanying symptoms may include nausea, vomiting, photophobia, depressed level of consciousness, and focal neurological signs [4]. Nearly half of patients will have a history a sudden, severe headache that often terminates within hours and may occur several weeks prior to the hemorrhage onset, termed *sentinal headaches* [5]. The presence of such headaches, especially in individuals without a known history of headache are commonly missed by medical personnel and should be investigated fully for the presence of subarachnoid hemorrhage. Patients may exhibit signs of meningeal irritation or low back pain due to irritation of the lumbar roots from dependent blood. Ocular hemorrhage may be apparent on funduscopic examination due to compression of retinal veins from elevated intracranial pressure. Findings on neurological examination may provide clues to aneurysm location (Table 2).

Table 2. Physical findings and aneurysm location

Finding	Likely location of aneurysm
Nuchal rigidity	Any
Diminished level of consciousness	Any (can result from hydrocephalus, Hematoma or ischemia)
Papilledema	Any
Retinal/subhyaloid hemorrhage	Any
Third-nerve palsy	Posterior communicating artery
Sixth-nerve palsy	Posterior fossa
Bilateral leg weakness, abulia	Anterior communicating artery
Nystagmus or ataxia	Posterior fossa
Aphasia, hemiparesis, neglect	Middle cerebral artery

Imaging

The initial study of choice for aSAH is non-contrast computed tomography (CT scan) with 95 % sensitivity if done within 48 hours of hemorrhage. CT is an efficient and rapid tool for making the diagnosis but also is invaluable in determining other features such as the presence of hydrocephalus, intracerebral or subdural hemorrhage, and global cerebral edema that may require additional emergent medical or surgical treatment. CT may also provide clues on aneurysm location based upon the distribution of hemorrhage [Table 3].

Table 3. Hemorrhage patterns from intracranial aneurysms

Site	SAH (cistern)	ICH	IVH (ventricle)	SDH
ICA				
Oph Seg	Ant suprasellar	Med inf frontal	Rare	Rare
PCom	Lat suprasellar, ambient	Med temporal	temporal	inf lat convexity
AChor				
Bifurc	Lat suprasella, prox sylvian	Basal ganglia	Lat vent	Rare
ACA				
ACom	Interhemisppheric, septal, ant suprasellar	Inf frontal	Ant III	Rare
Pericallosal	Interhemispheric	Med frontal	Rare	Falcine
MCA				
Bifurc	Sylvian	Temporal	Temporal	Convexity
Prox	Lat suprasellar, prox sylvian	Temporal, basal ganglia	Temporal or frontal	Rare
Distal	Distal sylvian	Frontal or temporal	Rare	Convexity
V-B				
Bas apex	interpeduncular, Suprasellar	Rare	Post III, lateral	Rare
PICA	Cerebellopontine angle	Cerebellar hemisphere	IV	Rare

It is important to note that the diagnostic sensitivity of CT diminishes over time with only 50% sensitivity at one week. Severe anemia, small volume SAH, and sentinal hemorrhage may all cause a falsely negative CT. If the clinical suspicion remains high, further investigations are warranted in the face of a negative CT. CT angiography (CTA) is a technology that is becoming more prevalent in its use as a diagnostic tool for the presence of intracranial aneurysms. Sensitivity rates have been comparable to conventional angiography and are increasingly being used prior to surgery without conventional angiography [6]. Certain limitations do exist for CTA such as technical error and reduced sensitivity for detection of small intracranial aneurysms. Regardless of CTA results, it is generally recommended that all patients with a rupture cerebral aneurysm undergoes a conventional angiogram at some point as up to 15% of patients may have multiple aneurysms present.

Cerebrospinal Fluid Analysis

In instances of a high clinical suspicion and negative CT, a lumbar puncture should be performed for cerebrospinal fluid analysis. The classic yellow discoloration of xanthochromia following centrifugation may be present within hours following hemorrhage but may be absent if done early. The typical appearance of non-clotting bloody fluid that does not clear with sequential tubes is characteristic. It is important to send multiple tubes for cell count as the red blood cell count should not vary significantly between tubes. In cases of equivocal results, conventional four-vessel angiography should be performed.

Conventional Four-Vessel Angiography

Conventional angiography remains the gold standard in diagnosis and identifies the source of aSAH in up to 85% of cases. In the presence of a negative angiogram, other etiologies such as vascular malformations, dissection, or perimesencephalic nonaneurysmal hemorrhage should be considered. A repeat angiogram increases the diagnostic yield and should be performed in 7 days following hemorrhage as the occult aneurysm may be obliterated by thrombosis at the time of initial angiography.

Grading Scales

Numerous grading scales exist for subarachnoid hemorrhage. The two more widespread clinical grading scales in use include the Hunt and Hess grading scale (HHG) and the World federation of Neurological Surgeons Scale (WFNS). These 2 clinical grading scales both consist of 5 categories of increasing clinical severity and are utilized to predict mortality following aSAH. The radiographic scales in use include the Fisher grading scale and the modified Fisher scale (mFS). These radiographic scales are used to predict risk for the development of delayed cerebral ischemia. The mFS, which accounts for thick cisternal blood and intraventricular hemorrhage was found to be more predictive of delayed cerebral ischemia than the Fisher scale [7]. Patients with mFS of 1 have a 10% risk while those with a mFS of 4 have a 40 percent risk for its development.

Table 4. Hunt and Hess Grading Scale

Grade	Clinical Description
1	Minimal headache and slight nuchal rigidity
2	Moderate to severe headache, nuchal rigidity, and no neurological deficit other than cranial nerve palsy
3	Confusion, drowsiness, or mild focal deficit
4	Stupor, moderate to severe hemiparesis, and possibly, early decerebrate rigidity and vegetative disturbances
5	Deep coma, decerbrate rigidity, and moribund appearance

Table 5. Modified Fisher Scale

Grade	Radiographic Description
0	No blood
1	Diffuse thin blood without IVH
2	Diffuse thin blood with IVH
3	Diffuse thick blood without IVH
4	Diffuse thick blood with IVH

Table 6. World Federation of Neurological Surgeons Grading Scale

Grade	Clinical Description
1	GCS 15, no motor deficit
2	GCS 13-14, no motor deficit
3	GCS 13-14, with motor deficit
4	GCS 7-12, with or without motor deficit
5	GCS 3-6, with or without motor deficit

Management of Asah (Figures 1 and 2)

Control of Intracranial Pressure (ICP)

Obstructive hydrocephalus is a common complication following SAH. In cases of diminished level of consciousness, an external ventricular drain should be placed for adequate treatment and monitoring of intracranial pressure. It is important that over-drainage is avoided in the presence of an unsecured aneurysm as a sudden drop in intracranial pressure may precipitate aneurysmal re-rupture. ICP maintained between 15-20mmHg acutely is reasonable.

Upwards of 20% of aSAH patients develop global cerebral edema following aneurysm rupture [8]. The etiology of this phenomenon is unknown but may be related to sudden ICP elevation and cerebral circulatory arrest. The presence of diffusion-weighted lesions on acute CT and MRI, *ictal infarction*, are often seen in its presence.

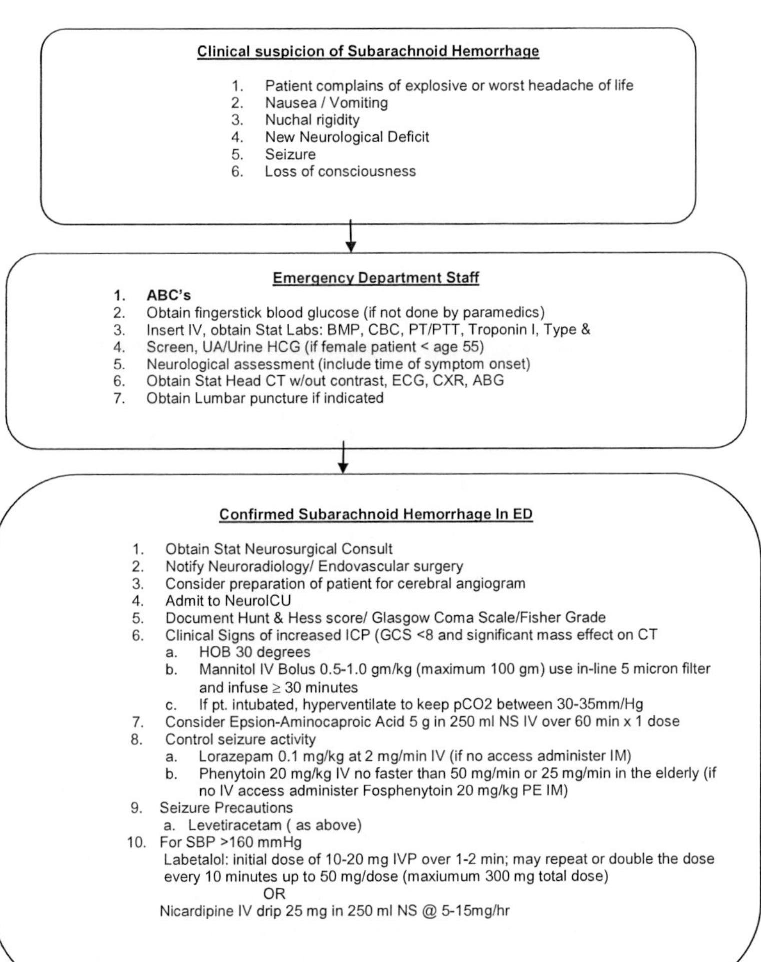

Figure 1. Management of Asah.

Guideline for Preoperative Neuro ICU Management SAH

1. Bedrest with HOB=30 degrees (unless post angiography)
2. Prepare for insertion of Arterial Line for continuous BP monitoring
   a. Maintain SBP < 160 mmHg with Labetolol or Nicardipine infusion as per NeuroICU protocol

3. Maintain oxygen saturation > 94%

4. Seizure Precautions

   a. Consider Levetiracetam for seizure prophylaxis
   b. If Hunt Hess grade 1-2, discontinue Levetiracetam on post-op day
   c. If Hunt-Hess grade 3-5, continue Levetiracetam
5. Consider placement of Swan Ganz / Central Line for monitoring PA / CVP pressures (especially in the presence of hemodynamic instability, CHF, or renal insufficiency)
6. Evaluate Swallow/ gag reflex
   a. Consider insertion of NG/Duo tube for poor gag reflex
7. Prepare patient for EVD placement if ventricular extension of hemorrhage with GCS < 8, posturing, or grade 3 with declining LOC; Refer to Nursing Standard for ICP Monitoring via EVD
   a. Cefazolin 1 gm IV before EVD insertion, (Penicillin allergy use Vancomycin 1 gm IV)

8. Strict I/O's

   a. Document I & O q 1 hour
   b. Foley Catheter
   c. Intravenous fluid: Normal Saline + 20 meq KCL/1 liter at 100ml/hr
9. If patient history positive for Warfarin

   a. Prepare to give 4 units FFP

   b. Administer IV Vitamin K 10 mg in 50 mL NS daily over 30 minutes x 3 days

10. If patient is unresponsive with pupillary asymmetry, motor posturing, or midline shift evident:

    a. Administer Mannitol 0.5-1.0 g/kg IV bolus (maximum 100 gm) use in-line 5 micron filter and infuse $\geq$ 30 minutes

    b. OR administer 23.4%NaCl 30cc over 20 min via CVC

    c. Consider changing baseline IVF to 1 ml/kg/hr of 3% Na Chloride/ Na Acetate (1:1) solution for target osmolarity of 300-320 and Na of 145-155 mmol/dL

11. Medications:

    a. Nimodipine 60 mg p.o./ NG q 4hr (hold for SBP < 120mm Hg
    b. Consider Epsilon-Aminocaproic Acid 5 g in 250 ml NS IV over 60 min x 1 dose (if not already administered in the ED), then 4 gm IV every 4 hrs. until aneurysm repair or up to 72 hrs after SAH onset.
    c. Consider treatment with rFVIIa (Heme Consult) for history of warfarin or coagulopathy for ongoing bleeding or neurosurgical intervention
    d. On ICU day 2, start Heparin 5,000 Units every 12 hours or Enoxaparin 30 mg every 12 hours subcutaneously (or 30 mg once daily for patients with CrCl < 30 mL/min).
12. Prepare patient for Neurosurgical/ Endovascular Intervention

13. Draw Toxicology Screen if not already done in ED

14. Consider Nicotine patch 21mg every day for current smoking history

15. Continue Levetiracetam as above

16. If patient is Hunt-Hess grade III-V and febrile, place surface cooling or endovascular heat-exchange catheter for Temp =37° C

17. Insulin & Hyperglycemia Management: Please refer to site specific protocols.

Figure 2. Management of Asah.

When seen, global cerebral edema should be treated aggressively as it is associated with increased mortality and cognitive disability among survivors [9]. A hyperosmolar state can be achieved with either Mannitol 20% 1 gram/kg IV every 6 hours or 3% saline at 1ml/kg/hr.

Prevention of Re-Bleeding

With a morbidity approaching 50%, aneurysm rebleeding is a major cause of morbidity and mortality [10]. After initial patient stabilization, securing the aneurysm is of paramount importance. Anticonvulsant therapy is administered to prevent seizures which may cause an increase in intracranial pressure. Due to recent evidence of impaired cognitive recovery following its use, phenytoin for seizure prophylaxis is becoming less in favor to other agents [11]. In patients who are of good clinical grade or who had no history of seizure, anticonvulsants can be stopped after aneurysm treatment. In high grade patients, it is reasonable to continue anticonvulsant therapy due to the higher frequency of nonconvulsive seizures in this patient population.

Hypertension should be treated prior to aneurysm treatment. Nitrates should be avoided due to their effect on intracranial pressure. In intubated patients, sedatives and analgesics such as propofol or fentanyl can be used for agitation. Pain control with narcotic analgesics are often necessary for pain control. Low dose dexamethasone can be considered for meningismus. Symptomatic treatment should also include antiemetics and stool softeners. A quiet environment without overstimulation is generally favored in patients awaiting treatment.

Should a delay occur with aneurysm treatment, antifibrinolytics can be used to prevent the risk for rebleeding. Although controversial, agents such as epsilon-aminocaproic acid have been shown to reduce the risk of rebleeding in unsecured aneurysms [12]. The benefit in patient outcome is lacking however, likely due to the increased risk of delayed cerebral ischemia following prolonged administration. Due to this risk, the use of antifibrinolytics beyond post–bleed day 3 should be avoided. A loading dose for epsilon-aminocaproic acid of 4 to 5 grams followed by 1 gram/hour can be used. The most effective treatment to prevent rebleeding is treatment of the underlying aneurysm. Controversy remains as to the mode of aneurysm treatment and is beyond the scope of this chapter. A multidisciplinary approach to aneurysm treatment is often necessary as patient factors, aneurysm size, morphology, and location are all important considerations.

Prevention and Treatment of Delayed Cerebral Ischemia (DCI)

The leading cause of morbidity and mortality from aneurysmal subarachnoid hemorrhage among survivors is DCI. DCI may occur in up to

46 percent of patients (between days 3 and 14 following hemorrhage and contributes to a high prevalence of cognitive impairment among survivors (13). Poor clinical condition on admission and amount of extravasated blood has been shown to be the strongest risk factors for its development. Other risk factors include intravascular volume depletion (14), hypertension and fever (15), and cigarette smoking (16). Aggressive fluid hydration is helpful in the prevention of delayed cerebral ischemia. Dehydration should be avoided and fever treated. Monitoring of central venous pressure with central venous access can be used to monitor volume status. Although unclear as to the optimal hemoglobin level to be maintained, it is generally agreed upon that anemia should be avoided. Oral nimodipine at a dose of 60mg every 4 hours for 21 days has been found to reduce poor oucome presumably by relaxation of vascular smooth muscle.

Despite extensive research, the pathogenesis of DCI has yet to be determined. It is widely believed that DCI is a result of angiographic vasospasm based upon studies showing a relationship between angiographic proven vasospasm and the presence of DCI. The delayed narrowing of both large and small intracranial arteries leads to cerebral ischemia and sometimes to infarction. A literature review including articles published after 1960 suggested that 67 % of 2,738 patients with aSAH had angiographic vasospasm during the second week after aSAH (17). While angiographic vasospasm is much more common in patients following aSAH than DCI, such neurological deterioration or focal deficits occurs only in a small proportion of patients with angiographic narrowing. When DCI does occur, about half of patients who experience it progress to significant cerebral infarction or death (18). Although the association with DCI and cerebral vasospasm has been shown in several studies [16], the fact that angiographic vasospasm may be found in the absence of DCI has lead to the differentiation of asymptomatic and symptomatic vasospasm. *Asymptomatic vasospasm*, which may occur in up to 70% of patients (19), is the finding of narrowing of the cerebral vessels on angiography in the absence of symptoms. *Symptomatic vasospasm* is defined as clinical features of DCI combined with radiologic vasospasm in the same region, and occurs in a much lower percentage of patients [2]. The pathogenesis of cerebral vasospasm and subsequent symptoms of DCI are still unknown. Theories range from microcirculatory arterial vasospasm from hemoglobin breakdown products within the subarachnoid space (20) to erythrocyte hemolysis evoking spreading cortical depressions which lead to microvascular spasm and cortical spreading ischemia (21). Regardless of the specific mechanism for its development, cerebral vasospasm has been shown to reduce cerebral blood flow below ischemic levels leading to disturbed brain metabolism and neurological dysfunction (22). Neurological dysfunction can potentially be reversed if adequate blood flow can be restored before infarction occurs.

The presence of DCI in patients is ascertained through the bedside neurological examination. In awake and alert patients, the neurological examination remains the most important clinical test for its detection (23). Symptoms may range from focal neurological signs such as hemiparesis or aphasia, depending upon the vascular territory affected. Symptoms such as depressed level of consciousness or inattention can result from distal vasospasm affecting small penetrating branches. It is in high-grade patients, where the clinical exam is difficult to perform, where detection may be problematic. It has been shown that 20% of SAH patients who meet the definition of DCI experience new infarction from spasm in the absence of clinically apparent deterioration, that this phenomenon occurs most commonly in comatose patients, and that these clinically "silent" infarcts independently contribute to poor outcome (24). Additional neuromonitoring techniques such as cerebral microdialysis, continuous EEG, brain tissue oxygen and cerebral blood flow monitoring are promising tools to detect and, in some cases, predict the onset of ischemia before it occurs in this population.

In addition to the neurological examination, daily transcranial doppplers ultrasound (TCD) examinations are performed and can provide an early clue to the onset of vasopasm through the measurement of blood flow velocities. Patient variability exists but velocities above 200cm/s are fairly accurate in the detection of cerebral vasospasm. Importantly, daily trends should be monitored as sudden increases may also signal its onset. Any sudden changes noted in TCD velocities should be correlated with the patient exam before changes in therapy are considered.

In the event that symptoms occur suggestive of DCI, a CT scan should be immediately performed to exclude alternate causes such as hemorrhage or hydrocephalus. Other mimics that should be quickly excluded include hyponatremia, hypoxia, or fever. An initial CT angiogram with perfusion is useful to correlate the clinical symptoms with radiographic regions of vasospasm. Findings of increased meant transit time with perfusion imaging can identify tissue at risk for infarction.

Hypertensive hypervolemic therapy (HHT) or hyperdynamic therapy is the mainstay of treatment of DCI. HHT involves inducing hypertension pharmacologically with vasopressors with the goal of improving cerebral perfusion pressure within regions affected by cerebral vasospasm. In addition, patients are placed in a hypervolemic state with the assistance of intravenous fluids and albumin in an effort to increase cerebral blood volume and flow to ischemic areas. The use of volume expansion in patients with DCI increases cerebral blood flow in ischemic areas as seen on positron emission tomography (PET) (25). Although clinical improvements can be dramatic with the use of HHT [26], the use of HHT has been associated with severe side effects. The use of pharmacological agents to induce hypertension such as dopamine, dobutamine, phenylephrine, and norepinephrine may result in arrhythmias and myocardial injury. The use of volume expansion may result in pulmonary edema and congestive heart failure. Despite these potential side effects, the use of HHT has become the mainstay of treatment for DCI.

The level of treatment varies on an individual level. Hemodynamic monitoring should be conducted with an arterial line and central line. Hematocrit levels are maintained above 30 to optimize oxygen delivery. Crystalloid fluids are administered and albumin administered to maintain central venous pressures between 8-12 and a pulmonary capillary wedge pressure of 18-20mmHg in those with a pulmonary artery catheter. Induced hypertension is accomplished with vasopressors such as dopamine or phenylephrine. In cases of myocardial dysfunction, inotropes such as milrninone can be used and titrated to cardiac indices. The endpoint of treatment is the resolution of symptoms or the development of complications.

In those patients who remain refractory to medical treatment or who develop complications, the use of intra-arterial papaverine or calcium channel blockers may enhance perfusion. The use of angioplasty may provide more sustained vasodilation but is without potential complications including arterial occlusion, dissection, or rupture.

Medical Complications

Cardiopulmonary

It has been estimated that up to 33% of aSAH patients will have a cardiac complication within 5 days of aneurysmal rupture [27]. Important complications range from ECG changes, arrhythmias, cardiac enzyme elevations, and pulmonary edema. Cardiac wall motion abnormalities have been well described after aSAH [27]. Abnormal wall motion can be focal or diffuse and frequently occur in the left ventricular apex and septum. Severe cardiac dysfunction leading to abnormal cardiac index and cardiogenic shock has been reported as well in association with aSAH. Higher myocardial enzymatic release has been associated with symptomatic delayed vasospasm and worse functional outcomes [28]. A sudden catecholaminergic surge has been implicated in the development of this syndrome. The effects of high catecholamines appear to induce important strain in the myocardial fiber which can be reflected by ventricular dysfunction, myocardial enzymatic release and evidence of contraction band necrosis in the myocardial wall [29]. This neurogenic stunned myocardium occurs within hours following hemorrhage and is typically transient lasting for 3-5 days after insult. Management can be problematic however due to systemic hypotension and pulmonary edema. Management involves use of inotropic agents such as dobutamine to augment cardiac performance. Demonstration of reversible wall motion abnormalities on repeat echocardiogram confirms the diagnosis.

Hyponatremia

Both cerebral salt wasting (CSW)and the syndrome of inappropriate secretion of antidiuretic hormone (SIADH)are important causes for hyponatremia following aSAH. The differentiation of the two can be challenging at times. Generally, CSW occurs more commonly and is manifested by a negative fluid balance and high urinary sodium levels. Treatment of hyponatremia should entail the use of isotonic crystalloid. Fluid restriction should be avoided due to the risk for causing symptoms of DCI. In cases of severe hyponatremia with soudium levels <125 mEq/L, hypertonic saline may be utilized. Other options include the use of fludrocortisone in a dose of 0.2mg IV or PO. It is important to monitor sodium levels frequently to avoid rapid correction. A rate of correction less than 10mEq/L in 24 hours is a reasonable target.

Prognosis

Due to advances in medical and surgical treatment of ruptured brain aneurysms, more patients are surviving and living longer. Case fatality rates have decreased by 17 percent between 1973 and 2002 and survivors have a reduced risk of death or dependency at 12 months. Despite these encouraging numbers, many survivors live with a significant level of disability. Among survivors, up to 12 percent are discharged to a nursing home and less than 60 percent will achieve functional independence (27). Admission Hunt and Hess grade remains the main primary driver of outcome. Other factors associated with poor functional outcome include age, fever, hyperglycemia, and delayed cerebral ischemia. With early surgical treatment and aggressive neurocritical care management, survivors

References

[1]   Rinkel GJ, Djibuti M, Algra A, van Gijn J. *Prevalence and risk of rupture of intracranial aneurysms: a systematic review.* Stroke. 1998;29:251-256.

[2]   Longstreth WT Jr, Nelson LM, Koepsell TD, van Belle G. *Clinical course of spontaneous subarachnoid hemorrhage:* A population based study in King County, Washington. Neurology. 1993;43:712-718.

[3]   Kassell NF, Torner JC, Haley EC Jr., et al. *The international cooperative study on the timing of aneurysm surgery. Part I: overall management results.* J. Neurosurg. 1990;73:18-36.

[4]   Hop JW, Rinkel GJ, Algra A, van Gijn J. *Initial los of consciousness and risk of delayed cerebral ischemia after aneurismal subarachnoid hemorrhage.* Stroke. 1999; 30:2268-2271.

[5]   Leblanc R. *The sudden leak preceeding subarachnoid hemorrhage.* J. Neurosurg. 1987;66:35-39.

[6]   Velthius BK, Rinkel GJ, Ramos LM, et al. *Subarachnoid Hemorrhage: Aneurysm detection and preoperative evaluation with CT angiography.* Radiology 1998;208:423-430.

[7]   Frontera JA, et al. *Prediction of Symptomatic Vasospasm after Subarachnoid Hemorrhage: the Modified Fisher Scale.* Neurosurgery. 2006 Jul;59(1):21-7.

[8]   Claassen J, et al. *Global cerebral edema after subarachnoid hemorrhage: frequency, predictors, and impact on outcome.* Stroke 2002 May;33(5):1225-32.

[9]   Kreiter KT, et al. *Predictors of cognitive dysfunction after subarachnoid hemorrhage.* Stroke 2002; 33:200-209.

[10] Kassell NF, Torner JC. *Aneurysmal rebleeding: A preliminary report from the cooperative study.* Neurosurgery 1983;13:479-481.

[11] Naidech AM, Kreiter KT, et al. *Phenytoin exposure is associated with functional and cognitive disability after subarachnoid hemorrhage.* Stroke 2005;36(12):2532

[12] Roos YB, Rinkel GJE, Vermeulen M, et al. *Antifibrinolytic therapy for aneurysmal subarachnoid hemorrhage.* Cochrane Database of Systematic Reviews 2000; Issue 2. Oxford: update software.

[13] Temes RE, Schmidt MJ, Mayer SA. *Prognosis and Outcomes Following Aneurysmal Saubarachnoid Hemorrhage.* Acute Stroke: Bench to Bedside 2006; 103-109.

[14] McGirt MJ, Blessing R, Nimjee SM, Friedman AH, Alexander MJ, Laskowitz DT, Lynch JR: *Correlation of serum brain natriuretic peptide with hyponatremia and delayed ischemic neurological deficits after subarachnoid hemorrhage.* Neurosurgery 2004; 54:1369–1374.

[15] Fergusen S, Macdonald RL: *Predictors of cerebral infarction in patients with aneurysmal subarachnoid hemorrhage.* Neurosurgery 2007; 60:658–667.

[16] Lasner TM, Weil RJ, Riina HA, King JT Jr, Zager EL, Raps EC, Flamm ES: *Cigarette smoking-induced increase in the risk of symptomatic vasospasm after aneurysmal subarachnoid hemorrhage.* J Neurosurg; 87:381–384.

[17] Dorsch NWC, King MT (1994) *A review of cerebral vasospasm in aneurysmal subarachnoid haemorrhage Part I: Incidence and effects.* J Clin Neurosci 1(1):19–26.

[18] Fisher CM, Kistler JP, Davis JM: *Relation of cerebral vasospasm to subarachnoid hemorrhage visualized by computerized tomographic scanning.* Neurosurgery 1980; 6(1):1-9.

[19] Vora YY, Suarez-Almazor M, Steinke DE, Martin ML, Findlay JM. *Role of transcranial Doppler monitoring in the diagnosis of cerebral vasospasm after subarachnoid hemorrhage.* Neurosurgery 1999; 44:1237–1247.

[20] Uhl E, Lehmberg J, Steiger HJ, Messmer K. *Intraoperative detection of early microvasospasm in patients with subarachnoid hemorrhage by using orthogonal polarization spectral imaging.* Neurosurgery 2003; 52:1307–1315.

[21] Shin HK, Dunn AK, Jones PB, Boas DA, Moskowitz MA, Ayata C. *Vasoconstrictive neurovascular coupling during focal ischemic depolarizations.* J Cereb Blood Flow Metab 2006; 26:1018–1030.

[22] Powers WJ, Grubb RL, Baker RP, Mintun MA, Raichle ME. *Regional cerebral blood flow in patients with ruptured aneurysms.* J Neurosurg 1985; 62:539-546.

[23] Munch E, Vajkoczy P. *Current advances in the diagnosis of vasospasm.* Neurol Res 2006; 28(7):703-12.

[24] Schmidt JM, Fernandez A, Rincon F, Claassen J, Ostapkovich ND, Badjatia N, Parra A, Connolly ES, Mayer SA. *Frequency and clinical impact of asymptomatic cerebral infarction due to vasospasm after subarachnoid hemorrhage.* J Neurosurg. 2008; 109: 1052–1059.

[25] Jost SC, Diringer MN, Zazulia AR, Videen TO, Aiyagari V, Grubb RL, Powers WJ. *Effect of normal saline bolus on cerebral blood flow in regions with low baseline flow in patients with vasospasm following subarachnoid hemorrhage.* J Neurosurg 2005;103(1):25-30.

[26] Miller JA, Dacey RG, Diringer MN. *Safety of Hypertensive Hypervolemic Therapy With Phenylephrine in the Treatment of Delayed Ischemic Deficits After Subarachnoid Hemorrhage.* Stroke. 1995; 26:2260-2266.

[27] Crago EA, Kerr ME, Kong Y, Baldisseri M, Horowitz M, Yonas H, Kassam A: *The Impact of Cardiac Complications on Outcomes in the SAH Population.* Acta Neurol Scand, 2000 Oct; 110(4): 248-53.

[28] Naidech, A.M., et al., *Cardiac Troponin Elevation, Cardiovascular Morbidity, and Outcome* After Subarachnoid Hemorrhage. 2005. p. 2851-2856.

[29] Cruickshank JM, Hayes Y, Neil-Dwyer G, Degaute JP, Hayes Y, Kuurne T, Kytta J, Vincent JL, Carruthers, ME, Patel, S. *Stress/catecholamine-induced cardiac necrosis. Reduction by beta 1-selective blockade.* Lancet. 1987 Sep 12; 2(8559): 585-589.

[30] Greebe P, Rinkel GJ, Algra A. *Long-term outcome of patients discharged to a nursing home after aneurysmal subarachnoid hemorrhage.* Arch Phys Med Rehabil. 2010; 91(2):247-51.

In: Handbook of Stroke and Neurocritical Care   ISBN: 978-61324-786-0
Editor: V. H. Lee   © 2012 Nova Science Publishers, Inc.

Chapter XIV

Other Stroke Like Conditions

Vivien Lee
Department of Neurological Sciences,
Section of Stroke and Neurocritical care,
Rush University Medical Center, Chicago, IL, USA

Posterior Reversible Encephalopathy Syndrome (PRES)

1) Other names- Reversible Posterior Leukoencephalopathy Syndrome (RPLS), eclampsia, hypertensive encephalopathy
2) Neuroimaging characterized by findings of reversible vasogenic subcortical edema without infarction
   a) As the name implies, PRES is classically associated the features of subcortical vasogenic edema, patchy symmetric bilateral involvement with preferential involvement of posterior head regions, and complete clinical and radiographic resolution.[1]
   b) Hemorrhage can occur in areas of injury, typically in patients with underlying coagulopathy or bleeding diathesis
3) Clinical presentation typically involves global encephalopathy, seizures, headache or visual symptoms.[1]

a)   Typically Reversible with withdrawal of offending agents, although Irreversible damage is possible

b)   Encephalopathy and seizures remain the major presenting symptom in RPLS, and RPLS can present as status epilepticus [2]

   1)   Anti-epileptic medication is typically necessary short term, and most patients do not develop epilepsy

4)   syndrome can be triggered by eclampsia, hypertensive emergency, and exposure to immunosuppresion (most notably the calcineurin inhibitors).[3,4,5,6,7,8]

5)   postulated to have a similar pathophysiology to hypertensive encephalopathy,[9,10]

   although correlation with elevated blood pressure has not been demonstrated.

a)   Schwartz suggested that the vertebrobasilar territory, due to its relative sparse sympathetic innervation, may suffer preferential disruption of autoregulatory mechanisms leading to increased perfusion and edema.[10] Regions of increased T2 signal on MRI have been reported to be associated with increased perfusion on SPECT, supporting a vasodilatory mechanism [10,11]

b)   Vasospasm theory

Reversible Cerebral Vasoconstriction Syndrome (RCVS)

1)   Benign Cerebral Angiopathy, Call-Fleming, drug-induced cerebral angiopathy, post-partum angiopathy [12]

2)   Clinical presentation- typically Thunderclap headache

a)   Can include neurological symptoms (if ischemic strokes develop)

3)   NeuroImaging

a)   Reversible segemental and multifocal vasoconstriction of cerebral arteries

b)   'string and beads' appearance on cerebral arteries, which resolves spontaneously in 1-3 months

c)   Similar angiographic appearance with vasculitis, and must be distinguished from CNS vascultis

4) Pathophysiology
   a) Not well understood, but felt to be a disturbance in the control of cerebral vascular tone
   b) Triggers
      (i) Sympathomimetics
      (ii) Serotonergic drugs and tumors
      (iii) Endocrine factors
      (iv) Uncontrolled hypertension
      (v) Neurosurgical trauma
5) Treatment/Prognosis
   a) Treatment is empiric
      (i) Calcium channel blockers have been used
   b) Prognosis- since condition is reversible, most patients do well with reversal of constriction seen in days to weeks
   c) Ischemic strokes can limit prognosis
6) A large series of 67 patients with angiographically confirmed RCVS[13]
   a) Early complications-
      (i) Cortical SAH (22%)
      (ii) ICH (6%)
      (iii) Seizures (3%)
      (iv) PRES (9%)
   b) Ischemic events occur later (2nd week)

Cerebral Venous Sinus Thrombosis (CVT)

1) Clinical presentation [14]
   a) Headache is the most common presenting symptom
   b) Other symptoms may include
      (i) Isolated Intracranial hypertension (may include headache, comiting, visual disturbances, papilledema, CN 6th palsy)
      (ii) Focal neurological symptoms (if parenchymal involvement with hemorrhagic venous infarct or edema)
      (iii) Encephalopathy
      (iv) Seizures

2) Natural history and prognosis
   a) Study of 624 adult patients with CVT[15]
   b) At end of follow-up (median 16 months), 57% mRS0, 22% mRS1, 8.3% died.
      (i) CVT low risk of death and good long-term prognosis
   c) Predictors of death/dependence were age >37, male sex, coma, mental status disorder, hemorrhage on admission CT, thrombosis of the deep cerebral venous system, CNS infection, and cancer.
   d) In acute phase, most patients (83%) were anticoagulated with IV heparin or LMWH.
3) 2 small randomized trials
   a) Einhaupl et al. [16]
      (i) adjusted dose IV heparin, randomized, blinded, placebo control
      (ii) 20 CVT patients (10 heparin group, 10 placebo group)
      (iii) Stopped early because of the efficacy of heparin
      (iv) In heparin group, 8 recovered completely and 2 had slight residual neurologic deficits at 3 months, compared to Placebo group with 1complete recovery, 6 neurologic deficits, 3 deaths (p < 0.01)
      (v) authors also reviewed retrospectively an additional 43 CVT patients with intracranial bleeding, 27 received dose-adjusted heparin. mortality rate was 15% in the heparin group compared with 69% in the nonheparin group.
   b) de Bruijn et al. [17]
      (i) 59 patients included (30 Nadroparin, 29 placebo)
      (ii) twice as many patients with isolated intracranial hypertension in placebo group (28% vs 13%)- a subgroup who typically have a good outcome.
      (iii) compared body-weight adjusted SQ nadroparin (180 anti-factor Xa U/kg per day) to placebo for 3 weeks followed by an unblinded comparison between 3 months of oral anticoagulation for patients who received nadroparin and no antithrombotic therapy for the placebo group.
      (iv) Patients with intracranial bleeding caused by the CVT were included

> (v) After 12 weeks, 13% (4 of 30 patients) in the anticoagulation group and 21% (6 of 29 patients) in the placebo group had a poor outcome
>
> (vi) absolute benefit of 7% and a RRR of 38% in the nadroparin group, a difference which did not reach statistical significance.
>
> (vii) no new symptomatic cerebral hemorrhages.

4) Chest guidelines[18]

a) heparin is firstline treatment, even in patients with hemorrhagic venous infarcts, followed by oral anticoagulation for a period of 3 to 6 months.

b) In patients who demonstrate progressive neurologic deterioration despite adequate anticoagulation, other options such as local intrathrombus infusion of a thrombolytic agent together with IV heparin are under investigation

References

[1] Hinchey J, Chaves C, Appignani B, Breen J, Pao L, Wang A, et al. *A reversible Posterior Leukoencephalopathy syndrome*. N Engl J Med 1996;334:494-500.

[2] Lee VH, Wijdicks EF, Manno EM, Rabinstein AA. *The Clinical spectrum of Reversible Posterior Leukoencephalopathy Syndrome*. Archives of Neurology. 2008;65:205-210.

[3] Schwaighofer BW, Hesselink JR, Healy ME. *MR demonstration of reversible brain abnormalities in eclampsia*. J Comput Assist Tomogr. 1989;13:310-2.

[4] Hauser RA, Lacey DM, Knight MR. Hypertensive encephalopathy. *Magnetic resonance imaging demonstration of reversible cortical and white matter lesions*. Arch Neurol. 1988;45:1078-83.

[5] Appignani BA, Bhadelia RA, Blacklow SC, Wang AK, Roland SF, Freeman RB. *Neuroimaging Findings in Patients on Immunosuppressive Therapy: Experience with Tacrolimus Toxicity*. AJR. 1996;166:683-688.

[6] Small SL, Fukui MB, Bramblett GT, Eidelman BH. *Immunosuppression-induced Leukoencephalopathy from Tacrolimus (FK506)*. Ann Neurol 1996;40:575-580.

[7]   Truwit CL, Denaro CP, Lake JR, DeMarco T. *MR Imaging of Reversible Cyclosporin A-induced neurotoxicity.* AJNR 1991;12:651-659.

[8]   Singh N, Bonham A, Fukui M. *Immunosuppressive-associated leukoencephalopathy in organ transplant recipients.* Transplantation. 2000;69;467-72.

[9]   Schwartz RB. *A reversible posterior leukoencephalopathy syndrome.* N Engl J Med. 1996;334:1743.

[10]   Antunes NL, Small TN, George D, Boulad F, Lis E. *Posterior leukoencephalopathy syndrome may not be reversible.* Pediatric Neurol. 1999;20:241-3.

[11]   Schwartz RB, Jones KM, Kalina P, et al. *Hypertensive encephalopathy: findings on CT, MR imaging, and SPECT imaging in 14 cases.* AJR 1992;159:379-83.

[12]   Calabrese LH, Dodick DW, Schwedt TJ, Singhal AB. *Narrative Review: Reversible Cerebral Vasoconstriction Syndrome.* Ann Intern Med. 2007;146:34-44.

[13]   Anne Ducros, Monique Boukobza, Raphael Porcher, Mariana Sarov, Dominique Valade and Marie-Germaine Bousser. *The clinical and radiological spectrum of reversible cerebral vasoconstriction syndrome. A prospective series of 67 patients.* Brain 2007;130,:3091-3101.

[14]   Filippidis A., Kapsalak E, Patrama G, Fountas KN. *Cerebral venous sinus thrombosis: review of the demographics, pathophysiology, current diagnosis,and treatment.* Neurosurg Focus 2009;27:E3.

[15]   José M. Ferro, MD, PhD; Patrícia Canhão, MD; Jan Stam, MD; Marie-Germaine Bousser, MD; Fernando Barinagarrementeria, MD; for the ISCVT Investigators. *Prognosis of Cerebral Vein and Dural Sinus Thrombosis Results of the International Study on Cerebral Vein and Dural Sinus Thrombosis (ISCVT).* Stroke. 2004;35:664-670.

[16]   Einhaupl KM, Villringer A, Meister W, et al. *Heparin treatment in sinus venous thrombosis.* Lancet 1991; 338:597–600.

[17]   de Bruijn SF, Stam J. *Randomized, placebo-controlled trial of anticoagulant treatment with low-molecular-weight heparin for cerebral sinus thrombosis.* Stroke 1999; 30:484–488.

[18]   Gregory W. Albers, MD, Chair; Pierre Amarenco, MD; J. Donald Easton, MD; Ralph L. Sacco, MD; and Philip Teal, MD. *Antithrombotic and Thrombolytic Therapy for Ischemic Stroke* American College of Chest Physicians Evidence-Based Clinical Practice Guidelines (8th Edition).* CHEST 2008; 133:630S–669S.

In: Handbook of Stroke and Neurocritical Care   ISBN: 978-61324-786-0
Editor: V. H. Lee   © 2012 Nova Science Publishers, Inc.

Chapter XV

Neuroimaging

Miral Jhaveri
Department of Diagnostic Radiology and Nuclear Medicine,
Rush University Medical Center, Chicago, IL, USA

Abbreviations

- NCCT - noncontrast CT
- CECT - contrast enhanced CT
- CTP   - CT perfusion
- CTA   - CT angiography
- MR   - magnetic resonance imaging
- MRA   - magnetic resonance angiography
- DWI   - Diffusion weighted imaging
- PWI   - Perfusion weighted MR imaging

15.1 Introduction

Comprehensive evaluation in acute stroke may be performed with a combination of computed tomography (CT) or magnetic resonance (MR) imaging techniques.

Imaging Protocols

- CT
- NCCT – non contrast CT performed with 5 mm axial sections.
- CECT - post contrast CT following intravenous injection of 75-100 ml iodinated contrast.
- CTA - fast thin section, volumetric spiral CT examination performed with a time optimized bolus of contrast material for opacification of vessels (volume 50-100 ml, rate 4-5 ml/sec). MIP (maximum intensity projection) reconstructions obtained in multiple planes, optional 3D volume rendered reconstructions.
- CTP –continuous cine axial images obtained every 1-2 secs for about 45 seconds over the same slab of tissue during dynamic administration of a small (40-50 ml) high flow contrast material bolus (injection rate 4-5 ml/sec).

MR

- MR – routine MR protocol for brain includes Diffusion, Sag and axial T1, axial T2 ,axial FLAIR , GRE images.
- MRA – 3D TOF (time of flight) sequence for circle of Willis, 2D TOF or postcontrast MRA for neck vessels.
- MR perfusion – either exogenous method of achieving perfusion contrast (ie, the administration of an MR contrast agent) or an endogenous method (ie, the labeling of hydrogen protons in water, also known as arterial spin labeling). Exogenous techniques are typically susceptibility based and depend on $T2^*$ effects or T1 weighted. Dynamic susceptibility-weighted $T2^*$ sequences most commonly used.

Table 1. MR signal characteristics of different tissues.

	MR – T1	MR – T2
Dense Bone	Dark	Dark
Air	Dark	Dark
Fat	Bright	Less Bright
Water(CSF)	Dark	Bright
Calcification	variable	Variable

Stroke has 4 Main Etiologies

- Ischemic stroke 80 %
- Non-tramatic intraparenchymal hemorrhage 15 %
- Non-traumatic subarachnoid hemorrhage 5 %
- Venous Infarction 1%

15.2 Ischemic Stroke

Goals of Acute stroke imaging can be summarized in Table 2.

Table 2.

Parenchyma	Assess early signs of acute stroke, rule out hemorrhage
Pipes	Assess extracranial and intracranial circulation for evidence of intravascular thrombus
Perfusion	Assess cerebral blood volume, blood flow and mean transit time
Penumbra	Assess tissue at risk of dying if ischemia continues without recanalization of intravascular thrombus

15.2.1 CT Findings in Ischemic Stroke

NECT

Acute Stage 0-2 Days

- Identify hemorrhage- contraindication to thrombolytic therapy.
- Use of stroke window settings (fig 1) – window width 8 HU/window level 32HU helps to demonstrate subtle abnormalities that suggest ischemia.

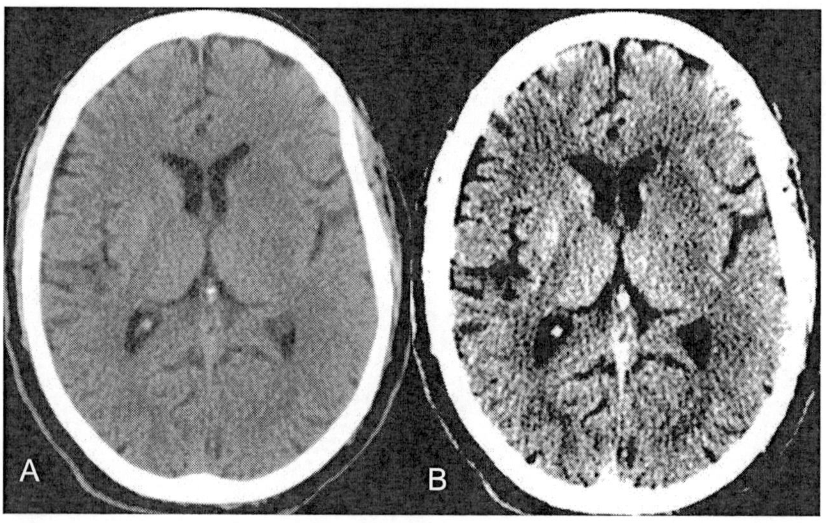

Figure 1A & B. Axial noncontrast CT images at the level of the basal ganglia with standard (A) and stroke window setting (B). The acute infarct involving the left lentiform and caudate nuclei is better visualized on image B (arrows).

- Detect early stage of acute ischemia
    1) Hyperdense vessel (high specificity, low sensitivity),represents acute thrombus in vessel
        o Hyperdense MCA (M1) (fig 2)
        o Hyperdense MCA 'dot' sign- occluded MCA branches in sylvian fissure (fig 3)
        o Hyperdense basilar artery (fig 4)

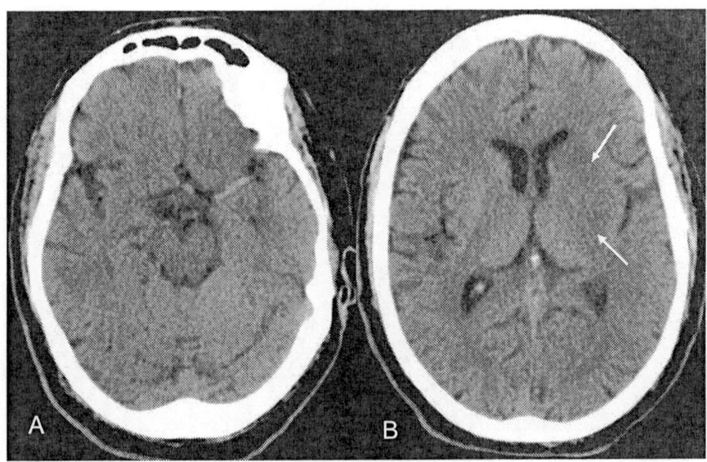

Figure 2. Axial CT images demonstrates a hyperdense MCA sign (red arrow, image A) representing acute thrombus, and the infarct in the left basal ganglia (white arrows, image B).

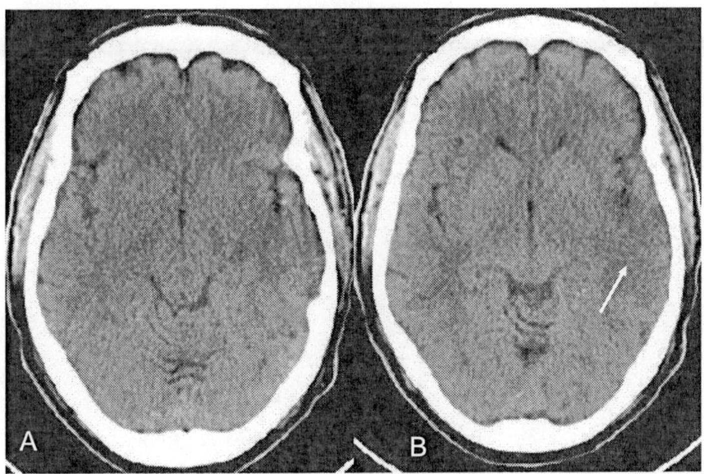

Figure 3. Axial CT image shows a hyperdense MCA 'dot' sign (red arrow) due to occluded MCA branch in the sylvian fissure. Image B shows subtle hypodensity in left temporal region consistent with an acute infarct in the left MCA distribution (white arrow).

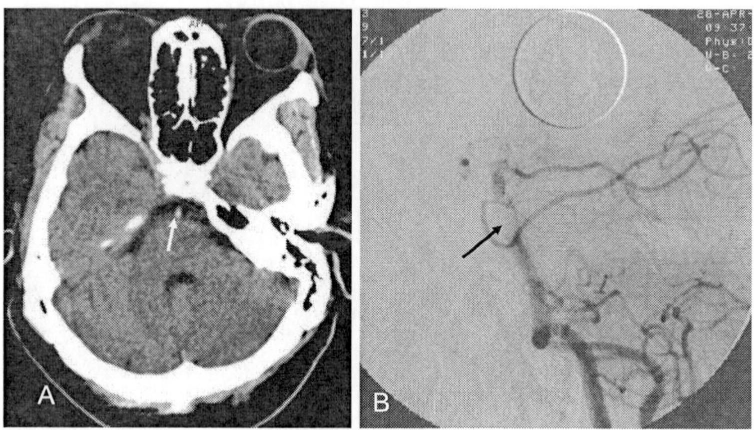

Figure 4. Axial CT image (A) demonstrates a hyperdense basilar artery (arrow) with subtle infarct in the left cerebellar hemisphere. Lateral projection of digital subtraction angiogram (B) demonstrates filling defect in the mid basilar artery (arrow) consistent with a thrombus.

2) Loss of gray-white matter differentiation
   o   Obscuration of lentiform nucleus (fig 5)
   o   Loss of insular cortical 'ribbon" Insular ribbon sign (fig 6)

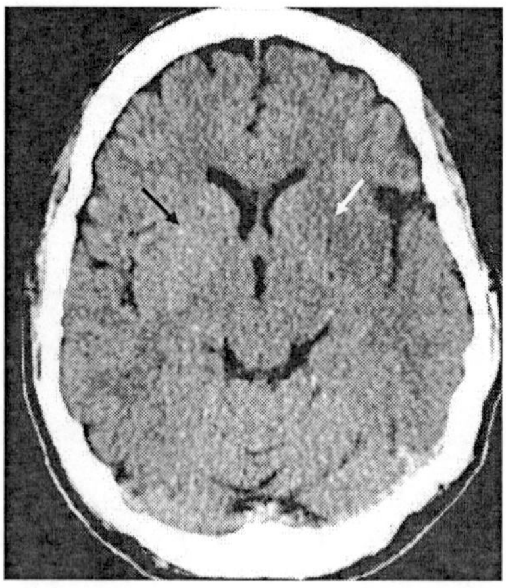

Figure 5. Axial CT demonstrates obscuration of the left lentiform nucleus due to an acute infarct (white arrow). Compare to the normal mildly hyperdense right lentiform nucleus (black arrow).

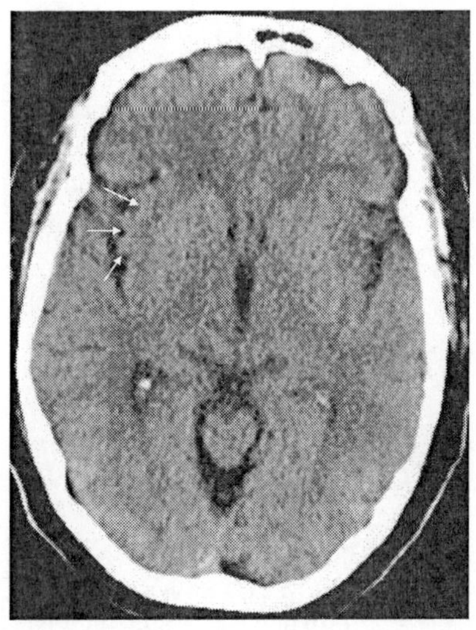

Figure 6. Axial CT demonstrates loss of insular cortical 'ribbon'on the left (red arrows) with a normal appearing right insular cortex (small white arrows).

- ASPECTS scoring system – Alberta Stroke Program Early CT Score (ASPECTS) proposed in 2001 as a means to quantitatively assessing acute ischemia on CT images using a 10-point scoring system (fig 7). Score of 0 translated into a finding of diffuse ischemia involving the MCA territory. The lower the score the greater the morbidity and mortality.
- Parenchymal hypodensity, gyral swelling, sulcal effacement
- Hemorrhagic transformation can be gross parenchymal or petechial (fig). Delayed onset 24-48 hrs most typical.

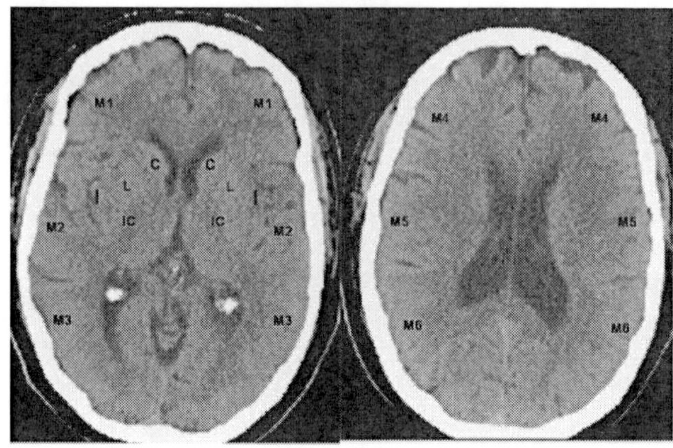

Figure 7. Axial CT images show the 10 regions of the MCA distribution, each of which accounts for one point in the ASPECTS system: M1, M2, M3, M4, M5, M6, the caudate nucleus (C), the lentiform nucleus (L), the internal capsule (IC), and the insular cortex (I).

Subacute Stage 2-14 Days

- Wedge shaped area of decreased attenuation involving gray and white matter
- ↓ mass effect by 7-10 days
- CT "fogging" – temporary transition to isodensity 2-3 wks post ictus.

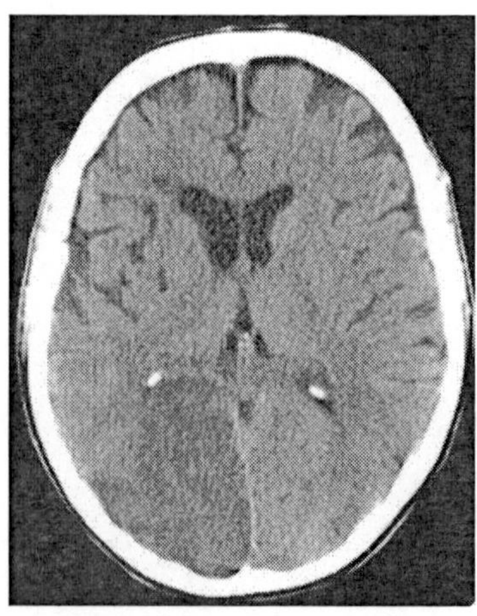

Figure 8. Axial CT showing a subacute right PCA infarct.

Chronic Stage (Months to Year)

- Volume loss, sulcal prominence, ipsilateral ventricular enlargement.
- Wallerian degeneration, dystrophic calcification.

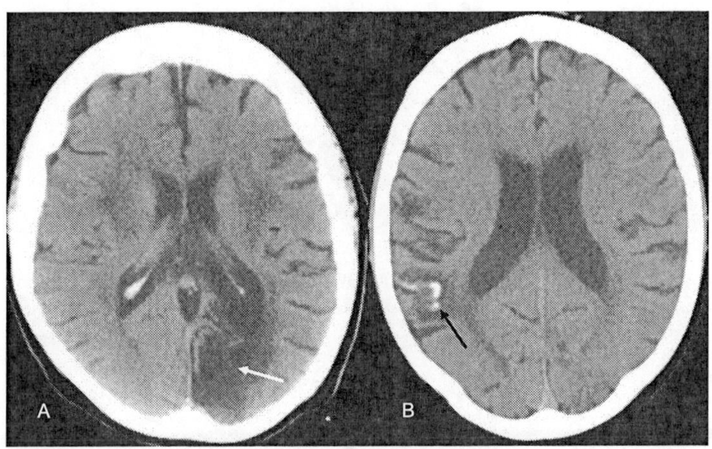

Figure 9. Axial CT (A) demonstrates a chronic left PCA infarct (white arrow) with attenuation similar to CSF, notice enlargement of left occipital horn due to volume loss. Image B shows dystrophic calcification in an old right MCA infarct (black arrow).

CECT

- Cortical vessel enhancement due to slow flow or collateral vessels
- Paucity of vessels due to proximal occlusion (fig 10)
- Subacute stage- enhancement which is patchy and gyral
- "2-2-2" rule – enhancement begins at 2 days, peaks 2 weeks and disappears by 2 months
- Chronic stage – no enhancement.

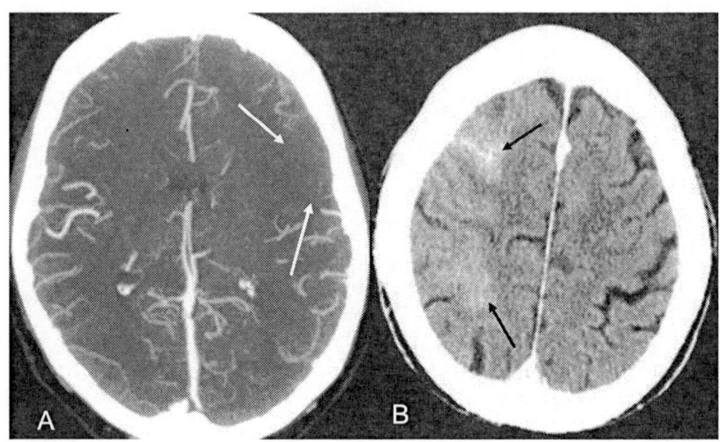

Figure 10. Axial CECT demonstrates paucity of vessels in an acute left MCA infarct (A). CECT image B demonstrates gyral enhancement in a subacute right MCA infarct.

CTA

- Evaluate status of large cervical and intracranial arteries.
- Help define occlusion site, depict arterial dissection, grade collateral blood flow, and characterize atherosclerotic disease. (fig 11)
- Useful in providing guidance prior to intraarterial thrombolysis
- Analyze extent of leptomeningeal collateral vessels beyond occlusion – patients with better collateral formation appear to have better prognosis.
- CT angiography source images more sensitive than NECT in detection of early irreversible ischemia and more accurate in predicting final infarct volume .

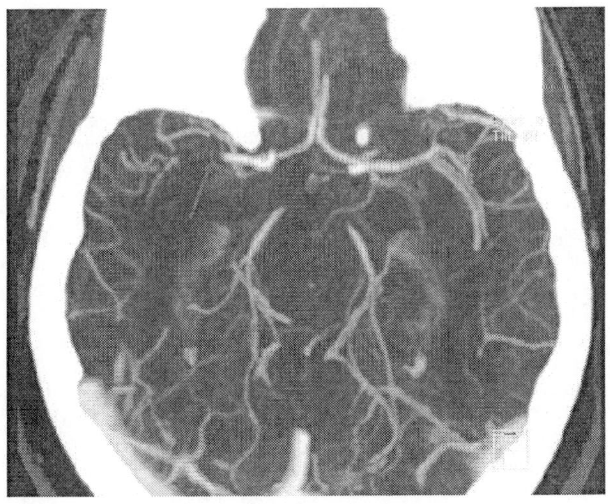

Figure 11. Axial CT angiogram maximum intensity projection (MIP) reconstruction demonstrates occlusion of the right MCA (red arrow) just distal to its origin in a patient presenting with dense left hemiparesis.

CTP

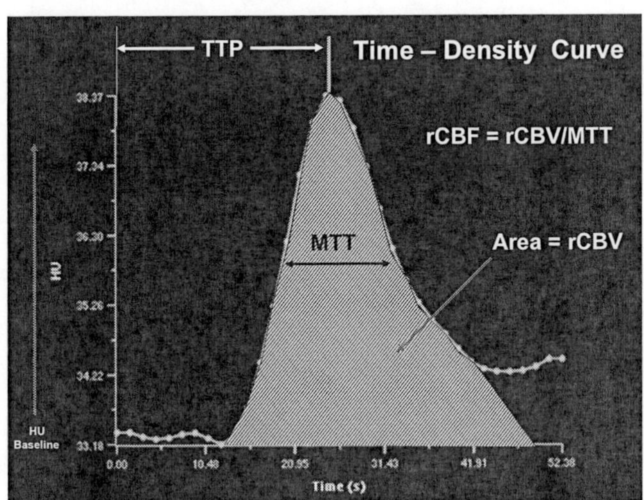

- Evaluation of perfusion CT data – values calculated for
- MTT – mean transit time
- TTP – time to peak
- CBV- cerebral blood volume ml/100 gm

- CBF – cerebral blood flow ml/100gm/min
- CBF = CBV/MTT
- Standard quantitative CTP values (table 3).
- Color coded maps of these parameters are displayed allowing quick visual assessment of possible infarction with a sensitivity of over 90 % in large ischemic lesions
- Perfusion CT can help distinguish penumbra from infarcted tissue in acute stroke patients (table 4) (fig 13)

Table 3. Standard Quantitative CTP Values.

	Grey matter	White matter	Infarct 'core'
CBF mL/100gm/min	60	25	< 12
CBV mL/100 gm	4	2	<1
MTT sec	4	4-4.8	>6

Ischemic penumbra

CT perfusion

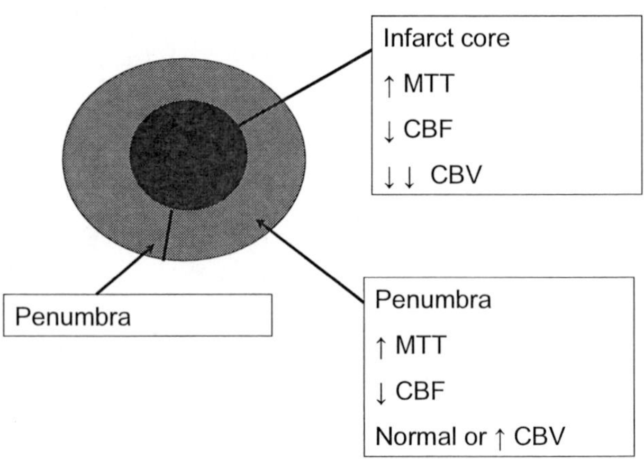

Table 4.

Ischemic tissue(penumbra)	↑ MTT	↓ CBF normal or mildly ↑ CBV
Infarcted tissue	↑ MTT	↓ CBF, ↓↓ CBV

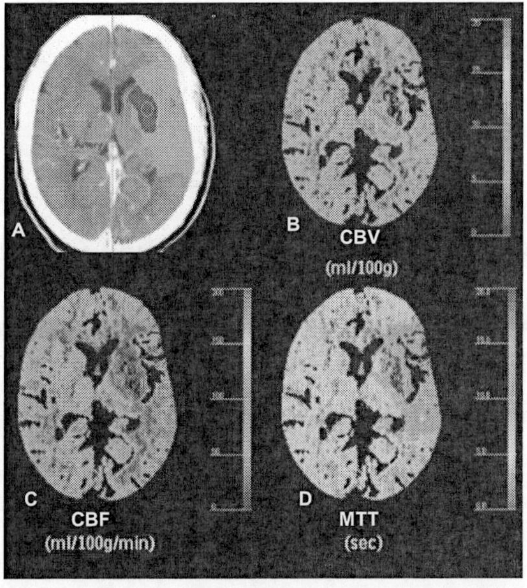

Figure 12. Axial post-processed images from CT perfusion study demonstrates infarct core (red shading image A) and penumbra (green shading image A). The infarct core shows decreased CBV (B), decreased CBF (C) and elevated MTT (D). The penumbra shows relative preservation of CBV with decrease CBF and elevated MTT.

15.2.2. MR Findings in Ischemic Stroke

Conventional MR Imaging

Acute Stage

- Early cortical swelling, FLAIR parenchymal hyperintensity approx 6 hrs post ictus while other sequences are normal.
- T2 hyperintensity develops by 12-24 hrs.
- Gradient echo T2* - detection of acute blood products (fig 13 a & b), 'blooming' artifact from thrombosed vessel due to clot susceptibility (reference) (fig 14).

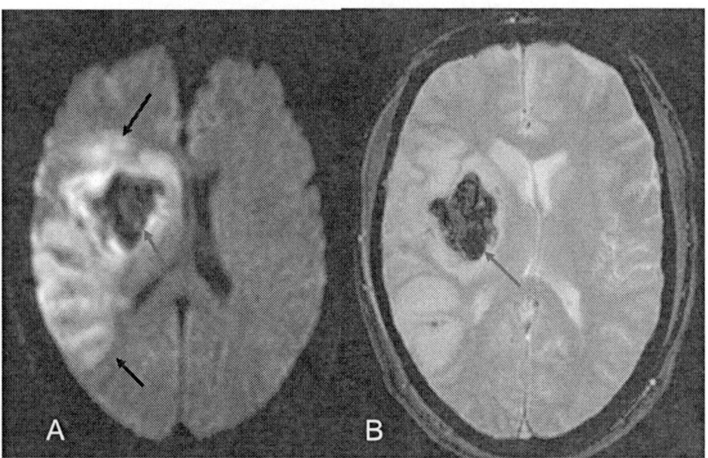

Figure 13a. Axial DWI (A) and GRE (B) demonstrates hemorrhagic conversion of a right MCA infarct.

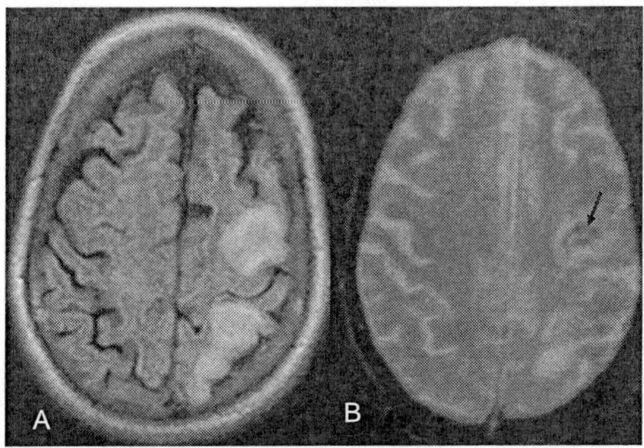

Figure 13b. Axial FLAIR (A) and GRE (B) images demonstrate petechial hemorrhage along the cortex in a patchy left MCA infarct.

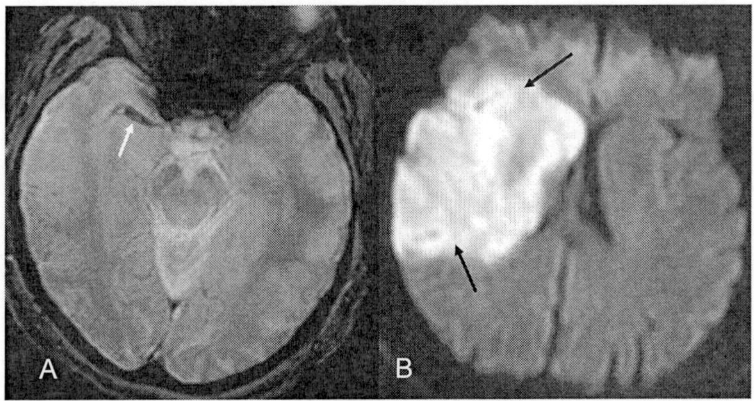

Figure 14. Axial GRE image (A) demonstrates susceptibility change (arrow) in the right sylvian fissure due to thrombus in the right MCA. Axial diffusion image (B) in the same patient demonstrates restricted diffusion due to an acute infarct in the right MCA distribution.

- Post contrast T1W – intravascular enhancement due to slow flow, meningeal enhancement due to leptomeningeal collaterals.(fig 15)

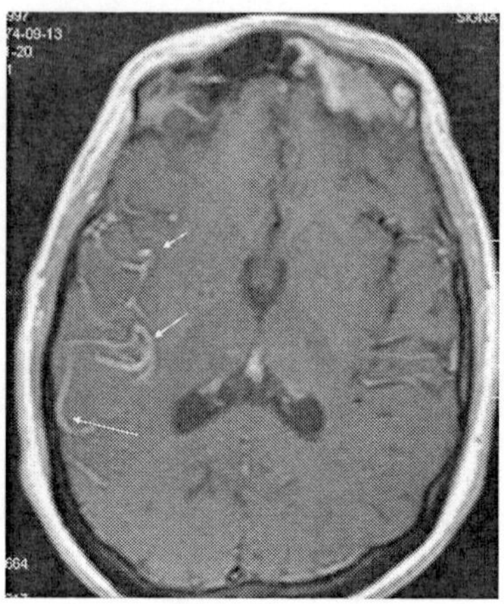

Figure 15. Axial post contrast T1W image demonstrates intravascular enhancement (arrows) due to slow flow in a patient with right MCA occlusion.

Subacute Stage

- T2 hyperintense edema with mass effect. " Fogging" effect – pseudonormalization on T2 with intense enhancement on post contrast T1 at 1-2 weeks following ictus.
- Early Wallerian degeneration may show T2 hyperintense signal along the corticospinal tract.
- Parenchymal enhancement in subacute stage is typically gyral and can persist up to 8-10 weeks (fig 16).

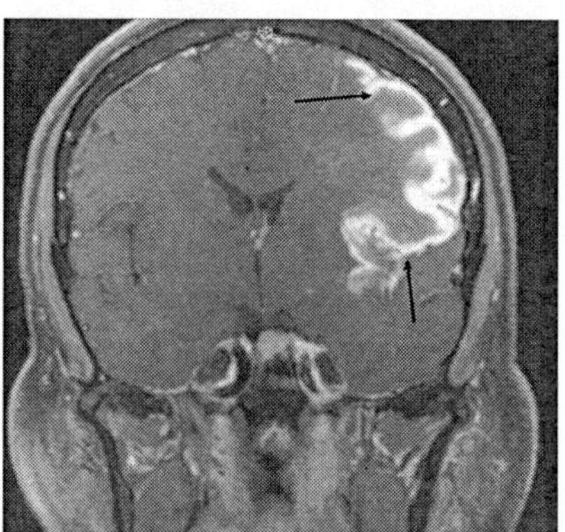

Figure 16. Coronal post constrat T1W image demonstrates extensive gyral enhancement (arrows) in a subacute left MCA infarct.

Chronic Stage

- Volume loss, atrophy, Wallerian degeneration (ipsilateral cerebral peduncle, pons shows atrophy). (fig 17)

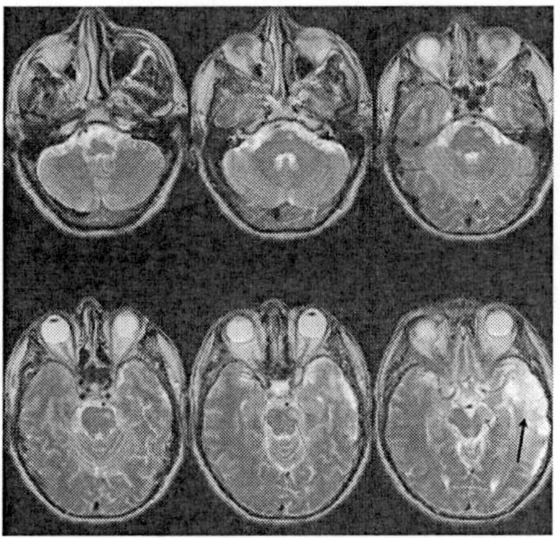

Figure 17. Axial T2W images demonstrate volume loss in the left temporal region due to an old MCA infarct (black arrow). There is high signal within the left cerebral peduncle, pons and medulla along the corticospinal tract (red arrows) consistent with Wallerian degeneration.

MRA

- Evaluate for major vessel occlusions, stenosis and status of collaterals (fig 18)

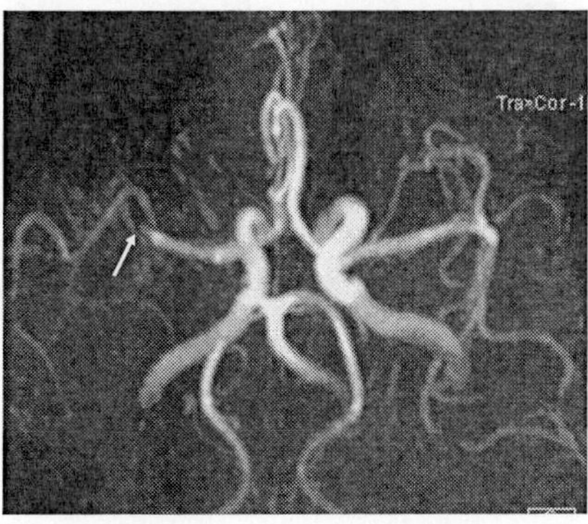

Figure 18. MR angiogram MIP image demonstrates abrupt termination of the right M1 segment (arrow).

DWI

- Restricted diffusion from cytotoxic edema – high signal on DWI with corresponding low signal on ADC maps (fig 19)
- Improves detection of hyperacute stroke
- Diffusion restriction with reduced ADC can be observed as early as 30 minutes after the onset of ischemia.
- Restricted diffusion typically lasts 7 -10 days
- Mildly hyperintense signal on diffusion with pseudonormal ADC values at 1-4 weeks
- Variable signal intensity on diffusion with increased ADC values several weeks to months after ictus.

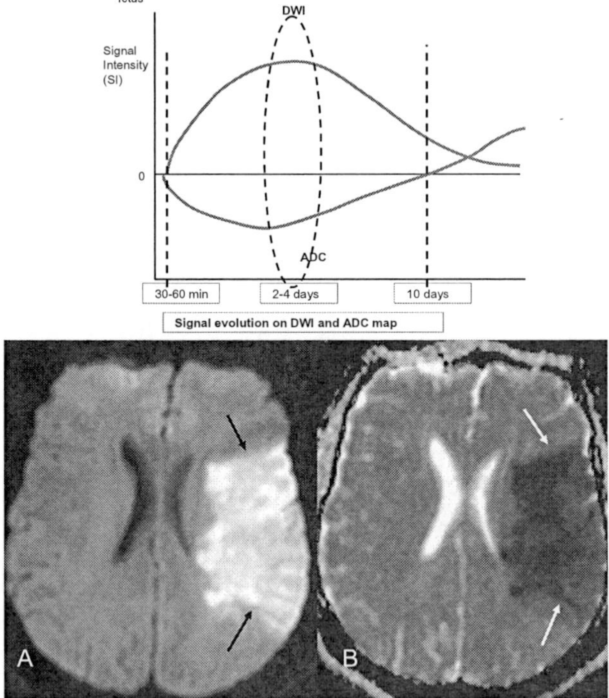

Figure 19. Axial diffusion image (A) shows high signal with corresponding low signal on ADC map (B) consistent with restricted diffusion in an acute left MCA infarct.

PWI

- Evaluate MTT (mean transit time), CBV (cerebral blood volume) and CBF (cerebral blood flow) maps.
- Look for areas of ↑ MTT. Maps of MTT generally show the largest area of abnormality and often reflect an overestimation of the final infarct.
- CBV maps tend to underestimate final infarct size.
- Cerebral blood volume maps closely correlate with changes in infarct size between initial and follow-up diffusion weighted MR imaging.

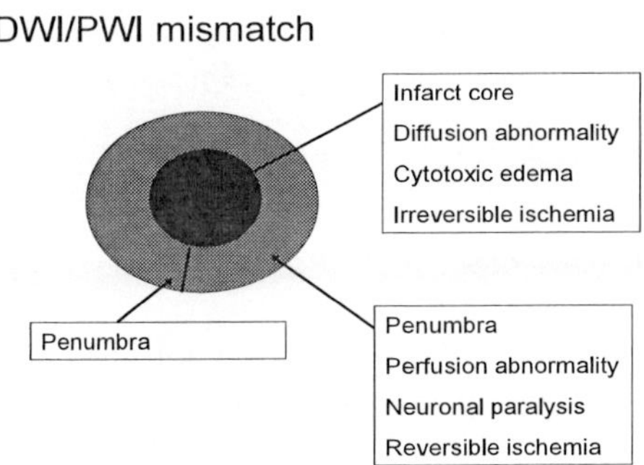

Comparison of DWI and PWI Abnormalities

- Lesion appears smaller on DWI than PWI – typically observed in large vessel strokes, suggests infarct core and penumbra. In acute stroke setting, a region that shows both DWI and PWI abnormalities is thought to represent irreversibly infarcted tissue. Regions that show PWI abnormalities with normal DWI likely represent viable ischemic tissue or penumbra.
- Lesion has same size on DWI and PWI – tissue is irreversibly infarcted and there is no penumbra. (fig 20)
- Lesion appears larger on DWI than on PWI – Usually associated with reperfusion of ischemic tissue. Size of the lesion on DWI does not usually change over time.

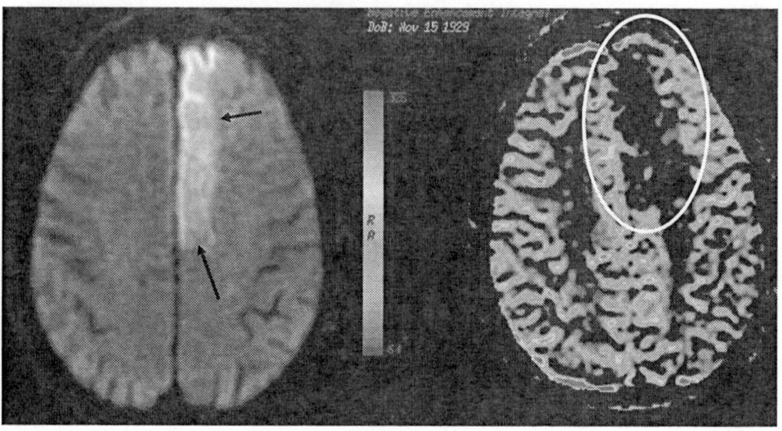

Figure 20. Axial DWI and PWI CBV map shows infarct in the left ACA territory with matching diffusion and perfusion abnormality.

15.2.3 Strokes in Specific Vascular Distributions

Supratentorial Infarcts

1) Middle cerebral artery (MCA)
    - 75-80 % of all strokes
    - Complete MCA infarct – basal ganglia, large wedge shaped area frontal, parietal and anterior temporal lobes extending from lateral ventricle to cortex.
    - MCA infarct distal to lenticulostriate arteries spare basal ganglia (fig 21).
    - Focal wedge shaped area involving cortex and subcortical white matter in branch occlusion.

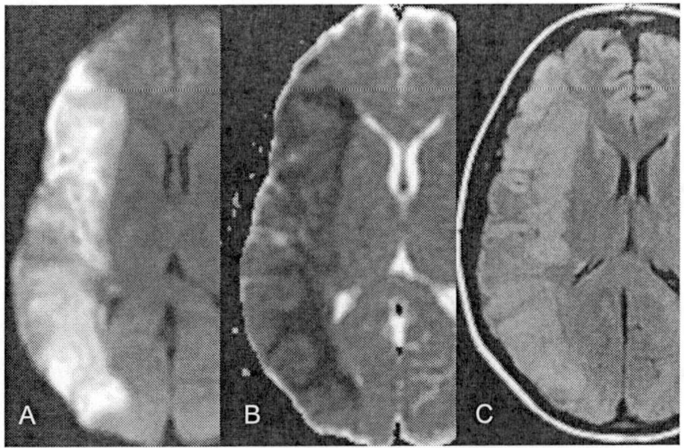

Figure 21. Axial DWI (A), ADC map (B) and FLAIR (C) in a right MCA infarct distal to the lenticulostriate arteries sparing the basal ganglia.

2) Posterior cerebral artery (PCA)
- Variable distribution, occipital and inferomedial temporal lobes, thalamus, posterior limb internal capsule, midbrain tegmentum (fig 22).

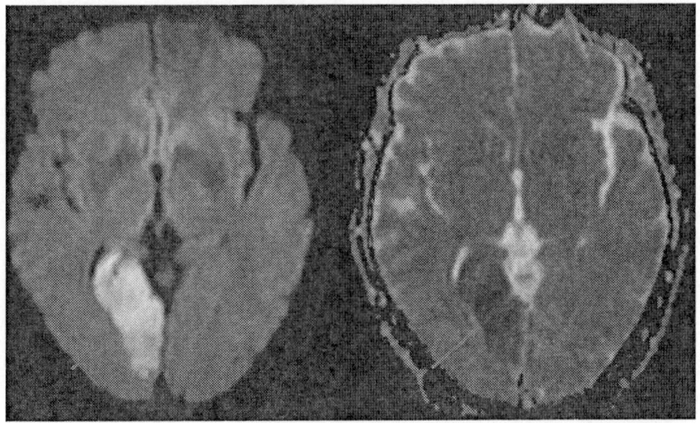

Figure 22. Axial DWI and ADC map demonstrates an acute right PCA infarct involving the occipital lobe.

3) Anterior cerebral artery (ACA)
- Less common, inferomedial frontal lobe, anterior 2/3 of medial hemisphere, corpus callosum (fig 23).

- Recurrent artery of Heubner, medial lenticulostriate arteries – septum pellucidum, genu corpus callosum, caudate head , anterior limb internal capsule.

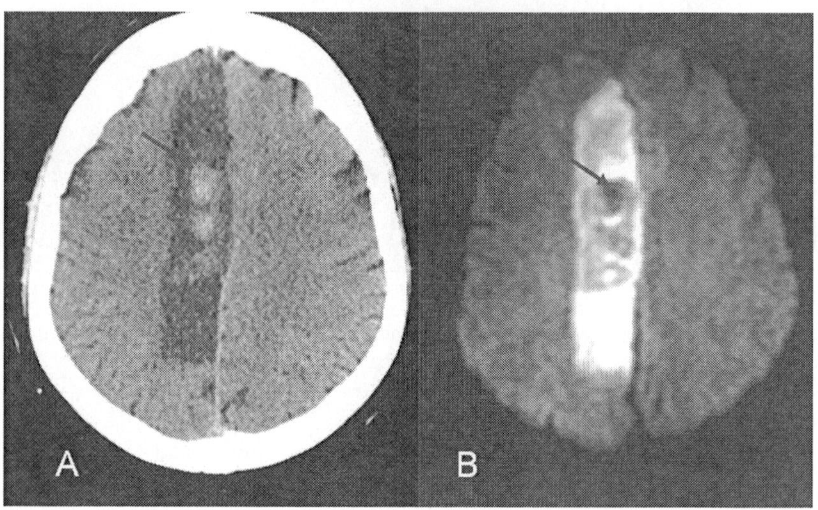

Figure 23. Axial CT (A) and DWI (B) demonstrates a classic ACA territory infarct. Note hyperdense areas on CT (arrow, low on Diffusion consistent with hemorrhagic conversion.

4) Lenticulostriate arteries
- Lacunar infarcts (< 1cm)
- Medial lenticulostriate arteries - from ACA, caudate head, anterior limb internal capsule.
- Lateral lenticulostriate arteries – from MCA, putamen, genu and superior aspect of posterior limb internal capsule.

5) Anterior choroidal artery
- Lateral midbrain, lateral thalamus, inferior posterior limb internal capsule

6) Thalamoperforating arteries
- Anterior thalamoperforating arteries – from posterior communicating artery, posterior hypothalamus, anterior thalamus.
- Posterior thalamoperforating arteries – from basilar bifurcation and posterior cerebral arteries, midbrain, posteromedial thalamus.

7) Watershed infarcts

- Peripheral – cortex between adjacent vascular territories, MCA/PCA, MCA/ACA.
- Deep – white matter between superficial cortical and deep perforating arteries in same vascular distribution.(fig 24)
- Caused by global/focal cerebral hypoperfusion secondary to decrease cardiac output, major vessel stenosis.

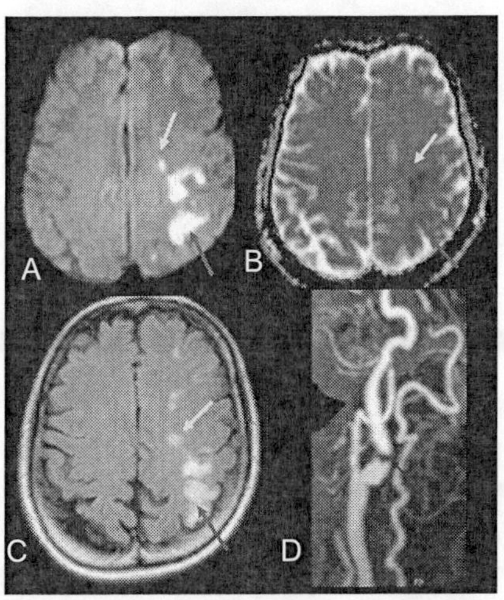

Figure 24. Axial DWI (A), ADC map (B), FLAIR (C) images demonstrate watershed infarcts which are peripheral in the cortex between MCA and PCA territories (red arrows) and deep white matter between superficial cortical and deep perforating arteries in same vascular distribution (yellow arrows). MIP reconstruction from carotid MRA shows high grade focal stenosis just distal to the origin of the left ICA (image D).

Infratentorial Infarcts

1) Basilar artery

- Pons, midbrain, mid/upper cerebellum, posteromedial thalami, occipital and medial temporal lobes (fig 25).
- "Top of basilar" infarct – posterior thalami bilateral, brainstem, occipital & medial temporal lobes
- Pontine perforating – small pontine infarcts

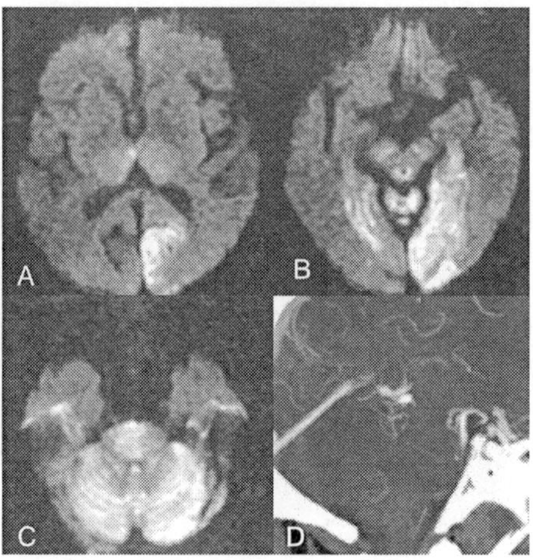

Figure 25. Axial DWI images (A,B &C) demonstrate acute infarcts involving the occipital lobes, medial temporal lobes, midbrain, pons and cerebellum due to basilar artery thrombosis. Sag MIP image (D) from CT angiogram study demonstrates non filling of the proximal and mid basilar artery (red arrow).

2) Superior cerebellar artery (SCA)
- Ipsilateral superior vermis, superolateral cerebellar hemisphere (fig 26).

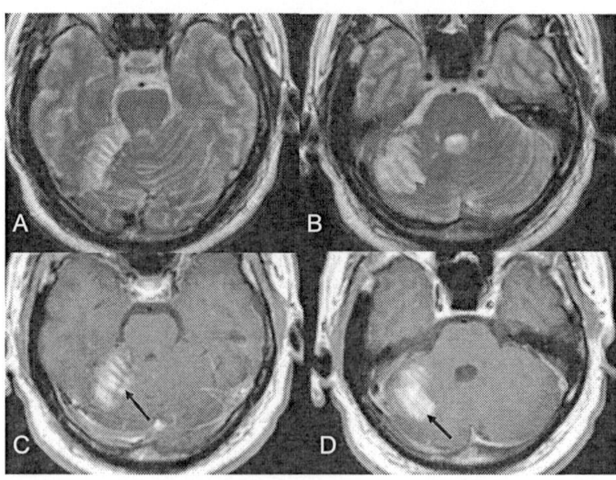

Figure 26. Axial T2 images (A & B) demonstrate a subacute right superior cerebellar artery territory infarct (red arrows). Axial post contrast T1 images (C & D) demonstrate characteristic gyral enhancement (black arrows).

3)   Posterior inferior cerebellar artery (PICA)
  •   May cause Wallenberg syndrome
  •   Dorsolateral medulla, posteroinferior cerebellum, inferior vermis(fig 27)

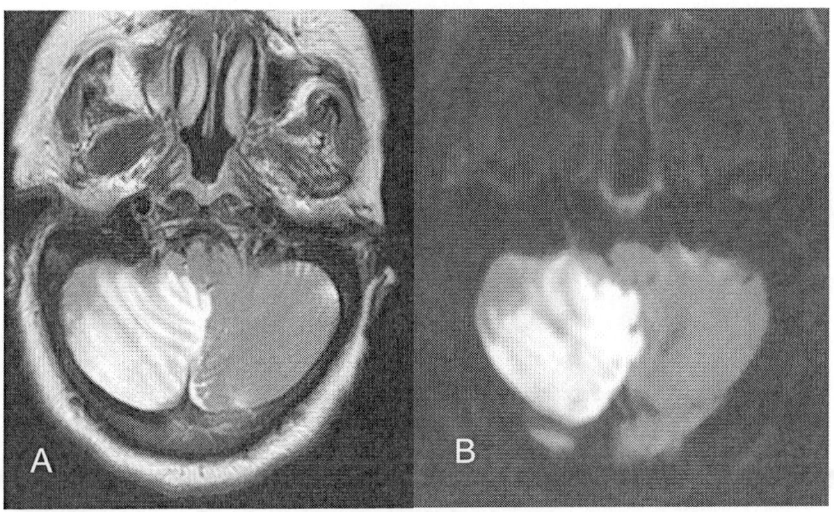

Figure 27. Axial FLAIR (A) and DWI (B) images demonstrate a right PICA territory infarct.

4)   Anterior inferior cerebellar artery (AICA)
  •   Anterolateral cerebellar hemisphere.

15.3 Intraparenchymal Hemorrhage

15.3.1 Evolution of Intracranial Hemorrhage on CT

- Hyperacute and acute – hyperdense mass with CT density increasing in the first few hours (fig 28). Average 60-80 HU. Isodense if low hemoglobin.
- Edema and mass effect initially mild.
- Active bleeding can give 'swirl' sign on NCCT – hypodense areas within hyperdense clot. On CECT active bleeding can cause contrast pooling.
- Subacute: 3-10 days – progressive decrease in attenuation. Edema peak around day 5.

- Chronic : > 10 days – decreasing attenuation approaching CSF, slit like residual cavity, calcification (fig 30).
- CECT – rim enhancement in subacute stage (fig 29).

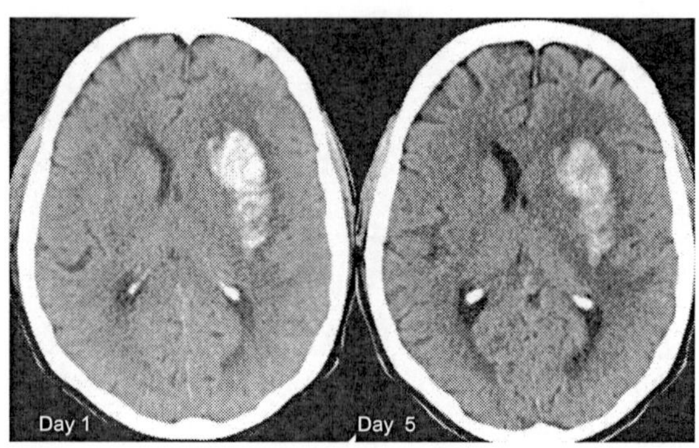

Figure 28. Axial CT images demonstrate an acute hematoma (day 1) involving the left external capsule and lateral putamen with minimal surrounding edema. On Day 5 notice some decrease in density of the hematoma with mild increase in surrounding edema which is typical in the subacute stage.

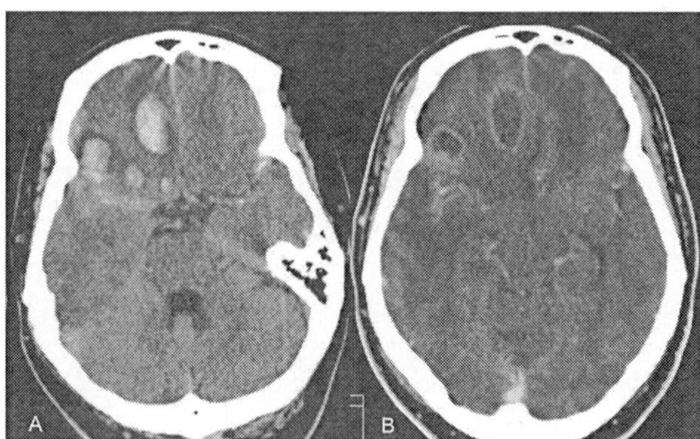

Figure 29. Subacute hemorrhage. Axial noncontrast CT (A) demonstrates post traumatic multiple hemorrhagic contusions in the right inferior frontal region. Followup CT with contrast (B) shows rim enhancement which can be seen in late subacute stage of the hemorrhage. This should not be mistaken for other ring enhancing lesions such as abscess, metastasis, granulomas.

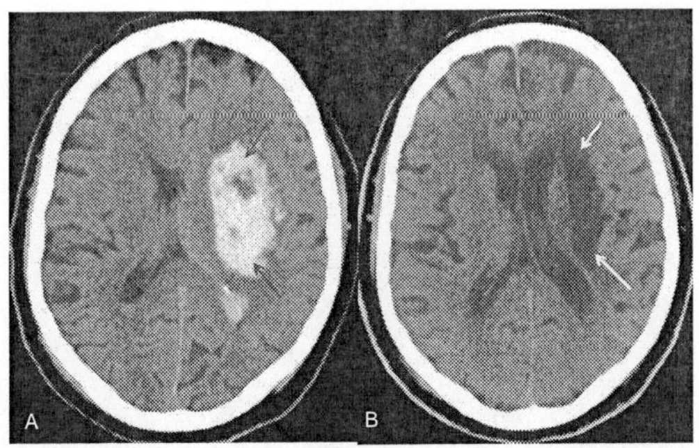

Figure 30. Axial CT demonstrates an acute hypertensive intracerebral hematoma in the left lentiform nucleus and external capsule (image A). Followup CT (image B) after 3 months demonstrates a slit like CSF density cavity in the region of the hemorrhage.

15.3.2 Evolution of Intracranial Hemorrhage on MR

- Different stages of intraparenchymal hemorrhage show variable signal intensity on T1 and T2 weighted images depending on the blood products (Table 5)
- T2* GRE (gradient echo) most sensitive for assessing acute intracerebral hemorrhage, hyperacute stage shows hypointense margin, becomes marked diffuse hypointense in acute stage. Late subacute/early chronic shows increasing low signal rim.
- DWI positive during subacute stage.
- Post infusion T1 images show peripheral enhancement within a few days and persist for months.

Table 5.

Stage	Time	Blood products	T1	T2
Hyperacute	< 24 hrs	Oxyhemoglobin	Isointense	Bright
Acute (fig 32)	1- 3 days	Deoxyhemoglobin	Isointense	Dark
Early subacute (fig 33)	> 3 days (days to 1 week)	Intracellular methhemoglobin	Bright	Dark
Late subacute (fig 34)	> 7 days (1 week to months)	Extracellular methhemoglobin	Bright	Bright
Chronic (fig 35)	> 14 days (months)	Hemosiderin	Dark	Dark

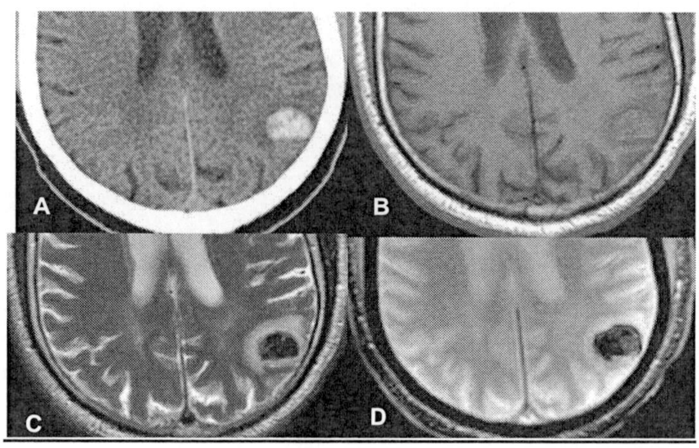

Figure 31. Acute intracerebral hemorrhage. Axial CT (A), T1 (B), T2 (C) and GRE (D) images demonstrate acute intracerebral hemorrhage which is hyperdense on CT. It is isointense on T1, hypointense on T2 and GRE due to deoxyhemoglobin.

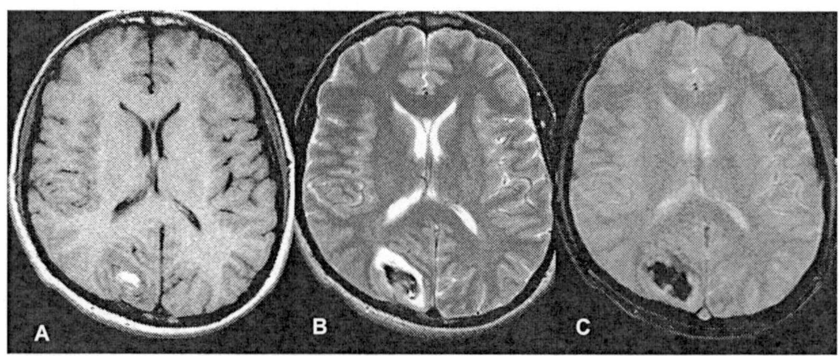

Figure 32. Early subacute hemorrhage. Axial T1 (A), T2 (B) and GRE (C) images demonstrates early subacute stage of hemorrhage which is hyperintense on T1, hypointense on T2 and GRE due to intracellular methmehomglobin.

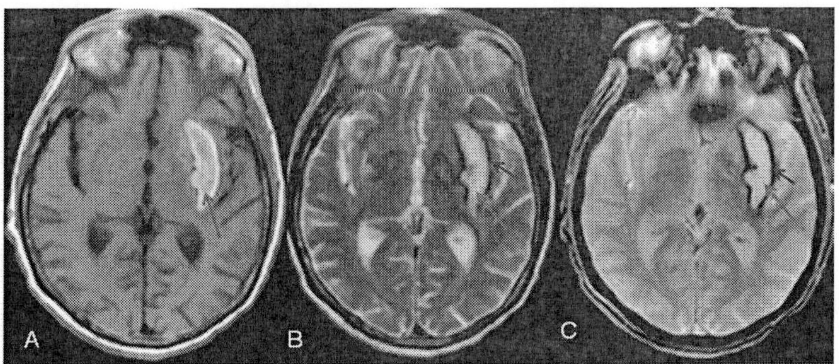

Figure 33. Late subacute hemorrhage. Axial T1 (A), T2 (B) and GRE (C) images demonstrate late subacute stage of intracerebral hemorrhage consisting of extracellular methhemoglobin. The hematoma is hyperintense on T1 and T2 (red arrows) and shows a hypointense rim on T2 and GRE (blue arrows).

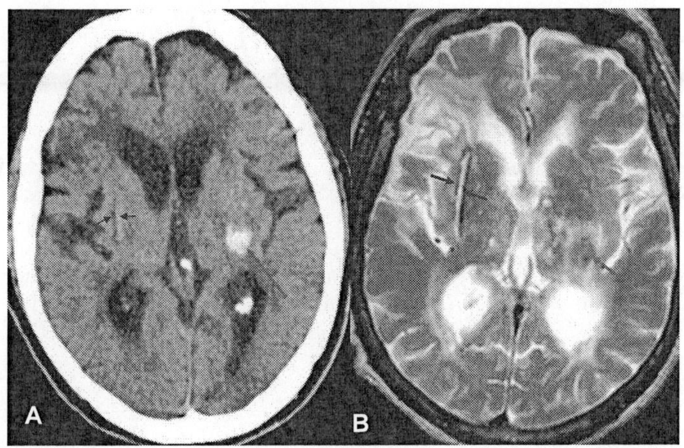

Figure 34. Axial CT (A) and T2 MR (B) images show a small acute hemorrhage in the left lentiform nucleus/internal capsule (red arrows). Note a slit like CSF density/intensity cavity in the right external capsule due to old hemorrhage. On T2 image there is a hypointense rim due to hemosiderin.

15.3.3 Causes of Spontaneous Nontraumatic Intracerebral Hemorrhage

1) Hypertension
   - Most common cause of nontraumatic ICH in adults
   - Putamen/external capsule most common site, other sites thalamus, pons, cerebellum, lobar (fig 35).
   - Small remote hemorrhages without correlative clinical events.

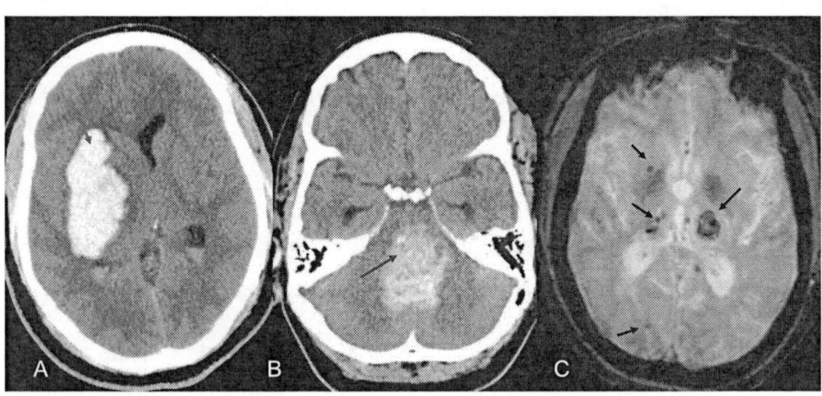

Figure 35 Hypertensive hemorrhage. Image (B) demonstrates a pontine hemorrhage with extension into fourth ventricle. Axial GRE (C) shows multiple small old hemorrhages predominantly in the thalami and basal ganglia in a patient with chronic poorly controlled hypertension.

2) Cerebral amyloid angiopathy
   - Common cause of nontraumatic ICH in normotensive adult.
   - Corticomedullary junction, lobar hemorrhages (fig 36).
   - Spares basal ganglia, brainstem.
   - Microbleeds on T2* GRE images.

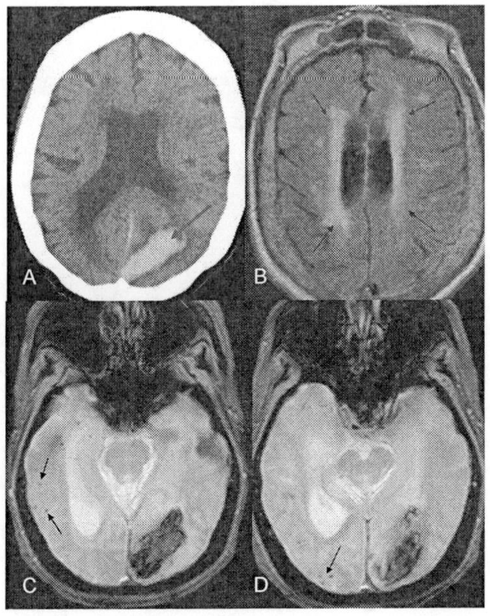

Figure 36 . Amyloid angiopathy. Axial CT (A) demonstrates lobar hemorrhage in the left occipital region. Axial FLAIR (B) shows periventricular white matter changes. Axial GRE images (C & D) demonstrates the lobar hemorrhage with multiple microhemorrhages in the subcortical region (black arrows)

3) Hemorrhagic infarction
   - Hemorrhagic transformation of initially ischemic infarct
   - May occur as complication of pregnancy, contraceptives, drug abuse, venous thrombosis.
4) Coagulopathies
   - Complication of anticoagulation therapy, blood dyscrasias
   - "growing" hematoma, fluid-fluid levels common (fig 37).

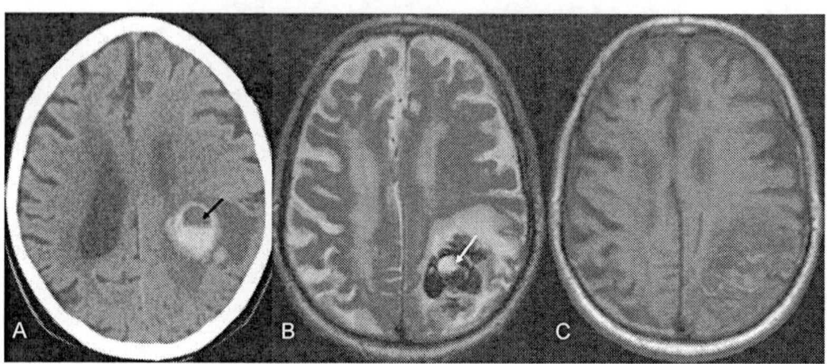

Figure 37. Axial CT (A), axial T2 (B) and axial T1(C) images show an acute hematoma with a fluid-fluid level (arrow).

5) Underlying neoplasm
- Primary tumors like anaplastic astrocytoma, glioblastoma multiforme.
- Metastatic tumors from lung and breast carcinoma, melanoma, choriocarcinoma, renal cell carcinoma (fig 38).
- Neoplastic hemorrhage often shows multiple stages of hematoma in same lesion, bizarre appearance, incomplete rim, nonhemorrhagic areas which enhance.

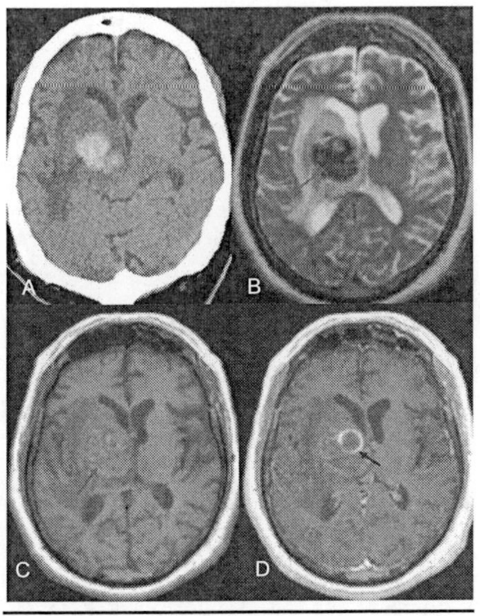

Figure 38. Hemorrhagic lung metastasis. Axial CT (A) demonstrates a lobular acute hemorrhage in the right basal ganglia and thalamus which is hypointense on T2 (B) and iso to hyperintense on T1 (C).There is extensive surrounding edema which is atypical for a primary acute intracerebral hemorrhage. Post contrast T1 (D) image demonstrates ring like enhancement (blue arrow) within the hemorrhage suggesting an underlying neoplasm.

6) Vascular malformation

- AVM- usually solitary, causes parenchymal hemorrhage (fig 39).
- Cavernous malformation – often multiple, MR shows clusters of hyperintensity on T1-weighted images with peripheral circumferential rim of hypointensity on T2. May have associated developmental venous anomaly, seen best after IV contrast.

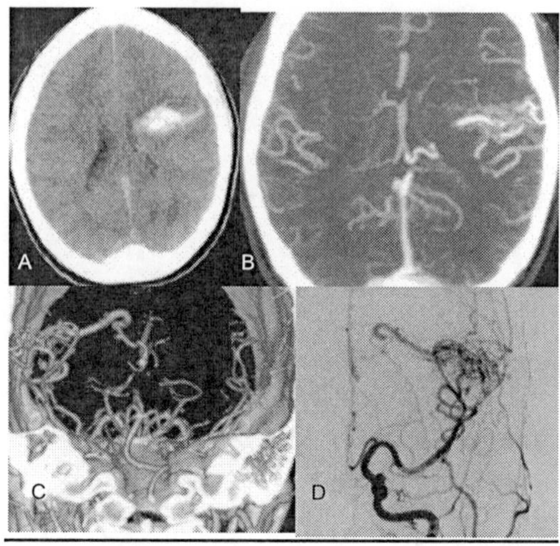

Figure 39. AVM rupture intracerebral hematoma. Axial CT (A) shows a lobulated hemorrhage in the left frontal region. Axial source images from CT angiogram study (B) shows a tangle of vessels in the region of the hemorrhage consistent with an AVM. 3D CTA image (C) and left ICA DSA study (D) show the nidus with the predominant arterial supply from the left MCA and a deep draining vein.

15.4 Nontraumatic Subarachnoid Hemorrhage

15.4.1 Etiologies of Nontraumatic Subarachnoid Hemorrhage

- Aneurysm, intracranial vascular malformations, benign perimesencephalic subarachnoid hemorrhage, bleeding diasthesis, iatrogenic coagulopathy
- Most common cause is a ruptured aneurysm.

15.4.2 Aneurysmal Subarachnoid Hemorrhage (SAH)

- Disribution depends on location of subarachnoid hemorrhage
- Anterior communicating artery – anterior interhemispheric fissure (fig 40)
- Middle cerebral artery – sylvian fissure

- Posterior communicating artery – suprasellar cistern, sylvian fissure, ambient cistern asymmetric to the side of ruptured aneurysm (fig 41)
- Basilar tip, superior cerebellar, posterior inferior cerebellar, vertebral artery – prepontine cistern, foramen magnum (fig 42).
- CT positive in 95 % of cases in 1st 24 hrs, hyperdense sulci, early hydrocephalus.
- CTA 90-95 % positive if aneurysm $\geq$ 2 mm.
- MR imaging – FLAIR most sensitive sequence. Difficult to see on T2 weighted images. CSF may appear isointense or midly hyperintense on T1.
- TOF MR angiogram 85-95 % sensitive for aneurysms $\geq$ 3 mm.
- Digitial subtraction angiogram (DSA) is gold standard.
- CT with CTA best initial imaging tool. DSA if CTA negative. MR if DSA and CTA negative.

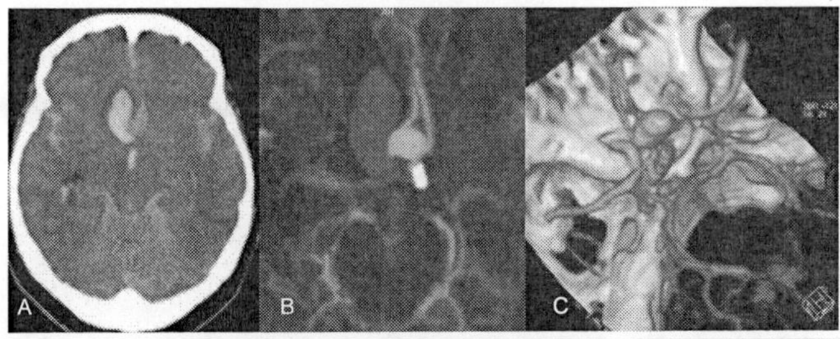

Figure 40. Acom aneurysm. Axial CT (A) shows acute right inferior frontal lobar hemorrhage and subarachnoid hemorrhage predominantly in the anterior interhemispheric fissure. Axial CTA MIP image (B) and 3D volume rendered image (C) show a well defined Acom aneurysm

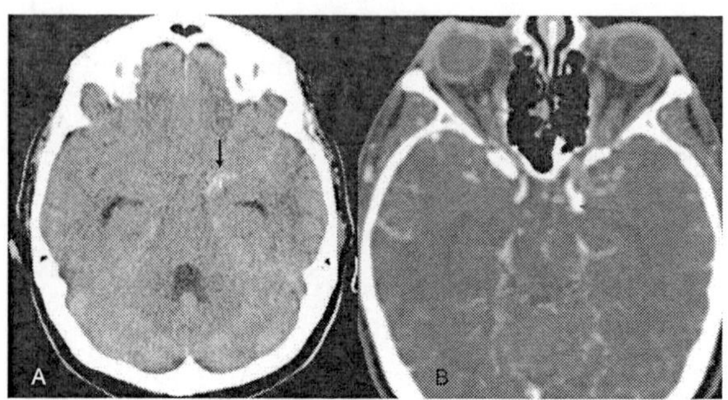

Figure 41. Pcom aneurysm. Axial CT (A) shows acute subarachnoid hemorrhage in the left lateral aspect of the suprasellar cistern and left sylvian fissue. Axial CTA MIP image (B) shows a saccular Pcom aneurysm (red arrow)

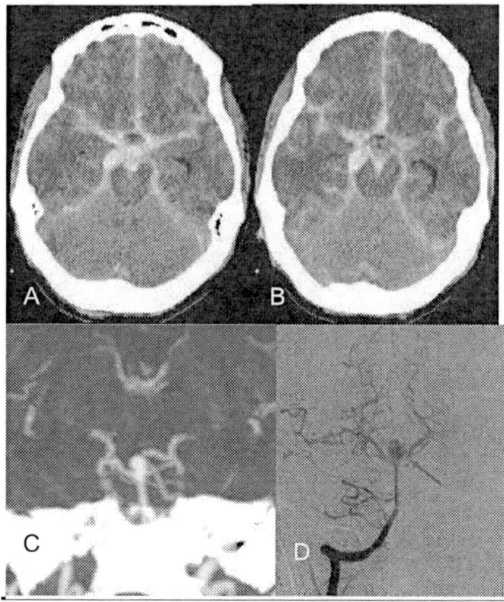

Figure 42. Basilar tip aneurysm. Axial CT (A & B) demonstrates extensive acute subarachnoid hemorrhage. Coronal CTA MIP image (C) and right vertebral injection DSA (D) show a saccular basilar tip aneurysm.

15.4.3 Benign Perimesencephalic Hemorrhage

- Small SAH localized to interpeduncular cistern (fig 43).
- Presumed venous in etiology
- CTA/DSA negative

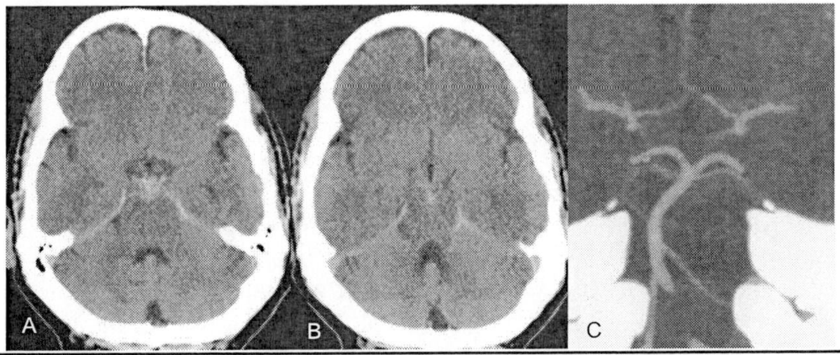

Figure 43. Benign perimesencephalic hemorrhage. Axial CT images (A & B) demonstrate small amount of acute subarachnoid hemorrhage restricted to the interpeduncular cistern. Coronal CTA MIP image C shows a normal basilar tip.

15.4.4 "Pseudo-Subarachnoid Hemorrhage"

- Severe diffuse cerebral edema causing basal cisterns to appear relatively hyperdense (fig 44).
- Intrathecal contrast and meningitis can cause increase attenuation of CSF mimicking SAH.

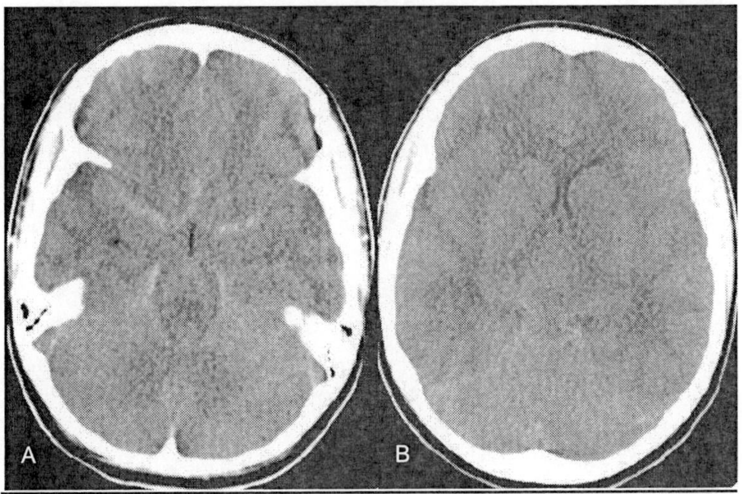

Figure 44. Pseudo subarachnoid hemorrhage. Axial CT images demonstrate diffuse cerebral edema with effacement of the basal cisterns and sulci. The cisterns appear relatively hyperdense to the brain parenchyma mimicking subarachnoid hemorrhage.

15.5 Venous Infarction

15.5.1 Dural Sinus Thrombosis

- Superior sagittal sinus more commonly involved than transverse and sigmoid.
- NECT hyperdense sinus, with or without venous infarct.
- "Empty delta" sign due to enhancing dura surrounding nonenhancing thrombus on CECT and post infusion T1 MR (fig 45).
- CT venogram filling defect due to thrombus in dural sinus.
- Variable signal intensity of thrombus on T1 and T2 weighted MR images depending on the stage. Acute thrombus is isointense on T1 and hypointense on T2, subacute thrombus is hyperintense on T1 and T2, chronic thrombus is isointense on T1 and hyperintense on T2 (fig 46).
- T2 * gradient echo images thrombus usually "blooms"
- MR venogram can be performed using Phase contrast, 2D TOF or postcontrast sequences. Absence of flow related signal in occluded sinus.
- Important pitfall – T1 hyperintense thrombus can mimic flow related signal on 2D TOF MR venogram.
- Venous infarction in adjacent brain parenchyma – gyral swelling, vasogenic edema, foci of hemorrhage.
- NECT, CECT and CT venogram as initial screening for dural sinus thrombosis
- If CT is negative then MR with MR venogram.
- Digital subtraction angiogram is gold standard.

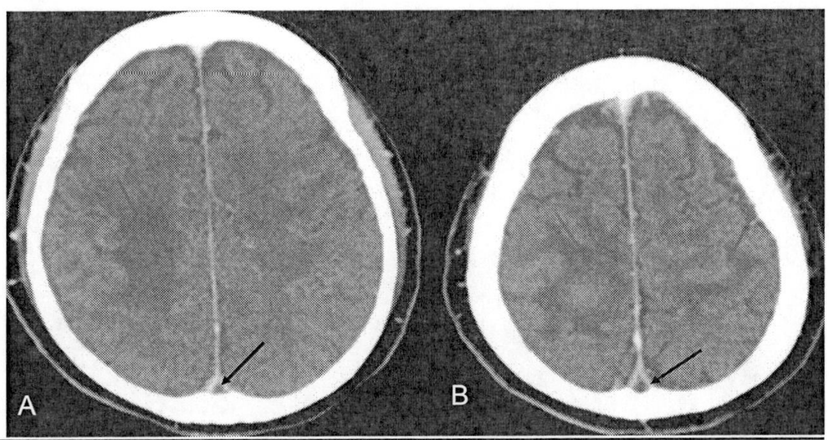

Figure 45. "Empty delta sign". Axial post contrast CT images demonstrate "empty delta sign". There is a filling defect in the superior sagittal sinus (black arrows) with enhancement of the adjacent dura. Note edema with subtle hemorrhage in the fronto-parietal white matter due to venous infarct (red arrows).

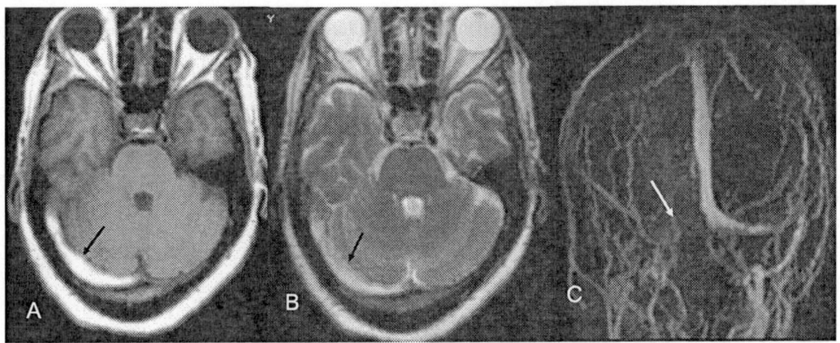

Figure 46. Axial T1 (A) and T2 (B) images demonstrate a subacute thrombus in the right transverse sinus (black arrows). Coronal MIP image MR venogram (C) shows absence of the normal flow related signal in the right transverse sinus (white arrow).

15.5.2 Cortical Venous Thrombosis

- Usually seen in presence of dural sinus thrombosis. Isolated cortical venous thrombosis less common.
- "Cord" sign – hyperdense vein on NECT (fig 47).

- T2* gradient echo most sensitive sequence for thrombus which appears hypointense cord like (fig 48).
- With or without venous infarction in adjacent brain parenchyma.
- Contrast enhanced MR venogram better than TOF MR venogram for smaller veins.

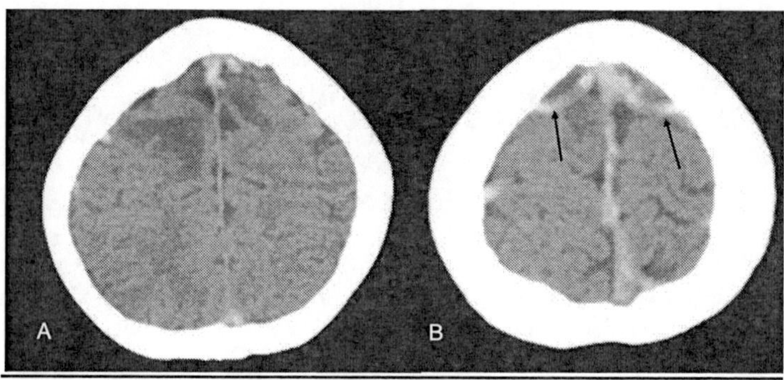

Figure 47. "Cord sign". Axial noncontrast CT images show hyperdense cortical veins due to thrombosis (black arrow). There is mild edema in the frontal subcortical white matter.

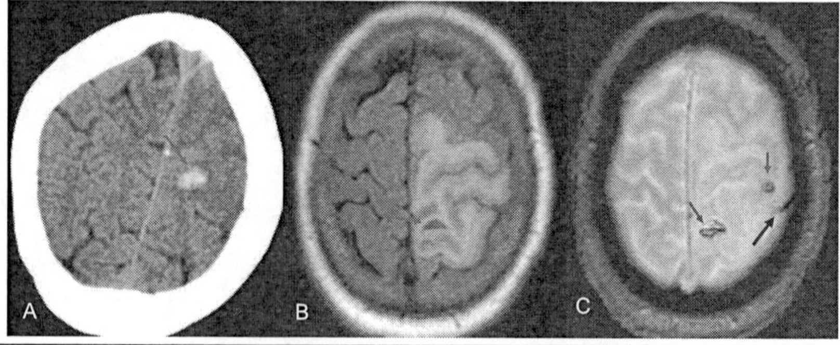

Figure 48. Axial CT image shows a small hemorrhage in the left frontoparietal subcortical region with surrounding edema. The vasogenic edema is better appreciated on the axial FLAIR image (B). Axial GRE image (C) shows small hemorrhages in the left fronto-parietal region (red arrows). Note thrombosed cord like cortical vein with susceptibility changes (blue arrow).

15.5.3 Deep Cerebral Venous Thrombosis

- Internal cerebral vein thrombosis which may extend into vein of Galen, straight sinus.
- NECT high density internal cerebral veins, low density thalami and basal ganglia with/without patchy petechial hemorrhages.
- CECT and post infusion MR shows filling defect in the involved deep venous system with dilated medullary and subependymal veins.

15.6 Imaging Arterial Dissection

15.6.1 Intracranial Dissection

- Dissection is intramural hematoma extending along the vessel wall
- Dissecting aneurysm is dissection with aneurysmal dilation contained by adventitia
- Pseudoaneurysm is lumen contained by thrombus outside vessel wall.
- Vertebral arteries most common
- May present as basal subarachnoid hemorrhage
- MR -Mural hematoma appears hyperintense with central flow void giving "Target" or "crescent" sign (fig 49).
- CT angiogram, MR angiogram or DSA may show mural thrombus or enlarged vessel due to dissecting aneurysm, long segment narrowing or tapered occlusion. Intraluminal flap best seen on DSA.

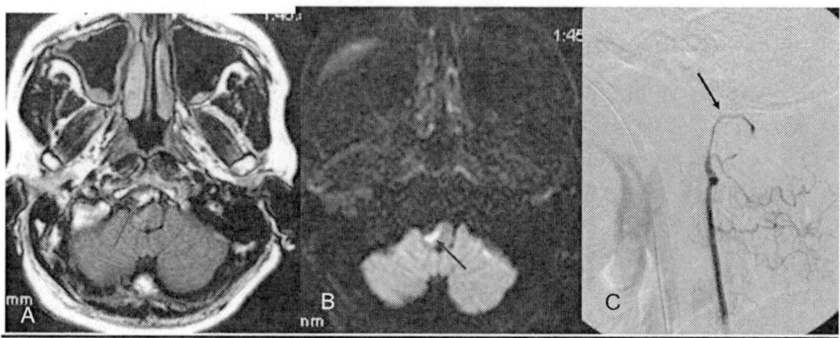

Figure 49. Axial T1 (A) demonstrates hyperintense signal along the distal right vertebral artery (red arrow) due to mural thrombus. Axial diffusion (B) shows acute lateral medullary infarct (blue arrow). Lateral DSA projection right vertebral injection shows gradual tapering and occlusion of the distal right vertebral artery due to dissection.

15.6.2 Extracranial Dissection

- Extracranial dissection occurs at sites unusual for atherosclerotic disease.
- Internal carotid artery from the distal carotid bulb to the skull base.
- Vertebral dissection most common at C1-2 level.
- CT brain may show infarcts in arterial territories(fig 50)
- Post contrast CT may show linear luminal filling defect due to intimal flap or false lumen.
- MR images with fat suppression show "target" or "crescent" sign due to intramural hematoma. Intramural hematoma is circumferential and eccentric.
- Acute dissection is isointense to slightly hyperintense on T1 and hypointense on T2.
- Subacute dissection is hyperintense on T1 and T2 (fig 51).
- CT angiogram, MR angiogram and DSA may show tapered narrowing "string" sign, pseudoaneurysm which may be oval and parallel to artery.
- Intimal flap may be seen at the proximal margin of dissection.
- CTA is more sensitive and specific than MR/MRA for vertebral dissections (fig 52).

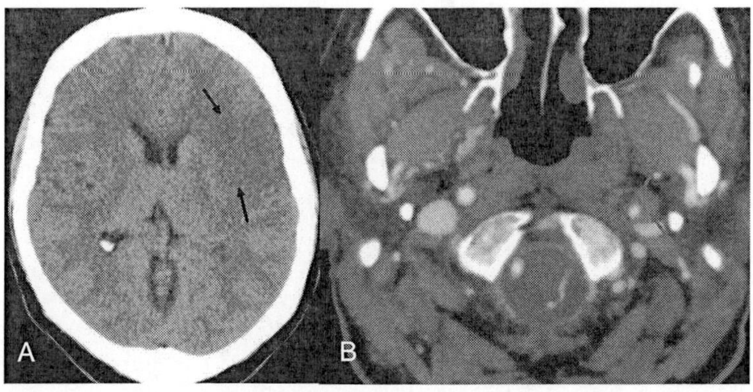

Figure 50. Axial noncontrast CT (A) shows an acute infarct in the left frontal region in the distribution of the left MCA. Axial CT angiogram image (B) shows eccentric soft tissue in the distal cervical carotid artery due to dissection (red arrows).

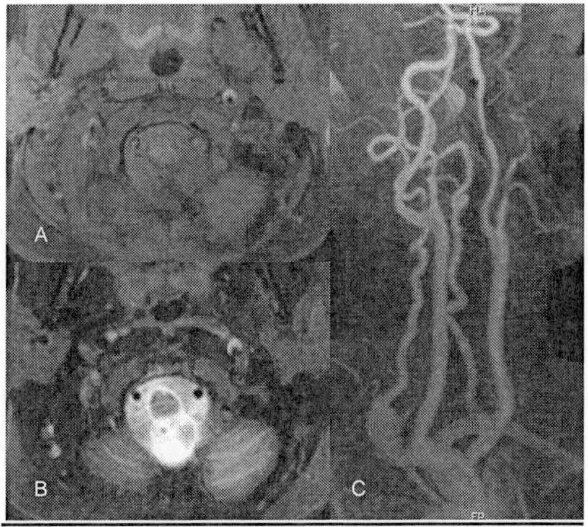

Figure 51. Axial MR T1 (A) and T2 (B) with fat suppression show hyperintense eccentric thrombus (blue arrows) surrounding the central flow void in this patient with traumatic distal cervical dissection. MR angiogram MIP image (C) shows narrowing with gradual tapering of the distal left cervical carotid artery (red arrow).

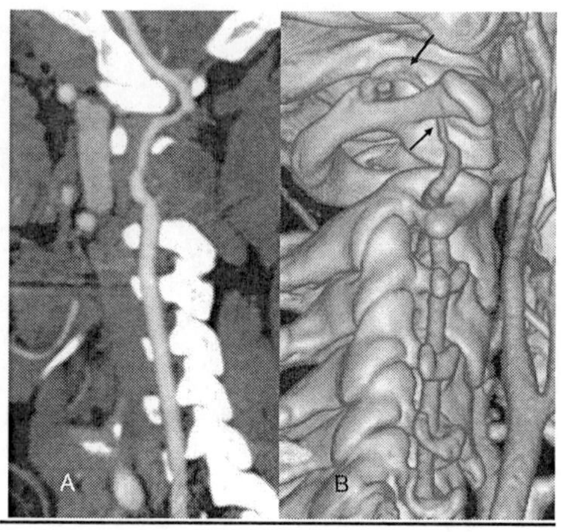

Figure 52. Vertebral dissection. Sagittal MIP image (A) and 3D VRT image (B) from CT angiogram study shows narrowing and irregularity of the V3 segment due to arterial dissection.

References

[1]   Rowley HA. *The four Ps of acute stroke imaging: parenchyma, pipes, perfusion, and penumbra.* AJNR Am J Neuroradiol. 2001 Apr;22(4):599-601.

[2]   Lev MH, Farkas J, Gemmete JJ, Hossain ST, Hunter GJ, Koroshetz WJ, Gonzalez RG. *Acute stroke: improved nonenhanced CT detection--benefits of soft-copy interpretation by using variable window width and center level settings.* Radiology. 1999 Oct;213(1):150-5.

[3]   Kim JJ, Fischbein NJ, Lu Y, Pham D, Dillon WP. *Regional angiographic grading system for collateral flow: correlation with cerebral infarction in patients with middle cerebral artery occlusion.* Stroke. 2004 Jun;35(6):1340-4. Epub 2004 Apr 15.

[4]   Camargo EC, Furie KL, Singhal AB, Roccatagliata L, Cunnane ME, Halpern EF, Harris GJ, Smith WS, Gonzalez RG, Koroshetz WJ, Lev MH. *Acute brain infarct: detection and delineation with CT angiographic source images versus nonenhanced CT scans.* Radiology. 2007 Aug;244(2):541-8. Epub 2007 Jun 20.

[5]   Barber PA, Demchuk AM, Hudon ME, Pexman JH, Hill MD, Buchan AM. *Hyperdense sylvian fissure MCA "dot" sign: A CT marker of acute ischemia.* Stroke. 2001 Jan;32(1):84-8.

[6]   Mullins ME. *The hyperdense cerebral artery sign on head CT scan.* Semin Ultrasound CT MR. 2005 Dec;26(6):394-403. Review.

[7]   Rodallec MH, Marteau V, Gerber S, Desmottes L, Zins M. *Craniocervical arterial dissection: spectrum of imaging findings and differential diagnosis.* Radiographics. 2008 Oct;28(6):1711-28. Review.

[8]   Dimmick SJ, Faulder KC. *Normal variants of the cerebral circulation at multidetector CT angiography.* Radiographics. 2009 Jul-Aug;29(4):1027-43. Review.

[9]   de Lucas EM, Sánchez E, Gutiérrez A, Mandly AG, Ruiz E, Flórez AF, Izquierdo J, Arnáiz J, Piedra T, Valle N, Bañales I, Quintana F. *CT protocol for acute stroke: tips and tricks for general radiologists.* Radiographics. 2008 Oct;28(6):1673-87. Review.

[10]   Srinivasan A, Goyal M, Al Azri F, Lum C. *State-of-the-art imaging of acute stroke.* Radiographics. 2006 Oct;26 Suppl 1:S75-95. Review.

[11]   Tomandl BF, Klotz E, Handschu R, Stemper B, Reinhardt F, Huk WJ, EberhardtKE, Fateh-Moghadam S. *Comprehensive imaging of ischemic stroke with multisection CT.* Radiographics. 2003 May-Jun;23(3):565-92. Review..

[12]   Provenzale JM. *Nontraumatic neurologic emergencies: imaging findings and diagnostic pitfalls.* Radiographics. 1999 Sep-Oct;19(5):1323-31.

[13]   Beauchamp NJ Jr, Ulug AM, Passe TJ, van Zijl PC. *MR diffusion imaging in stroke: review and controversies.* Radiographics. 1998 Sep-Oct;18(5):1269-83; discussion 1283-5. Review.

[14]   Leach JL, Fortuna RB, Jones BV, Gaskill-Shipley MF. *Imaging of cerebral venous thrombosis: current techniques, spectrum of findings, and diagnostic pitfalls.* Radiographics. 2006 Oct;26 Suppl 1:S19-41; discussion S42-3. Review.

In: Handbook of Stroke and Neurocritical Care   ISBN: 978-61324-786-0
Editor: V. H. Lee   © 2012 Nova Science Publishers, Inc.

Chapter XVI

Neurosonology

Vivien Lee

Department of Neurological Sciences,
Section of Stroke and Neurocritical care,
Rush University Medical Center, Chicago, IL, USA

Background Physics and Principles

1) Frequency (Hz) = number of complete sinusoidal waves (cycles) that occur during 1 second
2) Period = time it takes for one complete cycle to occur
   a) Period = $\dfrac{1}{\text{Frequency (Hz)}}$
3) Wavelength is the length of space over which one cycle occurs
   a) Wavelength (m) = $\dfrac{\text{propagation speed (m/sec)}}{\text{Frequency (Hz)}}$
4) Doppler effect is the change or shift in the frequency or wavelength of a wave due to relative movement between the sound source or scatterer and the receiver. This effect occurs for most waveforms, including sound. The change in frequency is called the Doppler frequency shift
5) When applied in vascular ultraonography, including TCD, to study moving red cells, the Doppler effect can be used to

         determine the speed and direction (velocity) of flow in blood vessels

6) Accurate estimation of the Doppler frequency shift and reflector speed requires knowledge of the angle formed between the sound beam and the flow direction, called the angle of insonation. The cosine of the angle of insonation (cos 0) is used to correct for the apparent decrease in the Doppler frequency shifrt when the direction of the ultrasonic beam is not identical to the flow direction

7) In current applications of TCD, a 0 degree angle of insonation is assumed

8) In extracranial carotid ultrasound, probe position is 60 degrees to skin.

Transcranial Doppler (TCD)

Introduction

1) Transcranial Doppler (TCD) is a noninvasive ultrasound technique that measures blood flow velocities in the basal cerebral arteries

2) In 1982 Dr. Rune Aaslid, a Norwegian physicist, demonstrated that by combining a lower emitting 2MHz frequency and pulsed Doppler technique, insonation of the cerebral vessels was possible through selected thin cranial foramina

3) Transcranial color imaging (TCI) was introduced by a German Neurologist, Dr. Ullrich Bogdahn in 1992. This advancement allows for visualization of the intracranial vessels and a spectral Doppler analysis. Color imaging allows for identification of structural landmarks that help locate and confirm the identity of vessels.

TCD Examination Technique [1]

1) Normal midline is considered to be 75mmm. Insonation at depths greater than this is considered contralateral. See Table 1.

Table 1. Summary of TCD Vessels characteristics

Vessel	Depth (mm)	Flow (towards tranducer)	Velocity (mean)	Window
MCA	45-65	towards	55 +/- 12	Transtemporal
ACA	65-70	away	50 +/-11	Transtemporal
PCA	65-70	towards	39 +/-10	Transtemporal
ACA/MCA bifurcation	55-65	bidirectonal	---	Transtemporal
OA	40-60	Toward	20-30	Transorbital
Carotid siphon	60-80	Bidirectional, away or toward	47 +/- 14	Transorbital
VA	60-70	Bidirectional or away	38 +/-10	Transoccipital
BA	75-100	away	41+/-10	Transoccipital

Transtemporal Window

1) temporal window can be localized above the zygomatic arch close to the vertical portion of the zygomatic bone or close to the pinna of the ear.
2) vessels that can be examined through this window include the MCA, PCA, and the terminal portion of the ICA.
   a) The ACOM or PCOM can be sampled at times, depending upon the hemodynamic variability of the circle of willis
3) Middle Cerebral Artery (MCA)
   a) found at depths of 45mm to 65mm.
   b) direction of flow is towards the transducer.
4) Anterior Cerebral Artery (ACA)
   a) found deeper than the point of the MCA/ACA bifurcation. It is usually insonated at depths of 65-70mm
   b) Flow direction is away from the transducer
5) bifurcation of the terminal internal carotid artery (ICA) and ACA
   a) usually be found between 65-75mm of depth
6) Posterior Cerebral Artery (PCA) can be found by redirecting the ultrasound transducer inferiorly and posteriorly from the point of the terminal bifurcation.
   a) signal is obtained at a depth of 65-70mm.
   b) flow direction is toward the transducer.

7) Considerations:
   a) depths of insonation describe above can vary slightly depending on skull size. The normal depth considered to be midline is 75mm. Insonation at depths greater than this is considered contralateral
   b) Absence of temporal windows due to hyperostosis is found to be 10%. This occurs in the elderly and African Americans.

Transorbital Window

1) power output of the doppler system is decreased to 10-20%
   a) This will reduce the ultrasonic exposure of the eye.
2) orbital window allows for direct insonation of the ipsilateral ophthalmic artery and ICA siphon
3) The Ophthalmic artery (OA) can be found beginning at shallow depths of 40-50mm with flow direction towards the probe.
   a) waveform is characterized by low diastolic velocities. This is because the vessel supplies a muscular capillary bed of very high resistance
4) internal carotid siphon consists of parasellar, genu & supraclinoid portions of the ICA.
   a) At a depth of 60-70mm flow may vary, depending on the segment of the vessel being sampled.
   b) lower portion of the siphon (parasellar) produces a signal towards the transducer.
   c) Sampling the genu will result in a bi-directional flow pattern.
   d) supraclinoid portion of the ICA siphon produces signal directed away from the transducer.
5) Transorbital window produces concern regarding adverse effects on the eye, specifically cataract formation.
   a) Limiting the length of exposure and decreasing the power to 10-25% of the maximum may help prevent this complication.
   b) No cases of cataract formation related to TCD have been reported
   c)

Transoccipital Window

1) naturally occurring window lies between the atlas and the base of the skull and is called the foramen magnum.
2) Insonation through the occiput allows for sampling of the intracranial vertebral arteries as well as the basilar artery, from its origin of the level of its bifurcation into the posterior cerebral arteries
3) Veretbral arteries (VA) are found at depths of 60-70mm and the direction of flow may be either bi-directional or away from the transducer.
   a) vertebral artery forms a genu at the cervical vertebra
4) Basilar artery (BA) can be found between 75-100mm.
   a) Flow velocities in the basilar artery are away from the transducer.

Tcd Interpretation

1) Velocities are measured in centimeters per second (cm/sec)
2) Measurement of peak systolic and end diastolic enable a mean flow velocity to be obtained
3) Mean flow velocity (MV) =_PSV + (EDV x 2)/3 (Figure 1)
4) Once a mean flow velocity is determined, a pulsatility index (PI) can be calculated
5) Pulsatility index refers to the relationship existing between the cardiac output and the peripheral vascular resistance
   a) Pulsatility index (PI) = (PV – EDV)/ MV
      (i) estimates downstream vascular resistance
   b) The normal PI throughout the entire circle of Willis is 0.8-1.2
      (i) Low resistance beds have low PI
      (ii) Increased PI is associated with
         1) distal resistance
         2) Increased ICP and decreased CPP
6) Flow Velocity Ratio (Vmca/Vica) of Aaslid and Lindegaard
   a) Lindegaard ratio compares extracranial ICA vs intracranial
   b) MCA vel/Caortid Vel
   c) <3 normal (or distal MCA vasospasm)
   d) 3-6 MCA proximal vasospasm
   e) 6 severe proximal MCA vasospasm

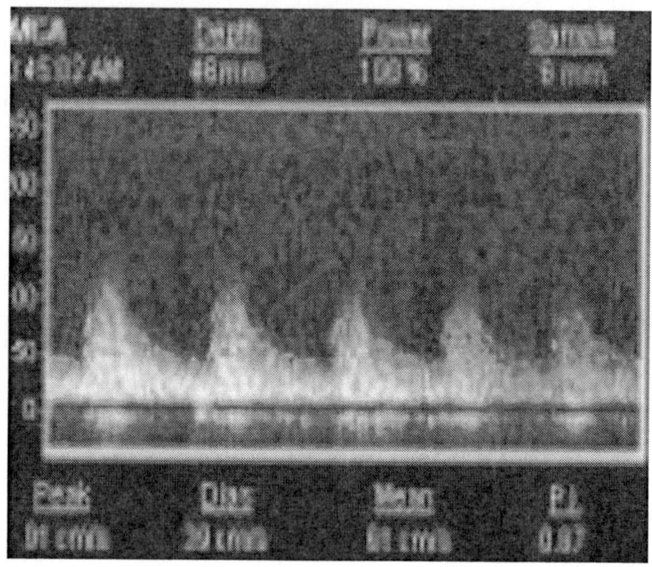

Figure 1. Normal MCA TCD waveform.

Table 2. TCD Table. Presumed Vasospasm

Vessel	Possible (cm/sec)	Probable (cm/sec)	Definite (cm/sec)
Intracranial ICA	80	125	>200
MCA	120	150	>200
VA	60	80	>105
BA	75	85	>140
PCA	80	120	>160

TCD Clinical Applications

1) Settings in which TCD clinical utility is established [2]
   a) Screening of children with Sickle cell screen (age 2-15) for assessing stroke risk3
   b) Detection and monitoring of angiographic vasospasm after SAH
2) Vasospasm

    a) Vasospasm predominates during the first 2 weeks of Subarachnoid hemorrhage (SAH) usually within 7-10 days.

    b) Spasm in the MCA is considered severe when mean blood flow velocities exceed 200 cm/sec.

        (i) 'Critical > 200cm/sec MCA is $\geq$50% angiographic spasm

3) Sickle cell disease

    a) STOP (Stroke Prevention Trial in Sickle Cell Anemia)- used prophylactic re-cell transfusions in children identified by TCD as being high risk for stroke [3]

    b) The use of TCD in sickle cell anemia has been validated in the STOP trial which demonstrated that transfusions greatly reduce the risk of a first stroke in children with sickle cell anemia when TCD MCA velocities > 200cm/sec [3]

    c) STOP 2 showed discontinuation of transfusion for the prevention of stroke in children with SCD results in a high rate of reversion to abnormal blood-flow velocities on dopple studies and stroke [4]

4) Cerebral Circulatory Arrest

    a) When intracranial pressure increases to a point at which blood flow into the peripheral circulation is prevented, a characteristic flow pattern emerges. The lack of peripheral perfusion results in a "to-and-fro" pattern, called oscillatory flow revereberation.

    b) AAN practice parameters accept the use of TCDs as *confirmatory* testing for brain death

    c) Brain death is a clinical diagnosis

        (i) any of the confirmatory tests may produce similar results in patients with catastrophic brain damage who do not (yet) fulfill the clinical criteria of brain death.

    d) 10% of patients may not have temporal insonation windows. Therefore, the initial absence of Doppler signals cannot be interpreted as consistent with brain death.

    e) Small systolic peaks in early systole without diastolic flow or reverberating flow, indicating very high vascular resistance associated with greatly increased intracranial pressure.

    f) Brain death testing with TCDs

(i)   Both anterior and posterior circulation must be evaluated (bilateral MCAs and BA)

(ii) Record measurements only after a stable MV and waveform are observed for more than 30 seconds

(iii) If flow velocity (FV) differs by more than 2 cm/sec during the initial period of observation or between the two trials, the study may be inadequate

(iv) Distal Cerebrovascular resistance is very high (as measured by PIs)

(v)   Patterns Seen with Brain Death

    1)   Short systolic spikes

        a)   The only detectable signals are brief anterograde spikes in the waveform that last for a brief portion of the cardiac cycle (without diastolic flow or reversal of blood flow in diastole)

5)   Absence of TCD signal

        a)   No intracranial TCD signal is detectable. Oscillating blood flow in the extracranial internal carotid artery is usually detectable with submandibular insonation

        b)   This pattern has been associated with extracranial angiographic arrest of flow in all vessels

        c)   Use of the absence of TCD signal to confirm intracranial circulatory arrest should be restricted to patients who previously have had demonstrable TCD waveforms. Otherwise, the absence of TCD signal could be the result of a thickened skull and inadequate cranial windows.

5)   Vasomotor Reactivity (VMR)

    a)   Vasomotor reactivity (VMR) measures autoregulatory response to a vasodilatory challenge with TCD

        (i)   Changes in BFV that accompany the rise in CO_2 associated with breath-holding (BH) are assessed distal to stenotic vessel

        (ii) Impaired VMR identifies a subgroup of patients at high-risk for stroke [6]

    b)   Breath holding (BH) method

(i) breath-holding method offers a convenient, well-tolerated screening method of assessing carbon dioxide reactivity BHI=_(MFV BH) – (MFV Baseline) X (100/ time of BH)

(ii) MFV Baseline

(iii) BHI of < 0.69 will be defined as impaired[7]

(iv) Protocol

1) If MCA is stenotic vessel, insonation should be distal to stenosis.

2) The patient should breathe normally until mean flow velocities (MFVs) have stabilized. Record MFV baseline values.

3) After a normal inspiration patient holds breath for 30 seconds.

4) No Valsalva maneuver should occur (observe the patient and flow velocities, which should not decrease). At the end of 30 seconds (or as soon as the patient breathe out if he/she cannot hold breath for 30 sec) the MFV values are recorded.

6) Intracranial lesions

a) The sonographic findings associated with intracranial stenosis are those of increased flow velocities across the narrowed segment of the lesion.

b) Flow distal to the stenosis sharply decreases with a decrease in pulsatility index

c) If the mean flow velocity in the MCA exceeds 200 cm/sec, the lesion is determined to be > 50% decreased lumen diameter reduction.

d) Sonia [8]

(i) Stenosis on TCD was identified using the mean of the maximum velocity. A positive test consisted of a mean velocity >100 cm/second in the MCA, >90 cm/second in the intracranial ICA, or >80 cm/second in the basilar artery BA or VAs.

(ii) PPV was 55%.

(iii) NPV was 93% for MCA 240, ICA 120, BA 130, VA 110

7) Extracranial lesions
   a) The characteristic findings of a proximal carotid system occlusion or severe stenosis include an ipsilateral low flow state in the MCA along with a low pulsatility index.
   b) Changes in the collateral flow patterns intracranially (i.e. across the ACOM) and extracranially (i.e. through the ophthalmic arteries) are identified
   c) In the presence of a competent ACOM, there is flow reversal in the ACA on the affected side
8) Cerebral MicroEmbolism detection
   a) TCD can be used to detect the passage embolic materials in to the intracranial vessels.
   b) Embolic signals (ES): random, unidirectional interruption in the Doppler signal with a characteristic acoustic chirp.
      (i) Emboli are usually transient (0.01- 0.1second) in duration, but may be seen in clusters, giving a prolonged rough signal similar to artifact.
   c) Larger air emboli produce so much signal reflection that TCD units show an overload on the visual display.

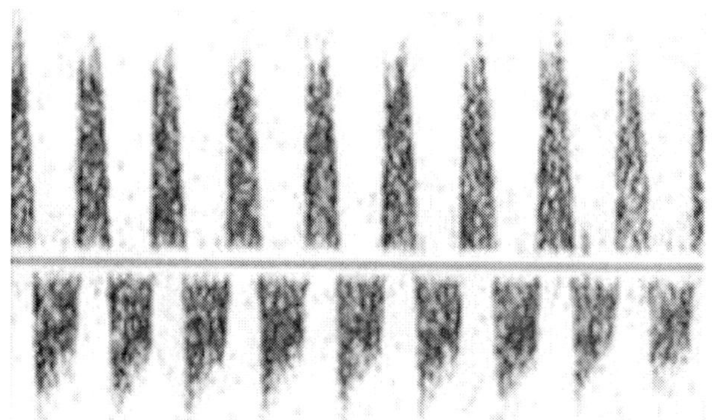

Figure 2. Short systolic spikes.

Carotid Ultrasound

1) Introduction
   a) Carotid ultrasound (CUS) is a screening test for carotid stenosis

b) Typically record transverse and sagittal views of bilateral neck arteries
  (i) ECA-
    1) High-resistance bed
  (ii) ICA'
    1) Low resistance bed
  (iii) Carotid Bifurcation
  (iv) Vertebral artery
2) Morphologic plaque classification
  a) Heterogenous – complex echogenic and echolucent material
  b) Homogenous –dense echogenic material
  c) Ulcerative- intraplaque hemorrhage
  d) Calcific- calcified with acoustic shadowing
3) Doppler velocities

Table 3. Rush velocity critieria for carotid stenosis

Stenosis	PSV (cm/sec)	EDV (cm/sec)	ICA/CCA PSV	Plaque
Normal	< 125	< 40	< 2	None
< 50%	<125	< 40	2	< 50% D R
50-69%	125-230	40-100	2-4	≥ 50% D R
> 70%	> 230	> 100	> 4	≥ 50% D R
occlusion	Undetectable	n/a	n/a	No lumen

DR= diameter reduction, PSV= Peak systolic velocity, EDV= End Diastolic velocity.

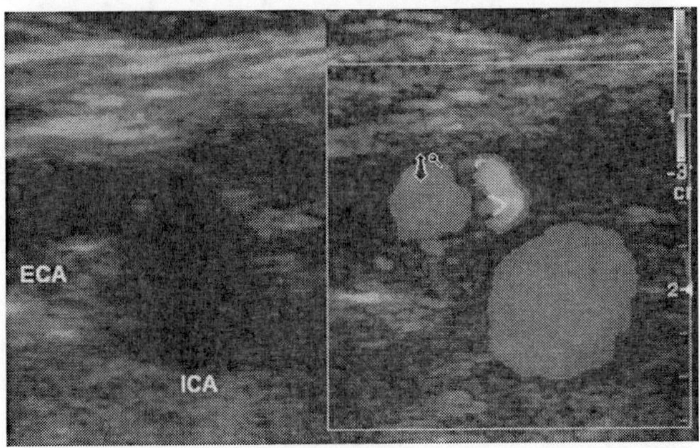

Figure 3. Transverse right carotid bifurcation.

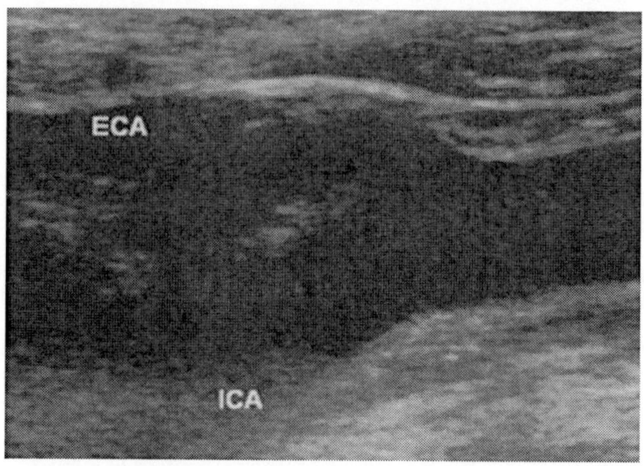

Figure 4. Sagittal right carotid bifurcation.

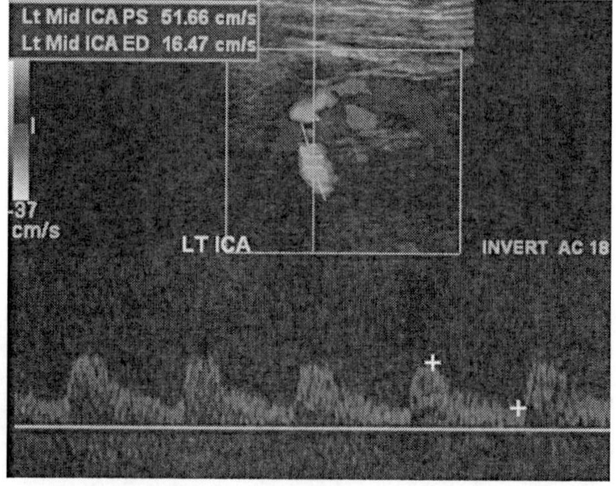

Figure 5. Left carotid Doppler.

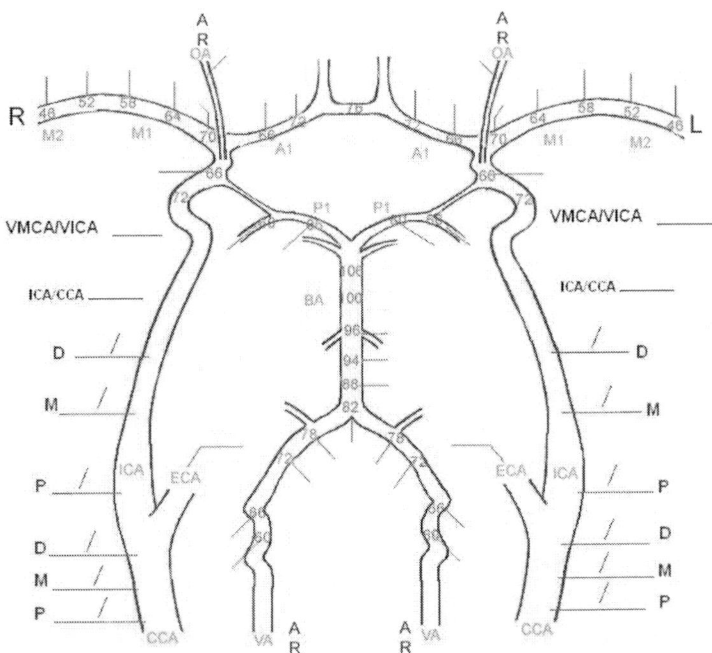

Figure 6. Sample Worksheet for TCD/CUS.

References

[1] *Cerebrovascular Ultrasound in Stroke Prevention and Treatment.* Edited by Andrei Alexandrov. 2004.

[2] Report of the Therapeutics and Technology Assessment Subcommitted of the American Academy of Neurology. Assessment: *Transcranial Doppler Ultrasonography.* Neurology 2004;62:1468.

[3] Adams RJ, McKie VC, Hsu L, et al. *Prevention of a first stroke by transfusions in children with sickle cell anemia and abnormal results on transcranial Doppler ultrasonography.* N Engl J Med 1998;339:5-11.

[4] The Optimizing Primary Stroke Prevention in Sickle Cell Anemia (STOP 2) Trial Investigators. *Discontinuing Prophylactic Transfusions Used to Prevent Stroke in Sickle Cell Disease.* N Engl J Med 2005;353:2769-78.

[5] Wijdicks EFM, Varelas RN, Gronseth GS, Greer DM. *Determining Brain Death in Adults. Neurology* 2010;74:1911–1918.

[6]   HS Markus and MJ Harrison. *Estimation of cerebrovascular reactivity using transcranial Doppler, including the use of breath-holding as the vasodilatory stimulus.* Stroke 1992;23;668-673.

[7]   *Silvestrini M, Troisi E, Matteis M, Cupini LM, Caltagirone C. Transcranial Doppler assessment of cerebrovascular reactivity in symptomatic and asymptomatic severe carotid stenosis.* Stroke 1996; 27: 1970–3.

[8]   E. Feldmann, J. L. Wilterdink, A. Kosinski, et al. *The Stroke Outcomes and Neuroimaging of Intracranial Atherosclerosis (SONIA) Trial.* Neurology 2007;68;2099-2106.

In: Handbook of Stroke and Neurocritical Care   ISBN: 978-61324-786-0
Editor: V. H. Lee   © 2012 Nova Science Publishers, Inc.

Chapter XVII

Cerebral Catheter Angiography

Michael Chen
Department of Neurological Sciences,
Section of Stroke and Neurocritical care,
Rush University Medical Center, Chicago, IL, USA

I.   Indications
   a)   Diagnosis of brain vascular disease
      (i)   Aneurysm, arteriovenous malformation, vasospasm, stenosis, occlusion, fistula or vasculopathy
   b)   Neurointerventional procedure planning.
   c)   Assistance with intraoperative aneurysm surgery.
   d)   Followup imaging after treatment
      (i)   Aneurysm, arteriovenous malformation
II. Neurologic Complications
   a)   Cerebral ischemic events are the most common of the serious complications associated with diagnostic cerebral angiography. Thromboemboli or air from catheters and/or wires, in addition to disruption of preexisting atherosclerotic plaque and vessel dissection are the usual etiologies.
   b)   Willinsky and colleagues reported on a series of 2,899 diagnostic cerebral angiograms with an overall neurologic complication rate of 1.3%, with 0.5% of complications permanent. They found higher rates of complications for

patients older than 55 years of age, those with cardiovascular disease, and those where fellows alone. [1]

c) The Asymptomatic Carotid Atherosclerosis Study (ACAS) reported a complication rate of 1.2% with cerebral angiography.[2]

d) Transient global amnesia has been reported and thought to be secondary to contrast reaction or vasospasm involving the medial temporal lobes and is usually transient. [3]

e) Temporary cortical blindness has been reported with contrast-mediated toxicity in the occipital visual areas related to excessive contrast runs in the posterior circulation. [4]

III. Non-Neurologic Complications

a) Groin and retroperitoneal hematoma, allergic reactions, femoral artery pseudoaneurysm, thromboembolism of the lower extremity, nephropathy, and pulmonary embolism.

b) Willinsky et al. reported on a series of 2,899 diagnostic cerebral angiograms and found 0.4% rate of groin hematoma, allergic cutaneous reactions of 0.1%, and pseudoaneurysm in 0.03%.[1]

c) Contrast-induced nephropathy

(i) Risk factors: serum creatinine >1.5 mg/dL, diabetes mellitus, dehydration, age > 60 years, paraproteinemia, hypertension, hyperuricemia.

(ii) Preventive measures:

1) Minimize use of contrast, including diluting syringes

2) Contrast agents with lower osmolarity

3) Aggressive hydration either orally or intravenously with normal saline

4) Administer acetylcysteine 600mg PO BID the day before and the day of the procedure. [5] This has never been proven with randomized trial though.

5) Sodium bicarbonate (150mEq/150cc added to 1000cc of D5W) at 3cc/kg/hour for one hour prior to procedure, then 1cc/kg/hour during the procedure and for 6 hours after the procedure. Thought to scavenge free radicals and shown to reduce the rate of contrast-nephropathy from 13.6% to 1.7%. [6]

(iii) Natural history
1) Renal insufficiency is usually transient
(iv) Metformin
1) Associated with lactic acidosis and a mortality rate of nearly 50%. [7]
2) Therefore, metformin should be held for 2 days after the procedure and restarted only after a serum creatinine has been checked and found to be unchanged.
3) Metformin, Glucophage, Avandamet, Glucovance, Metaglip
d) Contrast reactions
(i) Life threatening contrast reactions are considered very rare, estimated at < 0.1% [8] while cutaneous reactions can occur in about 1-2% of cases and often presents in a delayed fashion[Thomsen].
(ii) Risk factors: History of reaction to iodinated contrast, asthma, renal insufficiency, significant cardiac disease, anxiety.
(iii) History of previous reaction to contrast is the most important risk factor. Seafood allergies usually has no bearing on a reaction to ionic contrast.
(iv) Preventive measures:
1) Prednisone 50mg PO 13 hours, 7 hours and 1 hour prior to the procedure or hydrocortisone 200mg IV 1 hour prior to the procedure. [9]
2) Benadryl 50mg IV, IM or PO 1 hour prior to the procedure.

Performing the Catheter Cerebral Angiogram

I. Review the previous studies
a) Should not be overlooked. Helps the operator answer the pertinent clinical questions in the shortest amount of time, with the least amount of contrast and radiation, minimizing the risk of the study to the patient.

II. Preprocedure evaluation
   a) History and physical examination so any neurologic changes can be detected during or after the angiogram.
   b) Review allergies, particularly any prior reaction to iodinated contrast.
   c) The femoral pulse, dorsalis pedis and posterior tibial pulses should be evaluated and marked on the skin.
   d) Blood work, including hematocrit, coagulation parameters and serum creatinine should be reviewed.

III. Patient education
   a) A patient educated about the procedure is a more cooperative and relaxed patient.
   b) A step-by-step description of the procedure should be explained focusing on sensations the patient may experience when the anesthetic is used at the groin, and when contrast is injected.
   c) The importance of holding still such that the angiographic image is not degraded by motion artifact should also be emphasized.
   d) A cooperative patient results in decreased contrast usage from repeating runs as well as less catheter time, resulting in an overall safer procedure.

IV. Informed consent
   a) Written consent should be obtained prior to performing the procedure. Although the potential risks should be candidly discussed, as outlined above, they should not be overemphasized such that the patient is too frightened to pursue a procedure which may be in their best interest.

V. Reducing radiation exposure
   a) Make conscientious use of lead screens and shields
   b) Keep runs short when possible and use sparingly
   c) Minimize use of magnification if possible
   d) Collimate when possible
   e) Monitor others in the room for adequate lead protection
   f) Use lowest possible filming rates

VI. Patient sedation
   a) Usually consists of intravenous narcotic and sedative bolus
   b) Patient reassurance
   c) 1% lidocaine used for local anesthesia at incision site

VII. Angiographic Imaging

a) Biplane imaging allows for orthogonal images to be simultaneously obtained from a single injection of contrast and is considered the standard of care over monoplanar cerebral angiography.
   (i) Image interpretation
        1) Evaluate vessel morphology, contour and size
        2) Flow transit times
        3) Presence or absence of vascular blush
        4) Venous phase
        5) Bony anatomy
   (ii) Views
        1) Standard AP view: petrous ridges in the lower 1/3 of orbits
        2) Caldwell projection: petrous ridges with bottom of orbit
        3) Towne's view: petrous ridge with superior orbital rim, standard for imaging posterior fossa
        4) Water's view: inclined 45 degrees relative to skull base with petrous ridge some distance below orbit, used for imaging maxillary sinus
b) Three-dimensional rotational angiography
   (i) This anatomical imaging modality aims to recreate the in vivo status as close to its natural state as possible.
   (ii) Advantages:
        1) Provides critical information regarding depth, which is of particular importance when evaluating overlapping vessels. [10]
        2) Provides for greater understanding of aneurysm morphology, including the neck, takeoff of vacular branches and their relationship to the aneurysm wall and neck.
        3) Allows for imaging of the posterior walls of vessels, which either via planar imaging or even during operative procedures, was previously challenging to visualize.
        4) Enhances preoperative surgical planning.
   (iii) Limitations:
        1) Does not demonstrate well smaller branches of the arterial tree.

2) Does not allow for simultaneous visualization of background anatomy to provide spatial references.

VIII.   Plan the angiographic study
- a) 5F sheath used for most adults
- b) Choice of cerebral catheters
  - (i) For selection of internal carotid or vertebral
    - 1) Davis, Vert or Berenstein most often used
  - (ii) For particularly torturous vessels, Simmons 2 shaped catheter may be used
- c) Choice of manual double flush or continuous flush technique
- d) Heparinization is controversial
- e) External carotid angiographic studies may be needed for:
  - (i) Occlusive conditions such as Moyamoya disease
  - (ii) Giant cavernous, intracranial or otherwise unoperable aneurysms.
  - (iii) Brain arteriovenous malformations with possible extension to dural-pial anastomoses
  - (iv) Dural vascular disease as a possible cause for intracerebral hemorrhage
- f) Manual compression for 20 minutes after sheath removal is the gold standard, least expensive and most effective particularly for patients with significant atherosclerotic peripheral vascular disease.

IX.   Post-Angiogram Care
- a) Bed rest with accessed leg extended
- b) Head of bed <30 degrees for 5 hours, then out of bed for one hour. If closure device used, bed rest for 2 hours, out of bed for one hour.
- c) Vital signs: Every 15 minutes x 4, then every 30 minutes x 2, then every hour until discharge. Notify service for SBP <90 mmHg or decrease by 25mm Hg, or pulse >120.
- d) Check puncture site and distal pulses every 15 minutes x 4, then every 30 minutes x 2, then every hour until discharge. Notify service if bleeding or hematoma develops at puncture site, or distal pulses are no longer detectable beyond puncture site, or extremity becomes blue or cold.
- e) Normal saline at maintenance until patient is ambulatory

X.   Cerebral angiography related to specific diseases

a)   Atherosclerosis
  (i)   Aortic arch angiogram may help give broad overview of aortic atheroma and common carotid artery lesions.
  (ii) Simple curve catheters allow for selection of the proximal origin of the great vessels but allows further distal selection if the need arises.
  (iii) The diseased segment should be evaluated first.
  (iv) Vertebral artery origin arises off of posterior subclavian, therefore AP Townes view may be best.
  (v)   Multiple oblique views of carotid bifurcation may be necessary to truly determine degree of stenosis. (Figures 1 & 2).

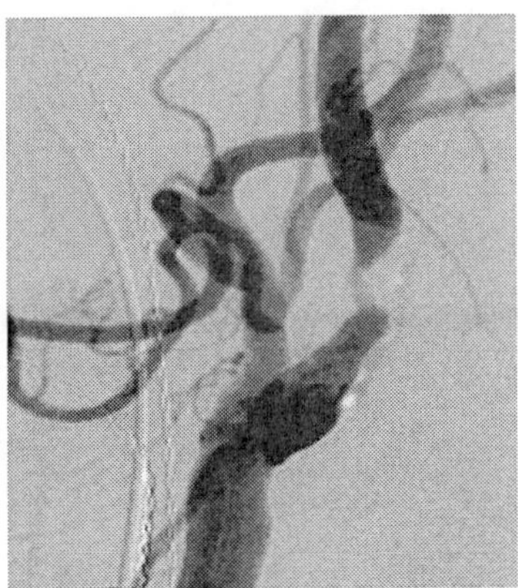

Figure 1.Left internal carotid artery stenosis.

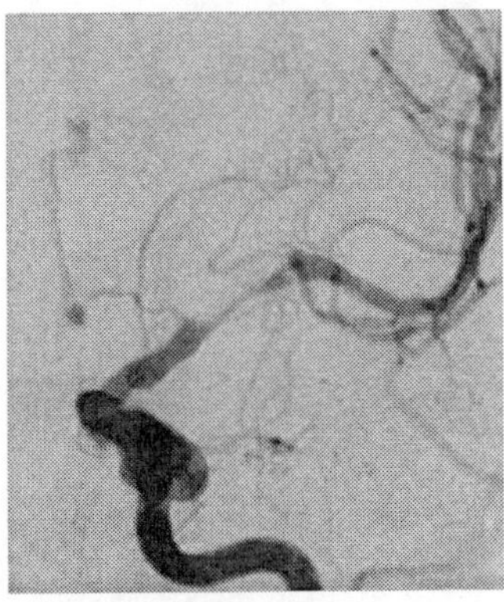

Figure 2. Left middle cerebral artery stenosis.

b) Cerebral aneurysm

    (i) Four vessel angiogram should be done in patients with subarachnoid hemorrhage because multiple aneurysms are seen in up to 20% of patients. [11]

    (ii) Selective internal carotid angiography will allow for unobstructed visualization of cerebral vessels.

    (iii) The anterior communicating artery should be well visualized and cross compression of the contralateral carotid artery may assist in opacifying this segment.

    (iv) External carotid angiography should be done if the intracranial vessels are normal and an arteriovenous fistula is entertained as a diagnosis for the intracerebral hemorrhage

    (v) Once an aneurysm is found, the size, neck, morphology, adjacent vessels and relationship to the parent vessel should be determined. (Figure 3).

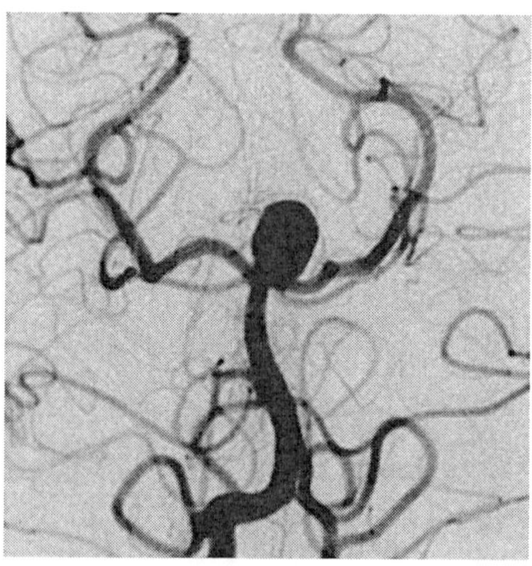

Figure 3. Basilar artery aneurysm.

    (vi) Three-dimensional angiography may be useful to determine best working angle and to understand in vivo anatomy in more detail (Figure 4).

    (vii) Microcatheter runs may be helpful in evaluation of large or giant aneurysms.

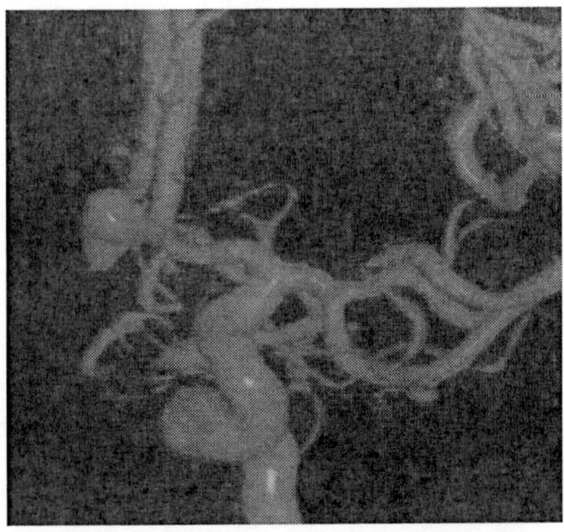

Figure 4. Three dimensional view of an anterior communicating artery aneurysm.

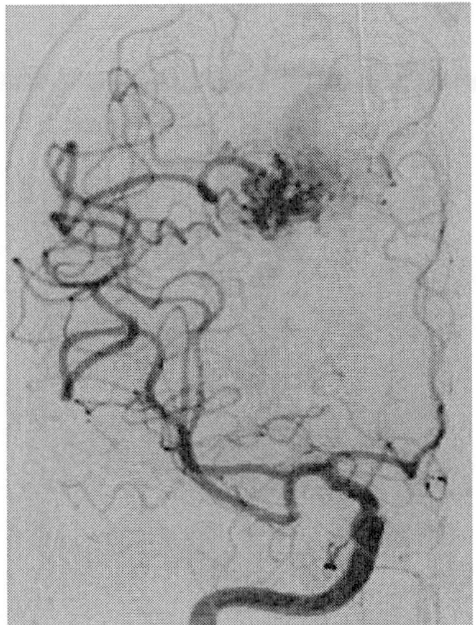

Figure 5. Right occipital brain arteriovenous malformation.

   c)   Brain arteriovenous malformations (Figure 5)
        (i) Six vessel cerebral angiogram is required to identify all feeding arteries and the nature of the venous drainage.

           (ii) Spetzler Martin scale should be calculated.

           (iii) High-speed runs of greater than 5 frames per second can help clarify the arterial, nidal and venous phase of the arteriovenous malformation.

d)   Dural arteriovenous fistula (Figure 6)

      (i)   Selective catheterization of the external carotid arteries are usually necessary

      (ii) The angiographic run should be carried out such that the venous phase is completely visualized

      (iii) It is critical to thoroughly evaluate the venous phases of the intracranial runs to look for any disturbance to normal venous drainage.

      (iv) High-speed runs greater than 5 frames per second may be useful.

      (v) Vertebral injection with compression of the carotid artery may allow for visualization of the carotid artery defect in the case of cavernous carotid fistula.

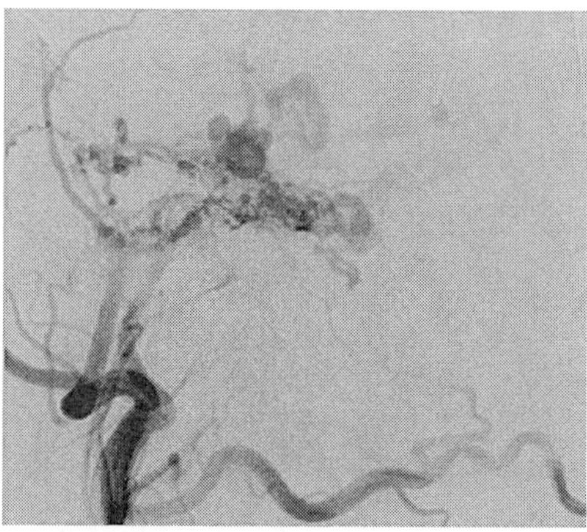

Figure 6. Left dural arteriovenous fistula.

Spinal Catheter Angiography

I.   Indications

a)   May be used to identify origin of spinal arteries prior to surgery

b) Evaluate spinal lesions prior to surgery for possible embolization

c) Evaluate for arteriovenous fistula or malformation

II. A complete spinal catheter angiogram

a) Must evaluate the following arteries:

(i) Vertebral arteries

(ii) External carotid arteries

(iii) Thyrocervical trunks

(iv) Costocervical trunks

(v) Supreme intercostal arteries

(vi) Segmental arteries from T4-L5

(vii) Median sacral artery

(viii) Lateral sacral arteries

References

[1] Willinsky, R.A., et al., *Neurologic complications of cerebral angiography: prospective analysis of 2,899 procedures and review of the literature.* Radiology, 2003. 227(2): p. 522-8.

[2] Young, B., et al., *An analysis of perioperative surgical mortality and morbidity in the asymptomatic carotid atherosclerosis study. ACAS Investigators. Asymptomatic Carotid Artheriosclerosis Study.* Stroke, 1996. 27(12): p. 2216-24.

[3] Wales, L.R. and A.A. Nov, *Transient global amnesia: complication of cerebral angiography.* AJNR Am J Neuroradiol, 1981. 2(3): p. 275-7.

[4] Studdard, W.E., D.O. Davis, and S.W. Young, *Cortical blindness after cerebral angiography.* Case report. J Neurosurg, 1981. 54(2): p. 240-4.

[5] Tepel, M., et al., *Prevention of radiographic-contrast-agent-induced reductions in renal function by acetylcysteine.* N Engl J Med, 2000. 343(3): p. 180-4.

[6] Merten, G.J., et al., *Prevention of contrast-induced nephropathy with sodium bicarbonate: an evidence-based protocol.* Crit Pathw Cardiol, 2004. 3(3): p. 138-43.

[7] Wiholm, B.E. and M. *Myrhed, Metformin-associated lactic acidosis in Sweden* 1977-1991. Eur J Clin Pharmacol, 1993. 44(6): p. 589-91.

[8] Thomsen, H.S. and W.H. Bush, Jr., *Adverse effects of contrast media: incidence, prevention and management.* Drug Saf, 1998. 19(4): p. 313-24.

[9]   Lasser, E.C., et al., *Pretreatment with corticosteroids to prevent adverse reactions to nonionic contrast media*. AJR Am J Roentgenol, 1994. 162(3): p. 523-6.

[10]   Borden, N.M. and J.K. *Costantini, 3D angiographic atlas of neurovascular anatomy and pathology*. 2007, Cambridge [England]; New York: Cambridge University Press. x, 273 p.

[11]   af Bjorkesten, G. and V. *Halonen, Incidence of intracranial vascular lesions in patients with subarachnoid hemorrhage investigated by four-vessel angiography*. J Neurosurg, 1965. 23(1): p. 29-32.

In: Handbook of Stroke and Neurocritical Care   ISBN: 978-61324-786-0
Editor: Vivien H. Lee   © 2012 Nova Science Publishers, Inc.

Chapter XVIII

Pharmacology

Amy Green

Department of Pharmacy, Rush University Medical Center,
Chicago, IL, USA

Intravenous Antihypertensive Agents

Clevidipine Butyrate Injectable Emulsion (Cleviprex®)

Dosing: Initiate at 1-2 mg/hr, initially titrate by doubling dose at 90 second intervals, as BP approaches goal dose increase should be less than double previous rate and time between dose adjustments should be lengthened to every 5-10 mins. Usual maintenance dose 4-6 mg/hr. Maximum dose (due to lipid load restriction) 1000 mL (average 21mg/hr) over 24 hr period.

Mechanism of action/indication: Dihydropyridine calcium channel blocker which reduces mean arterial blood pressure by decreasing systemic vascular resistance (afterload)

Contraindications:

- Allergies to soy products, eggs, or egg products
- Defective lipid metabolism (pathologic hyperlipemia, lipoid nephrosis, acute pancreatitis accompanied by hyperlipidemia

- Severe aortic stenosis

Adverse effects: Hypotension, reflex tachycardia.
How supplied: 0.5 mg/mL injectable emulsion, single-use 50mL and 100mL glass vials.

Nicardipine HCL Injection (Cardene®I.V.)

Dosing: IV: Initiate at 5mg/hr, titrate by 2.5mg/hr every 5 to 15 minutes up to 15mg/hr.
Mechanism of action: Dihydropyridine calcium channel blocker which reduces mean arterial blood pressure by decreasing systemic vascular resistance (afterload.)
Contraindications: Severe aortic stenosis
Precautions: Congestive heart failure, renal failure, hepatic failure
Adverse effects: Hypotension, reflex tachycardia, headache
How supplied: Ampules 25mg/10mL, Premixed iso-osmotic intravenous solution 40mg/200/mL and 20mg200/mL.

Sodium Nitroprusside

Dosing: Use with extreme caution, understand mechanisms of cyanide and thiocyanate accumulation and toxicity before initiating. Use should be limited to situations where no other IV antihypertensive agents are available or appropriate. Initiate infusion at 0.3mcg/kg/min, titrate to achieve desired goal, up to maximum of 10mcg/kg/min. Do not continue maximum rate of 10mcg/kg/min for more than 10 minutes due to risk of cyanide and thiocyanate toxicity. Rates > 2mcg/kg/min generate cyanide faster than the body can eliminate it. Follow cyanide or thiocyanate levels if used for > 24hrs, or in patients with renal or hepatic insufficiency.
Mechanism of action: Rapid-acting vasodilator of peripheral veins and arteries (veins > arteries.) Venous dilation decreases venous return, left ventricular end-diastolic pressure and pulmonary capillary wedge pressure (preload reduction). Arteriolar dilation reduces systemic vascular resistance, systolic arterial pressure, and mean arterial pressure (afterload reduction.) Dilation of coronary arteries also occurs.

Precautions: May raise ICP in patients with intracranial mass lesions.[1] Use with caution in patients with hepatic insufficiency or renal insufficiency. Protect from light.

Adverse effects: Cyanide and thiocyanate toxicity can occur with higher dose and/or prolonged use (may consider sodium thiosulfate co–infusion to increase the rate of cyanide processing). Methemoglobinemia can also occur after large doses.

Nitroglycerin

Dosing: Initiate infusion at 5mcg/min, titrate by 5 to 10 mcg/min every 3 to 5 mins until desired response is obtained (up to 200mcg/min)

Mechanism of action: Relaxation of vascular smooth muscle of peripheral arteries and veins, including dilation of coronary arteries.

Contraindications: Conditions when cardiac output is dependent on venous return (pericardial tamponade, restrictive cardiomyopathy, constrictive pericarditis)

Precautions: May further compromise cerebral perfusion pressure in patients with intracranial mass lesions.[2] Requires the use of supplied non-PVC tubing to avoid absorption issues.

Adverse effects: Severe headache, lightheadedness

Labetalol HCL

Dosing: Repeated IV injection: 10 to 20 mg IVP over 2 mins, every 10 minutes (up to 300mg). Peak effect of each bolus after approx 5 mins. Loading with a slow continuous infusion: Prepare 200mg labelalol in 200mL NS or D5W (final concentration 1mg/mL) administer at a rate of 2mg/min until desired blood pressure is achieved, then start oral and stop infusion.

Mechanism of action: Adrenergic receptor blocker with both selective alpha1 and nonselective beta blocking actions. Ratio of alpha to beta blockade 1:7 for IV formulation. (1:3 for oral formulation)

Contraindications: Severe bradycardia, overt cardiac failure, greater-than-first degree heart block.

Precautions: Bronchospastic disease, severe hepatic dysfunction

Adverse effects: Bradycardia, hypotension, dizziness, nausea, elevated LFTs

How supplied: 5mg/mL inj. 20mL(100mg) or 40mL(200mg) multidose vials.

Esmolol HCL (Brevibloc®)

Dosing: For supraventricular tachycardia or hypertension: Load 500mcg/kg over one min, followed by maintenance infusion of 50mcg/kg/min may titrate by 50mcg/kg/min every 5 mins to max of 200mcg/kg/min. It will take 30 mins to reach steady state if the infusion is titrated without giving boluses. If more rapid results are desired, reload with 500mcg/kg over one min before every up titration of the infusion.

Mechanism of action: β_1 selective adrengeric receptor blocking agent with rapid onset and very short duration of action (elimination t1/2 ~ 9mins) Hydrolyzed by red blood cell esterases

Contraindications: Sinus bradycardia, heart block greater-than-first-degree, overt heart failure.

Precautions: Bronchospastic disease, impaired renal function

Adverse effects: Bradycardia, hypotension, thrombophlebitis, dizziness

How supplied: Ready-to-use bags 2500mg/250mL and double strength 2000mg/100mL. Ready-to-use vial 100mg/10mL and double strength 100mg/5mL. Concentrated ampules for dilution 2500mg/10mL.

Hydralazine

Dosing: 10 to 20 mg IVP every 1 to 2 hours.

Mechanism of action: Causes relaxation of arteriolar vascular smooth muscle, peripheral vasodilation and decreased systemic vascular resistance

Precautions: Coronary artery disease, mitral valve rheumatic heart disease

Adverse effects: Headache, nausea, vomiting, tachycardia, angina, antipyridoxine effect (peripheral paresthesia, numbness, tingling). Rare: reduction in hemoglobin and red blood cell count, leucopenia, agranulocytosis, rash, eosinophilia, hepatitis

How supplied: 20mg/mL single dose vial 1mL.

Enalaprilat

Dosing: 0.625 to 1.25mg slow IVP every 6 hours.

Mechanism of action: Inhibition of ACE resulting in decreased plasma angiotensin II, decreased aldosterone secretion and increased bradykinin.

Contraindications: Pregnancy

Precautions: May cause severe hypotension in volume depleted patients, may worsen acutely impaired renal function

Adverse effects: Angioedema, cough, hypotension, orthostatic hypotension renal dysfunction, neutropenia (rare), thrombocytopenia (rare)

How supplied: 1.25 mg/mL injection 1mL and 2mL vials.

Antiplatelet Agents

Aspirin

Dosing: 75 – 325mg daily.

Mechanism of action: Inhibits platelet aggregation by irreversibly inhibiting platelet cycloxygenase and thus the generation of thromboxane A2.

Contraindications: Patients with hemophilia, gastric or duodenal ulcers, thrombocytopenia, or other bleeding tendencies, hypersensitivity to salicylates or other non-steroidal anti-inflammatory agents, or patients receiving other anticoagulant therapy, use with caution in patients with severe renal impairment.

Adverse effects: gastric irritation and bleeding, peptic ulceration, melena, dizziness, tinnitus, nausea, vomiting, hypersensitivity reactions including angioedema

Clopidogrel (Plavix)

Dosing: Recent stroke, MI, or established peripheral arterial disease (PAD): 75mg daily. Non-ST elevation ACS: 300mg load, then 75mg daily. Endovascular cerebral stenting procedures: 300 – 600mg load, then 75mg daily.

Mechanism of action: Clopidogrel is a prodrug which is metabolized by P450 enzymes to an active metabolite which irreversibly inhibits the binding of ADP to its platelet receptor and subsequently inhibits activation of the GPIIb/IIIa complex and platelet aggregation.

Contraindications: Active pathological bleeding such as a peptic ulcer or intracranial hemorrhage.

Precautions: Patients with genetically reduced CYP2C19 have diminished antiplatelet responses. Drugs that inhibit CYP2C19 may decrease effectiveness of clopidogrel.

Adverse effects: Rare: thrombotic thrombocytopenic purpura, increased LFTs, hyperuricemia, edema, GI hemorrhage, aplastic anemia, rash, agranulocytosis, leucopenia, neutrapenia, thrombocytopenia.

How supplied: 75mg and 300mg tablets

Abciximab (ReoPro)

Dosing: 0.25mg/kg IV bolus, followed by a continuous infusion 0.125mcg/kg/min (to a maximum of 10mcg/min) for 12 to 24 hours.

Mechanism of action: Inhibits platelet aggregation by binding to platelet GPIIb/IIIa receptors.

Contraindications: Active bleeding, known hypersensitivity to murine proteins.

Adverse effects: Thrombocytopenia, bleeding.

How supplied: 10mg/5mL single-use vials

Prasugrel (Effient)

Dosing: 60mg loading dose, followed by 10mg once daily. For patients weighing less than 60 kg, consider 5mg once daily.

Mechanism of action: The active metabolite of prasugrel irreversibly inhibits the binding of ADP to its platelet receptor and subsequently inhibits activation of the GPIIb/IIIa complex and platelet aggregation.

Contraindications: History of stroke or transient ischemic attack, active pathological bleeding such as a peptic ulcer or intracranial hemorrhage, or hypersensitivity to prasugrel.

Precautions: Use with caution in patients greater than or equal to 75 years of age, do not initiate in patients likely to undergo urgent CABG.

Adverse effects: Bleeding, thrombocytopenia, anemia, abnormal hepatic function, angioedma, leukopenia, rash, Rare: thrombotic thrombocytopenic purpura.

How supplied: 5mg and 10mg tablets.

Anticoagulants

Dabigatran Etexilate Mesylate (Pradaxa)

Dosing: To reduce the risk of stroke and systemic embolism in patients with non-valvular atrial fibrillation: 150mg twice daily. For patients with CrCL 15-30 mL/min use 75mg twice daily (do not chew, break or open capsules) Start dabigatron at the time of stopping IV UFH or 0-2 hours prior to the next scheduled dose of parenteral anticoagulant (LWMH, fondaparinux, etc.).For patients currently taking dabigatron wait 12 hours (if CrCL>30) or 24 hour if (if CrCL<30) after the last dose of dabigatron before starting a parenteral anticoagulant.

Mechanism of action: Prevents thrombus development by competitive direct thrombin inhibition.

Contraindications: Active pathological bleeding such as a peptic ulcer or intracranial hemorrhage, history of serious hypersensitivity reaction to dabigatran.

Precautions: Avoid coadministration with P-glycoprotein inducers (rifampin)

Adverse effects: bleeding, gastritis-like symptoms.

How supplied: 75mg and 100mg capsules

Dalteparin (Fragmin®)

Dosing	Normal renal function		CrCL < 30mL/min
DVT prophylaxis	5000 IU SC Daily		Use with caution, consider monitoring anti-Xa levels
DVT/PE Treatment	First 30 days	Months 2 to 6	Dose determined by anti-Xa monitoring. Monitor anti-Xa levels 4-6 hours after the 3rd or 4th dose. Target anti-Xa range 0.5-1.5 IU/mL
	Approx 200 IU/kg total body weight SC once daily (round to the nearest prefilled syringe size) Max dose 18000 IU SC daily	Approx 150 IU/kg total body weight SC once daily (round to the nearest prefilled syringe size) Max dose 18000 IU SC daily	

Mechanism of action: A low molecular weight heparin that enhances the inhibition of factor Xa and thrombin by antithrombin.

Contraindications: Active major bleeding, history of heparin-induced thrombocytopenia, hypersensitivity to heparin or pork products

Precautions: Significant increased risk of epidural or spinal hematomas in patients receiving neuroaxial anesthesia or spinal puncture, use with caution in patients with severe renal impairment

Adverse effects: Pain and hematoma at the injection site, thrombocytopenia, bleeding, elevated serum aminotransferase (AST/ALT)

How supplied: Single-dose prefilled syringes 2500 IU/0.2mL, 5000 IU/0.2mL, 7500 IU/0.3mL, 10000 IU/0.4mL, 12500 IU/0.5mL, 15000 IU/0.6mL, 18000 IU/0.72mL. Single-dose graduated syringe 10000 IU/1mL. Multiple dose vials: 95000 I/U.3.8mL, 95000 IU/9.5mL

Enoxaparin (Lovenox®)

Dosing	Normal to moderate renal dysfunction (CrCL >30mL/min)	Severe renal dysfunction (CrCL < 30mL/min)
DVT prophylaxis	40mg SC q24h [3] 30mg SC q12h (spinal cord injury) [4,5,6]	Use with caution, consider monitoring anti-Xa levels
DVT/PE Treatment	1mg/kg SC q12h 1.5mg/kg SC q24h (inpatient treatment only)	1mg/kg SC q24h, consider monitoring anti-Xa levels

Mechanism of action: A low molecular weight heparin that enhances the inhibition of factor Xa and thrombin by antithrombin

Contraindications: Active major bleeding, allergy to heparin or pork, severe renal impairment, history of heparin-induced thrombocytopenia

Precautions: Significant increased risk of epidural or spinal hematomas in patients receiving neuroaxial anesthesia or spinal puncture, use with caution in patients with severe renal impairment

Adverse effects: Pain and hematoma at the injection site, thrombocytopenia, bleeding, anemia, elevated serum aminotransferase (AST/ALT)

How supplied: Prefilled syringes 30mg/0.3mL, 40mg/0.4mL. Graduated pre-filled syringes 60mg/0.6mL, 80mg/0.8mL, 100mg/1mL, 120mg/0.8mL, 150mg/1mL. Multiple-dose vial 300mg/3mL

Warfarin (Coumadin®)

Dosing: Initiate with 2 – 5mg daily. Monitor INR and adjust dose as necessary to achieve goal INR. Begin with lower doses in the elderly. If an oral route is temporarily unavailable, an equivalent IV dose may be given. There is no benefit of intravenous administration if oral access is available.

Mechanism of action: Warfarin inhibits vitamin K epoxide reductase, and thereby reduces synthesis of the vitamin K dependent clotting factors and the anticoagulant proteins C and S. Based on the half-life (hrs) of the factors and proteins inhibited, warfarin causes a sequential depression of the activity of Factor VII (4-6), Protein C (8), Factor IX (24), Protein S (30), Factor X (48-72), and Factor II (60.) The effects of a single dose of warfarin generally last for 2 – 5 days.

Contraindications: Any circumstance in which the hazard of hemorrhage may outweigh the potential benefits of anticoagulation such as: pregnancy, hemorrhagic tendencies or blood dyscrasias, recent or contemplated surgery, active ulceration or disease state with high risk of overt bleeding, inadequate ability to monitor INR, unsupervised senile patients, spinal puncture, major regional, lumbar block anesthesia, malignant hypertension.

Precautions: Due to variable vitamin K intake, high protein binding (99%), and metabolism by hepatic P450 is enzymes 2C9, 2C19, 2C8, 2C18, 1A2, and 3A4, a large amount of significant drug-drug and drug-disease interactions exist that may affect the INR. The INR should be closely monitored whenever medication regimens (including botanicals) or dietary habits, are initiated, discontinued, or are taken with irregularly.

Adverse effects: Increased risk of bleeding, purple toe syndrome, skin necrosis, gangrene, elevated LFTs,

How supplied: 1mg, 2mg, 2.5mg, 3mg, 4mg, 5mg, 7.5mg, 10mg scored tablets, 5mg/2.5mL injection single-use vial

Fibrinolysis

Tissue Plasminogen Activator (TPA)/ Alteplase (Activase®)

Dosing: Acute ischemic stroke - total dose = 0.9mg/kg (up to a max of 90mg) Give 10% of total dose as a bolus over 1 min, administer the remainder as an infusion over 60 mins.

Mechanism of action: Tissue plasminogen activator is an enzyme which binds to clot bound fibrin and converts plasminogen to plasmin, initiating local fibrinolysis.

Contraindications (for use in acute ischemic stroke): recent intracranial and/or spinal surgery, head trauma, or previous stroke within past 3 months; evidence or history of intracranial hemorrhage; suspicion of subarachnoid hemorrhage; uncontrolled hypertension at time of treatment (systolic BP >185 or diastolic BP > 110); known intracranial neoplasm, AVM, or aneurysm; known bleeding diathesis; INR > 1.7 or PT > 15; administration of heparin within 48 hours of preceding onset of stroke and elevated aPTT; platelet count < 100,000/mm^3;

Precautions: Seizure at the onset of stroke.

Adverse effects: Bleeding, anaphylaxis, extravasation may cause ecchymosis and/or inflammation at the site.

How supplied: 50mg and 100mg powder for injection vials with diluent, final concentration after reconstitution 1mg/mL. Stable 8 hours after reconstitution.

Hemostatic Agents

Coagulation Factor VIIa (Recombinant) rFVIIa (Novoseven®)

Dosing: For acute INR reduction: Doses of 5 − 90 mcg/kg slow IVP over 2 -5 mins have been used in emergent situations. However recombinant FVIIa is not routinely recommended as a sole agent for warfarin reversal in ICH.[7] The effects on INR are temporary and other modalities such as fresh frozen plasma and intravenous vitamin K administration should be given concomitantly for warfarin reversal with life-threatening hemorrhage.[8]

Mechanism of action: Promotes hemostasis by activating the extrinsic pathway of the coagulation cascade. When recombinant factor VIIa is complexed with tissue factor can activate factor X, which complexed with other factors converts prothrombin to thrombin which leads to the conversion of fibrinogen to fibrin and the formation of a local Hemostatic plug.

Adverse effects: Arterial and venous thrombotic and thromboembolic events, anaphylaxis, rash, angioedema.

How supplied: 1mg, 2mg, 5mg lyophilized powder for injection single-use vials with specific histidine diluent, administer within 3 hrs of reconstitution.

Aminocaproic Acid (Amicar®)

Dosing: To prevent rebleeding in aneurysmal subarachnoid hemorrhage (SAH): 4gm (diluted) IV bolus over 60 minutes, followed by 1gm/hr (diluted) continuous infusion, with cessation 4 hours before angiography or surgery for a maximum duration of 72 hours after SAH onset.[9]

Mechanism of action: Inhibits plasminogen activators and plasmin activity and subsequently fibrinolysis, thereby enhancing hemostasis when fibrinolysis contributes to bleeding.

Contraindications: Do not use when the cause of bleeding is disseminated intravascular coagulation (DIC)

Precautions: Avoid rapid IV administration

Adverse effects: Thrombosis, hypotension, bradycardia, thrombophlebitis, myalgias, myopathy, increased CPK, rhabdomyolysis, seizures, intracranial hypertension, injection site reactions, agranulocytosis, leucopenia, thrombocytopenia, renal failure.

How supplied: 250mg/mL injection 20mL vial (dilute before use), 250mg/mL oral solution, 500mg tablets

Phytonadione – Vitamin K

Dosing: Reversal of oral anticoagulants in patients with life-threatening hemorrhage: 10mg (diluted) IV by slow infusion repeat if necessary q12h for persistently elevated INR. Reversal of oral anticoagulants in patients with mild to moderately elevated INR without major bleeding: 2.5 to 5mg orally, may repeat dose in 24 hours if INR is persistently elevated.[8]

Vitamin K deficiency: 2.5-10mg PO/ SC daily.

Mechanism of action: Phytonadione is an essential cofactor necessary for the biosynthesis of active coagulation factors II, VII, IX and X.

Precautions: May cause temporary resistance to prothrombin-depressing anticoagulants, especially when larger doses of phytonadione are used.

Adverse effects: Anaphylaxis, hypotension, flushing sensations during infusion.

How supplied: 5mg tablets, 1mg/0.5mLampule for injection, 10mg/1mL ampule for injection

Protamine Sulfate

Dosing:

1) Reversal of unfractionated heparin: Because heparin half-life is 60 - 90 mins, Protamine dose should be calculated from the estimated amount of active heparin in plasma at the time of Protamine administration. Protamine 1mg will neutralize approximately100 units of active heparin. Max dose = 50mg in any 10 min time period. A prolonged infusion of Protamine may be necessary to reverse subcutaneously administered heparin.[10]
2) Reversal of low molecular weight heparin: Protamine only reverses a variable portion of the anti-Xa activity of LMWH. If less than 8 hours has elapsed since time of LMWH administration, give 1mg Protamine per 100 anti-Xa units of LMWH. Smaller doses should be considered if 8 to 12 hours have elapsed since LMWH administration.[10]

Mechanism of action: Protamine is a basic protein derived from fish sperm that binds to heparin and forms a stable salt, interfering with the action of heparin with antithrombin III. Protamine also has weak anticoagulant activity.

Precautions: Avoid rapid administration, use with precaution in patients with fish allergy or previous exposure to Protamine sulfate.

Adverse effects: Flushing, nausea, vomiting, dyspnea, hypotension, bradyarrhythmia, bronchoconstriction, anaphylaxis, circulatory collapse.

How supplied: 10mg/mL injection 5mL vial

Hyperosmotic Agents

Mannitol

Dosing: Elevated ICP: 0.25 – 2gm/kg IV over 30-60 mins using 15 - 20% solution with a filter. Inspect solution for crystallization before infusing [11]

Mechanism of action: Expands circulating volume, decreases blood viscosity and therefore increases cerebral blood flow and cerebral oxygen delivery, osmotic dieresis resulting in reduction of cerebral water content.

Contraindications: Well established anuria due to severe renal disease.

Precautions: Congestive heart failure, pulmonary edema.

Adverse effects: Pulmonary congestion, fluid and electrolyte imbalance, acidosis, dry mouth, urinary retention, edema, headache, blurred vision, nausea, vomiting, extravasation, skin necrosis, thrombophlebitis, hypotension, tachycardia, urticaria, fever, angina-like chest pains

How supplied: 15% (75gm/500mL) flexible container, 20% (50gm/250mL and 100gm/500mL) flexible container, 25% (12.5gm/50mL) fliptop vial

Hypertonic Saline

Dosing: Many dosing strategies exist for both correction of hyponatremia and management of elevated intracranial hypertension [11, 12]

- 1.5 – 3% continuous infusion for hyponatremia treatment or elevation of serum osmolarity: Starting dose 0.5 – 1mL/kg/hr titrate to desired serum sodium and/or serum osmolarity (solutions greater than 2% should be administered via central venous access)
- 23.4 % bolus for acutely elevated intracranial pressure: 30mL IV over 15 to 20 mins (central venous catheter required for administration)

Mechanism of action: May decrease intracranial pressure by optimization of blood viscosity and cerebral blood flow (early effects), in addition to osmotic mobilization of water across the intact blood brain barrier which reduces cerebral water content (latter effect). May have a favorable immunomodulatory effect on brain tissue after traumatic brain injury.[13]

Precautions: Use with caution in patients with congestive heart failure, pulmonary edema, and preexisting chronic hyponatremia (risk of central pontine myelinolysis)

Adverse effects: Pulmonary congestion, volume overload, fluid and electrolyte imbalance, hyperchloremic acidosis, rebound intracranial hypertension, prolonged prothrombin time and activated partial thromboplastin time, phlebitis, potential for increased risk of infectious complications.

How supplied: Compounded intravenous solutions vary per institution. Commercially available as:

- 3% sodium chloride 500mL bag
- 5% sodium chloride 500mL bag
- 14.6% sodium chloride 20mL and 40mL vials
- 23.4% sodium chloride 30mL vial

Anticonvulsant Agents

Carbamazepine (Tegretol®)

Dosing: Tablets: Initiate at 100-200mg bid, titrate up by 200mg/day (in divided dose 3 to 4 times daily) every week up to a maximum of 1600mg/day. Oral suspension: Initiate 100mg qid, titrate up by 200mg/day (in divided doses, 4 times daily.) XR tablets: initiate at 200mg bid, titrate up by 200mg/day (in divided doses) every week.

Therapeutic range: 4 – 12 mcg/mL

Mechanism of action: Prolongs sodium channel inactivation.

Contraindications: Do not use in patients with history of bone marrow suppression, or known sensitivity to tricyclic antidepressants (TCAs)

Precautions: Increased risk of serious dermatologic reactions, aplastic anemia, agranulocytosis

Adverse effects: Common: nausea, vomiting, diarrhea, rash, puritus, hyponatremia, drowsiness, blurred vision, ataxia, transient elevation of LFTs, transient thrombocytopenia and/or leukopenia. Severe: agranulocytosis, aplastic anemia, SJS, TEN, hepatic failure, dermatitis, pancreatitis.

How supplied: 200mg tablets, 100mg chewable tablets, 100mg/5mL oral suspension, 100mg, 200mg, 400mg extended-release (XR) tablets, 100mg, 200mg, 300mg extended-release capsules (Equetro®)

Felbamate (Felbatol®)

Dosing: Initiate at 1200mg/day in divided doses 3 to 4 times per day. Increase by 600mg every 2 weeks up to 3600mg/day.

Mechanism of action: Precise mechanism unknown, potentially blocks NMDA receptors, potentiates GABA-mediated responses, blocks L-type calcium channels, and possibly also prolongs sodium channel inactivation.

Contraindications:

Precautions: Recommended only for use in patients who respond inadequately to alternative treatments and whose epilepsy is so severe that a substantial risk of aplastic anemia and/or hepatic failure is considered to be acceptable.

Adverse effects: Common: nausea, vomiting, anorexia, dizziness, headache. Severe: aplastic anemia, hepatic failure.

How supplied: 400mg, 600mg tablets, 600mg/5mL oral suspension.

Fosphenytoin (Cerebryx®)

Dosing: Loading dose 15 to 20 mg/kg IV/IM no faster than 150mg/min. Maintenance dose 5 to 7mg/kg/day IV/IM in 2 to 3 divided doses.

Therapeutic concentrations: phenytoin total level 10-20mcg/mL, free level 1-2mcg/mL

Mechanism of action: Fosphenytoin is a prodrug which is hydrolyzed by phosphatases to yield phenytoin. Phenytoin prolongs the inactivation of voltage-gated sodium channels.

Contraindications: Sinus bradycardia, sino-atrial block, second and third degree AV block.

Adverse effects: Burning, itching, and/or tingling predominantly in the groin area, hypotension (related to infusion rate), hypertension, bradycardia, fever, nausea, vomiting, nystagmus, dizziness, headache, somnolence, ataxia, atrial and ventricular conduction depression, rash, hepatotoxicity, thrombocytopenia, leucopenia, granulocytopenia, agranulocytosis, pancytopenia, pseudolymphoma.

How supplied: 50mg PE (phenytoin equivalents)/mL injection 2mL and 10mL vials.

Lacosamide (Vimpat®)

Dosing: Initiate at 50mg bid, titrate by 100mg/day at weekly intervals, up to 400mg daily in divided doses. Reduce dose for patients with mild to moderate hepatic impairment and severe renal impairment (CrCl < 30 mcg/mL.)

Mechanism of action: Selectively enhances slow inactivation of voltage-gated sodium channels.

Precautions: Use with caution in patients with known cardiac rhythm and conduction abnormalities, may cause PR interval prolongation.

Adverse effects: Dizziness, ataxia, nausea, diplopia, and headache.

How supplied: 50mg, 100mg, 150mg, 200mg film-coated tablets, 200mg/20mL single-use vial for intravenous use

Lamotrigine (Lamictal®)

Dosing: Starting dose: 25mg every other day to 50mg daily (starting dose dependent on current treatment with valproic acid, phenytoin, phenobarbital, primidone, carbamazepine, or estrogen.) Titrate by increasing dose 25mg to 50 mg per day every two weeks. For doses greater than 50mg/day divide twice daily. Usual maximum dose: 400mg daily, in divided doses.

Mechanism of action: Inhibits voltage-sensitive sodium channels.

Adverse effects: Common: Rash, nausea, dizziness, somnolence, blurred vision, headache. Rare: SJS, hypersensitivity reaction, neutropenia, thrombocytopenia, and pancytopenia.

How supplied: 25mg, 100mg, 150mg, 200mg tablets, 2mg, 5mg, 25mg chewable dispersible tablets, 25mg, 50mg, 100mg, 200mg oral disintegrating tablets, 25mg, 50mg, 100mg, 200mg extended-release tablets (XR) for once daily dosing

Levetiracetam (Keppra®)

Dosing: Initiate at 500mg q12h, titrate by increasing dose 1000mg/day in divided doses every two weeks. Recommended maximum dose 3000mg daily. XR formulation should be given once daily.

Dosing in renal impairment: mild (CrCL 50 – 80 mL/min) 500mg to 1000mg q12h, moderate (CrCl 30 – 50 mL/min) 250 to 750mg daily, severe

(CrCL <30 mL/min) 250 to 500mg q12h, ESRD patients receiving dialysis 500 to 1000mg q24h with 250mg to 500mg supplemental dose following dialysis.

Mechanism of action: Precise mechanism unknown. Binds to synaptic vesicle protein SV2A, involved in the regulation of vesicle exocytosis.

Adverse effects: Agitation, anxiety, fatigue, somnolence, dizziness.

How supplied: 500mg/5mL injection single-use vial, 250mg, 500mg, 750mg, 1000mg scored, film-coated tablets, 100mg/mL oral solution, 500mg, 750mg extended-release tablets (XR) for once daily dosing

Pentobarbital (Nembutal®)

Dosing for pentobarbital coma (requires ventilatory support): For refractory status epilepticus [14] or refractory elevated intracranial pressure (ICP) (note: many dosing strategies exist)

1) Loading dose 10mg/kg over 30 mins, followed by 5mg/kg every hour x3 doses, followed by a maintenance infusion of 1mg/kg/hr [15, 16]
2) Loading dose 3-5mg/kg over one hour, followed by a maintenance infusion of 1-3mg/kg/hr May rebolus with 1.5gm/kg and titrate maintenance dose to achieve EEG burst suppression [17]

Mechanism of action: Potentiates GABA-induced chloride conductance at GABA-A receptors leading to CNS depression, and burst suppression. A decrease in cerebral metabolic rate is accompanied by a reduction in cerebral blood flow, causing cerebral vasoconstriction, which decreases cerebral edema and ICP. [17]

Precautions: May require invasive cardiovascular monitoring, may require fluid and vasopressor support to maintain desired mean arterial pressure and/or cerebral perfusion pressure.

Adverse effects: respiratory depression, bradycardia, hypotension, liver damage,

How supplied: 1gm/20mL injection, multiple-dose vial (Contains propylene glycol 40%v/v), 2.5gm/50mL injection, multiple-dose vial (Contains propylene glycol 40%v/v)

Phenobarbital

Dosing:

1) Status epilepticus (may require ventilatory and blood pressure
    support): 20mg/kg IV infusion at a rate of 50 – 75 mg/min [16]
2) Maintenance anticonvulsant dosing: 60 – 250mg IV or oral
    daily (may be divided bid or tid) Target plasma concentration
    15 – 40 mcg/mL.

Mechanism of action: Potentiates GABA-induced chloride conductance
at GABA-A receptors, enhancing the inhibition of neurotransmission.

Contraindications: Severe liver function impairment.

Precautions: patients with renal function impairment and mild liver
function impairment may require increased monitoring and dosage
adjustments

Adverse effects: respiratory drive depression, decreased level of
consciousness, dizziness, drowsiness, hypotension

How supplied: 15mg, 16.2mg, 30mg, 60mg, 64.8mg, 97.2mg, 100mg
tablets, 30 mg/mL, 60mg/mL, 65mg/mL, 130mg/mL injection, 20mg/5mL
oral elixir

Phenytoin

Dosing: IV: Loading dose 15-20 mg/kg IV no faster than 50mg/min.
Maintenance dose 5-7mg/kg/day IV in 2 or 3 divided doses. Oral chewable
tablets/suspension: usual maintenance dose 5-7mg/kg/day in 2 or 3 divided
doses. ER capsules: usual maintenance dose 5-7 mg/kg/day.

Therapeutic concentration: total level 10-20 mcg/mL, free level 1-
2mcg/mL

Mechanism of action: Prolongs the inactivation of voltage-gated sodium
channels.

Contraindications: Sinus bradycardia, sino-atrial block, second and third
degree AV block.

Adverse effects: Hypotension (related to infusion rate), hypertension,
bradycardia, fever, nausea, vomiting, nystagmus, dizziness, headache,
somnolence, ataxia, atrial and ventricular conduction depression, rash,
hepatotoxicity, thrombocytopenia, leucopenia, granulocytopenia,
agranulocytosis, pancytopenia, pseudolymphoma.

How supplied: 50mg chewable infatabs (not intended for once-a-day dosing)

30mg and 100mg ER capsules, 125mg/5mL oral suspension (not intended for once-a-day dosing), 50mg/mL injection 2mL and 10mL vials

Topiramate (Topamax®)

Dosing: Initiate at 25mg bid, titrate up by 25-50mg/day every week up to a usual max of 400mg/day in divided doses. Higher doses (300 – 1600mg/day) have been used in the treatment of refractory status epilepticus. [18]

Mechanism of action: Prolongs inactivation of voltage-gated sodium channels, potentiates the activity of GABA at GABA-A receptors, has weak inhibitory effect against carbonic anhydrase, and may cause inactivation of the AMPA/kainate subtype of glutamate receptor.

Adverse effects: Common: metabolic acidosis, weight loss, paresthesias, kidney stones, fatigue, somnolence, confusion, difficulty concentrating, depression, language problems, anxiety, tremor. Rare: risk of acute myopia and secondary angle closure glaucoma, oligohidrosis and hyperthermia,

How supplied: 25mg, 50mg, 100mg, 200mg tablets, 15mg, 25mg sprinkle capsules.

Valproic Acid/ Divalproex Sodium/ Valproate Sodium

Dosing:

- Oral: Initiate at 10-20mg/kg/day in divided doses. Titrate by 5-10mg/kg/day each week until clinical response is obtained. Doses above 60mg/kg/day have not been evaluated.
- Intravenous: Loading dose for status epilepticus 20 – 40 mg/kg at a rate no greater than 3mg/kg/min. maintenance starting dose 10 -20 mg/kg/day divided every 6 to 8 hours. [16]

Therapeutic range: total level 50 – 100mcg/mL, free level 5-10mcg/mL

Mechanism of action: Multiple mechanism of action may exist including prolonged recovery of voltage-activated sodium channels from inactivation, reduction of current through T-type calcium channels, increased GABA synthesis and/or decreased GABA degradation.

Contraindications: Severe hepatic dysfunction, urea cycle disorders

Precautions: Multiple serious drug interactions, evaluate potential reactions for all patients on concomitant medications (including but not limited to, meropenem, doripenem, ertapenem, erythromycin, amikacin, phenytoin, carbamazepine, Lamotrigine, oxcarbazepine, phenobarbital, rifampin, etc.)

Adverse effects: Somnolence, nausea, GI irritation, tremor, weight gain. Rare adverse effects: hyperammonemia, elevated LFTs, hepatic failure, thrombocytopenia, hyponatremia, SIADH. Severe adverse effects: Stevens Johnson Syndrome, toxic epidermal necrosis, pancreatitis, hyperammonemic encephalopathy

How supplied:

- Valproic acid
  - 250mg liquid-filled gelatin capsules
  - 250mg/5mL oral syrup
- Divalproex sodium
  - 125mg, 250mg capsules (delayed release pellets)
  - 125mg, 250mg, 500mg delayed release tablets
  - 250mg, 500mg extended release tablets
- Valproate sodium
  - 100mg/mL injection

Zonisamide (Zonegran®)

Dosing: Initiate at 100mg bid, titrate up by 100mg/day every 2 weeks up to a maximum of 600mg/day.

Mechanism of action: Prolongs inactivation of voltage-gated sodium channels and reduces voltage-dependent T-type calcium currents.

Contraindications: Contraindicated in patients who have demonstrated hypersensitivity to sulfonamides.

Precautions: Weak carbonic anhydrase inhibitor (may contribute to development of renal calculi.)

Adverse effects: Common: Somnolence, fatigue, ataxia, anorexia, nervousness. Rare: renal calculi, rash, Stevens Johnson Syndrome, toxic epidermal necrosis, aplastic anemia, agranulocytosis, oligohidrosis and hyperthermia.

How supplied: 25mg, 100mg capsules.

Aquaretics

Conivaptan HCL (Vaprisol®)

Dosing: Loading dose: 20mg IV infused over 30 minutes through large vein. Followed by 20mg continuous infusion over 24 hours for 1 to 4 days. Dose may be titrated up to 40mg/day if necessary. Change infusion site every 24 hours to minimize risk of vascular irritation.

Mechanism of action: Arginine vasopressin (AVP) V_{1A} and V_2 receptor antagonist, indicated for the treatment of euvolemic and hypervolemic hyponatremia.

Contraindications: hypovolemic hyponatremia

Precautions: Monitor for overly rapid correction of hyponatremia (>12mEq/L/24 hours) – may result is osmotic demyelination syndrome, monitor serum sodium and volume status frequently during use. Conivaptan is a substrate of CYP3A4. Do not administer with potent CYP3A4 inhibitors (ketoconazole, itraconazole, clarithromycin, ritonavir, indinavir)

Adverse effects: Injection site reactions/phlebitis, hypokalemia, headache, thirst, constipation

How supplied: 20mg/4mL injection ampule. (must be diluted in at least 100mL D5W only prior to administration), Premixed IV infusion 20mg/100mL D5W

Tolvaptan (SAMSCA®)

Dosing: 15mg daily. May titrate every 24 hours to max of 60mg daily.

Mechanism of action: Selective vasopressin V_2-receptor antagonist, indicated for the treatment of euvolemic and hypervolemic hyponatremia in hospitalized patients.

Contraindications: Hypovolemic hyponatremia. Anuric patients are expected to have no benefit. If urgent increase in serum sodium is required to prevent or treat serious neurological symptoms tolvaptan should not be used.

Precautions: Monitor for overly rapid correction of hyponatremia (>12mEq/L/24 hours) – may result is osmotic demyelination syndrome, monitor serum sodium and volume status frequently during use. Tolvaptan is a substrate of CYP3A4. Do not administer with potent CYP3A4 inhibitors (ketoconazole, itraconazole, clarithromycin, ritonavir, indinavir) or moderate inducers of CYP3A4.

Adverse effects: dry mouth, constipation, thirst, polyuria,
How supplied: 15mg, 30mg tablets

Acid-Inhibitors

H$_2$ Blockers	Usual Dosing	Dosage forms
Cimetidine (Tagamet®)	300 – 800mg once to four times daily (max 2400mg/day) Reduce dose for CrCL < 30mL/min Reduce dose by 50% for severe liver disease	- 200mg, 300mg, 400mg, 800mg tablets - 300mg/5mL oral solution - 300mg/2mL injection
Famotidine (Pepcid®)	20mg q12h, if CrCL < 50mL/min give 20mg q24h	- 10mg, 20mg, 40mg tablet - 20mg chewable tablet - 40mg/5mL oral suspension - 10mg/mL injection
Nizatidine (Axid®)	75mg to 300mg once or twice daily Reduce dose for CrCL < 50mL/min	- 75mg tablet - 150mg, 300mg capsule - 15mg/mL oral solution
Ranitidine (Zantac®)	150mg q12h Reduce dose for CrCL < 50mL/min	- 75mg, 150mg, 300mg tablets - 150mg, 300mg capsules - 15mg/mL oral syrup, - 25mg/mL injection

Mechanism of action: Inhibit histamine action at the histamine H(2) receptors of the parietal cells, lowering basal gastric acid secretion.

Precautions: Increased number of drug interaction with cimetidine

Adverse effects: Generally well tolerated. May cause abdominal pain, constipation, or diarrhea. Rare adverse effects include confusion, hallucinations, thrombocytopenia, rash, and angioedema.

Proton pump inhibitors	Usual dosing	Dosage forms
Esomeprazole (Nexium®)	20 to 40 mg daily	- 20mg, 40mg capsule (delayed release pellets) - 10mg, 20mg, 40mg packets for oral suspension (delayed release) - 20mg/vial, 40mg/vial injection

Lansoprazole (Prevacid®)	15 to 30 mg daily	- 15mg, 30mg capsule (delayed release pellets) - 15mg, 30mg packets for oral suspension (delayed release) - 15mg, 30mg orally disintegrating tablet (delayed release) - 30mg/vial injection
Dexlansoprazole (Dexilant®)	30 to 60 mg daily	- 30mg, 60mg delayed release capsule
Omeprazole (Prilosec®)	20 mg daily	- 10mg, 20mg, 40mg capsule (delayed release pellets) - 2.5mg, 10mg packets for oral suspension (delayed release) - 20mg delayed release tablet
Pantoprazole (Protonix®)	40 mg daily	- 20mg, 40mg delayed release tablets - 40mg packet for oral suspension (delayed release) - 40mg /vial injection
Rabeprazole (Aciphex®)	20 mg daily	- 20mg delayed release tablet

Mechanism of action: Irreversibly inhibit active proton pumps, thereby inhibiting the final common pathway of gastric acid secretion.

Adverse effects: Generally well tolerated. Events occurring in >2% of treatment group patients in placebo-controlled clinical trials: headache, diarrhea, and abdominal pain

Miscellaneous Agents

Nimodipine (Nimotop®)

Dosing: 60mg orally q4h for 21 days after aneurysmal subarachnoid hemorrhage (SAH).

Mechanism of action: Nimodipine is a highly lipophilic dihydropyridine calcium channel blocker, which decreases calcium influx into vascular smooth muscle cells leading to inhibition of vascular smooth muscle contraction. No arteriographic evidence exists to suggest that Nimodipine reduces cerebral vasospasm following SAH, however clinical studies have demonstrated a favorable effect of nimodipine on the severity of neurological deficits following aneurysmal SAH. [19]

Contraindications: Concomitant use with rifampin, phenytoin, phenobarbital, and carbamazepine (may induce hepatic metabolism and reduce effectiveness of nimodipine)

Precautions: Avoid inadvertent intravenous or parenteral administration, ensure administration via oral route.

Adverse effects: hypotension, abnormal liver function tests, nausea, headache

How supplied: 30mg liquid-filled gelatin capsules

Antihypertensive Agents

Thiazide Diuretics

	Usual daily dose	Usual frequency	How supplied
Chlorthalidone (Hygroton®)	12.5 – 25 mg	Once daily	Tablet 25mg, 50mg
Chlorothiazide (Diuril®)	Oral: 125 – 500 mg IV: 500mg	Once daily or divided bid	Tablet 250mg, 500mg IV Injection 500mg/vial
Hydrochlorothiazide (Hydrodiuril®)	12.5 – 50 mg	Once daily	Tablet 25mg, 50mg
Indapamide (Lozol®)	1.25 – 2.5 mg	Once daily	Tablet 1.25mg, 2.5mg
Metolazone (Zaroxolyn®)	2.5 – 10 mg	Once daily	Tablet 2.5mg, 5mg, 10mg

Mechanism of action: Inhibits the sodium-chloride symporter in the distal convoluted tubules of nephrons, leading to increased excretion of sodium and chloride and water.

Contraindications: Avoid in gout

Precautions: Minimally effective GFR < 30mL/min

Adverse effects: Fluid balance and electrolyte abnormalities, hypokalemia, hyperuricemia, hypochloremia, hypomagnesemia, hypercalcemia, metabolic alkalosis, extracellular volume depletion, hypotension

Loop Diuretics

	Usual daily dose	Usual frequency	How supplied
Furosemide (Lasix®)	20 – 80 mg	Divided bid to qid	Tablet 20mg, 40mg, 80mg Oral Solution 10mg/mL, 40mg/5mL IV Injection 10mg/mL
Torsemide (Demadex®)	2.5 – 10 mg	Once daily	Tablet 5mg, 10mg, 20mg, 100mg IV Injection 10mg/mL
Bumetanide (Bumex®)	0.5 – 2 mg	Once daily or divided bid	Tablet 0.5mg, 1mg, 2mg IV Injection 0.25mg/mL
Ethacrynic acid (Edecrin®)	Oral: 25-200mg	Once daily or divided bid	Tablet 25mg IV Injection 50mg/vial

Mechanism of action: Inhibits the reabsorption of sodium, potassium, and chloride in the thick ascending loop of Henle, leading to increased excretion of sodium, potassium, chloride and water.

Contraindications: Anuria, severe electrolyte depletion

Precautions: Use with caution in patients with sulfonamide allergy (except ethacrynic acid), systemic lupus erythematosus (may exacerbate), avoid concomitant use of aminoglycosides

Adverse effects: Electrolyte imbalances including hypokalemia, hypomagnesemia, hyponatremia, hypocalcemia, hypochloremic alkalosis, hyperuricemia, ototoxicity, metabolic alkalosis, muscle cramps, volume depletion, hypotension

Potassium-Sparing Diuretics

	Usual daily dose	Usual frequency	How supplied
Amiloride (Midamar®)	5 – 10 mg	Once daily or divided bid	Tablet 5mg
Triamterene (Dyrenium®)	50 – 100 mg	Once daily or divided bid	Capsule 50mg, 100mg

Mechanism of action: Block sodium channels in the late distal tubule and collecting duct leading to decreased potassium and hydrogen ion excretion. Provide only mild naturesis therefore normally used in combination with loop or thiazide diuretics to offset the kaluretic effects of the other diuretics.

Contraindications: Hyperkalemia

Precautions: Use with caution in patients with renal dysfunction, severe cirrhosis, renal stones, or patients receiving concomitant potassium supplements or potassium-containing medications, ACE inhibitors, aldosterone antagonists, or blood

Adverse effects: Hyperkalemia, metabolic acidosis, hypotension, dizziness, fatigue, rash, gynecomastia, nausea, vomiting, leg cramps.

Aldosterone Receptor Blockers

	Usual daily dose	Usual frequency	How supplied
Eplerenone (Inspra®)	50 – 100 mg	Once daily	Tablet 25mg, 50mg
Spironolactone (Aldactone®)	25 – 50 mg	Once daily	Tablet 25mg, 50mg, 100mg

Mechanism of action: Competitively antagonize aldosterone at mineralcorticoid receptors in the late distal tubule and collecting duct leading to increased sodium, chloride, and water excretion and decreased potassium and hydrogen ion excretion

Contraindications: Hyperkalemia, anuria

Precautions: Renal insufficiency, hepatic disease, hyponatremia, or patients receiving concomitant potassium supplements or potassium-containing medications, ACE inhibitors, other potassium-sparing diuretics or blood

Adverse effects: Hyperkalemia, dizziness, fatigue, rash, nausea, vomiting, gynecomastia

Combination Diuretics

	Usual frequency	How supplied
Hydrochlorothiazide + spironolactone (Aldactazide®)	Once daily	Tablet 25mg H/25mg S, 50mg H/50mg S

Hydrochlorothiazide + triamterene (Dyazide®, Maxzide®)	Once daily	Dyazide® Capsule 25mg H/37.5mg T Maxzide® Tablet 25mg H/37.5mg T, 50mg H/75mg T Capsule 25mg H/50mg T
Hydrochlorothiazide + amiloride (Moduretic®)	Once daily	Tablet 50mg H/5mg A

Beta-Blockers

	Usual daily dose	Usual frequency	How supplied
*Acebutolol (Sectral®)	200 – 800 mg	Divided bid	Capsule 200mg, 400mg
Atenolol (Tenormin®)	25 – 100 mg	Once daily	Tablet 25mg, 50mg, 100mg
Betaxolol (Kerlone®)	5 – 20 mg	Once daily	Tablet 10mg, 20mg
Bisoprolol fumarate (Zebeta®)	2.5 – 10 mg	Once daily	Tablet 5mg, 10mg
Metoprolol tartrate (Lopressor®)	50 – 100 mg	Divided bid	Tablet 25mg, 50mg, 100mg
Metoprolol succinate (Toprol-XL®)	25 – 100 mg	Once daily	Extended release tablet 25mg, 50mg, 100mg, 200mg
Nadolol (Corgard®)	40 – 120 mg	Once daily	Tablet 20mg, 40mg, 80mg
Nebivolol HCl (Bystolic®)	5 – 40 mg	Once daily	Tablet 2.5mg, 5mg, 10mg, 20mg
	Usual daily dose	Usual frequency	How supplied
*Penbutolol sulfate (Levatol®)	10 – 40 mg	Once daily	Tablet 20mg
*Pindolol (Visken®)	10 – 40 mg	Divided bid	Tablet 5mg, 10mg
Propranolol HCl (Inderal®)	40 – 160 mg	Divided bid	Tablet 10mg, 20mg, 40mg, 60mg, 80mg Oral solution 20mg/5mL, 40mg/5mL
Propranolol HCl (Inderal LA®)	60 – 180 mg	Once daily	Extended release capsule 60mg, 80mg, 120mg, 160mg
Timolol maleate (Blocadren®)	20 – 40 mg	Divided bid	Tablet 5mg, 10mg, 20mg

* partial β receptor agonists which possess intrinsic sympathomimetic activity.

Mechanism of action: Block adrenergic β_1 receptors in the myocardium leading to a reduction in cardiac output, may also block β_2 receptors in vascular smooth tissue leading to vasodilation, and inhibit the release of renin by juxtaglomerular apparatus in the kidney

Contraindications: Severe bradycardia, second or third degree heart block, cardiogenic shock, severe decompensated heart failure, sick sinus syndrome (in patients without a pacemaker)

Precautions: Bronchspastic disease, severe hepatic dysfunction, severe peripheral vascular disease, diabetes mellitus (may mask signs of hypoglycemia), hypotension, thyrotoxicosis (may mask sign of hyperthyroidism), avoid abrupt withdrawal

Adverse effects: Bradycardia, hypotension, rash, diarrhea, fatigue, dizziness, weakness, depression

Angiotensin Converting Enzyme Inhibitors (ACE –Inhibitors)

Mechanism of action: Reduce the formation of angiotensin II from angiotensin I by inhibiting angiotensin converting enzyme, also inhibit the inactivation of bradykinin thereby stimulating the synthesis of nitric oxide resulting in vascular smooth muscle relaxation and increased fibrinolysis

Contraindications: Bilateral renal artery stenosis, previous ACE inhibitor associated angioedema, pregnancy

Precautions: Use with caution in patients with aortic stenosis, hypovolemia, impaired/worsening renal function, avoid in women who are likely to become pregnant

Adverse effects: Dry cough, Hyperkalemia, taste disturbance, rash, dizziness, increased liver function tests, deterioration of renal function, neutropenia/agranulocytosis, angioedema

	Usual daily dose	Usual frequency	How supplied
Benazepril HCl (Lotensin®)	10 – 40 mg	Once daily	Tablet 5mg, 10mg, 20mg, 40mg
Captopril (Capoten®)	25 – 100 mg	Divided bid to tid	Tablet 12.5mg, 25mg, 50mg, 100mg
Enalapril maleate (Vasotec®)	5 – 40 mg	Once daily or divided bid	Tablet 2.5mg, 5mg, 10mg, 20mg

	Usual daily dose	Usual frequency	How supplied
Fosinopril sodium (Monopril®)	10 – 40 mg	Once daily	Tablet 10mg, 20mg, 40mg
Lisinopril (Zestril®, Prinivel®)	5 – 40 mg	Once daily	Tablet 2.5mg, 5mg, 10mg, 20mg, 30mg, 40mg
Moexipril HCl (Univasc®)	7.5 – 30 mg	Once daily	Tablet 7.5mg, 15mg
Perindopril erbumin (Aceon®)	4 -8 mg	Once daily	Tablet 2mg, 4mg, 8mg
Quinapril HCl (Accupril®)	10 – 80 mg	Once daily	Tablet 5mg, 10mg, 20mg, 40mg
Ramipril (Altace®)	2.5 – 20 mg	Once daily	Tablet 1.25mg, 2.5mg, 5mg, 10mg Capsule 1.25mg, 2.5mg, 5mg, 10mg
Trandolapril (Mavik®)	1 – 4 mg	Once daily	Tablet 1mg, 2mg, 4mg

Angiotensin II Receptor Blockers (ARBs)

	Usual daily dose	Usual frequency	How supplied
Candesartan cilexetil (Atacand®)	8 – 32 mg	Once daily	Tablet 4mg, 8mg, 16mg, 32mg
Eprosartan mesylate (Teveten®)	400 – 800 mg	Once daily or divided bid	Tablet 400mg, 600mg
Irbesartan (Avapro®)	150 – 300 mg	Once daily	Tablet 75mg, 150mg, 300mg
Losartan potassium (Cozaar®)	25 – 100 mg	Once daily or divided bid	Tablet 25mg, 50mg, 100mg
Olmesartan medoxomil (Benicar®)	5 – 40 mg	Once daily	Tablet 5mg, 20mg, 40mg
Telmisartan (Micardis®)	20 – 80 mg	Once daily	Tablet 20mg, 40mg, 80mg
Valsartan (Diovan®)	80 – 320 mg	Once daily or divided bid	Tablet 40mg, 80mg, 160mg, 320mg

Mechanism of action: Specifically antagonize the binding of angiotensin II to angiotensin receptors (AT_1-R) resulting in relaxation of vascular smooth muscle

Contraindications: Bilateral renal artery stenosis, pregnancy

Precautions: Use with caution in patients with hypovolemia, impaired/worsening renal function, hepatic dysfunction, avoid in women who are likely to become pregnant

Adverse effects: Hyperkalemia, headache, dizziness, hypotension, deterioration of renal function, rash

Dihydropyridine Calcium Channel Blockers

Mechanism of action: Block voltage-gated calcium channels causing a decrease in calcium influx leading to smooth muscle relaxation, peripheral arterial vasodilation, and a decrease in peripheral vascular resistance

Contraindications: Clinically significant aortic stenosis, cardiogenic shock, acute myocardial infarction, unstable angina

Precautions: Hepatic dysfunction

Adverse effects: Flushing, headache, peripheral edema, tachycardia, hypotension, dizziness, rash, gingival hyperplasia

	Usual daily dose	Usual frequency	How supplied
Amlodipine besylate (Norvasc®)	2.5 – 10 mg	Once daily	Tablet 2.5mg, 5mg, 10mg
Felodipine (Plendil®)	2.5 – 20 mg	Once daily	Extended release tablet 2.5mg, 5mg, 10mg
Isradipine (DynaCirc®, DynaCirc CR®)	2.5 – 10 mg	Divided bid	Capsule 2.5mg, 5mg Extended release capsule 5mg, 10mg
Nicardipine HCl (Cardene®, Cardene SR®)	60 – 120 mg	Divided bid	Capsule 20mg, 30mg Extended release capsule 30mg, 45mg, 60mg
Nifedipine (Adalat CC®, Procardia XL®)	30 – 90 mg	Once daily	Extended release tablet 30mg, 60mg, 90mg

Non-Dihydropyridine Calcium Channel Blockers

Mechanism of action: Inhibit the influx of calcium across the cell membrane of arterial smooth muscle and in conducible and contractile myocardial cells

Contraindications: Severe LV dysfunction, hypotension, sick sinus syndrome and/or 2nd or 3rd AV block (except in patients with pacemaker), atrial fibrillation or flutter with an accessory bypass tract

Precautions: Hepatic dysfunction

Adverse effects: Peripheral edema, dizziness, headache

	Usual daily dose	Usual frequency	How supplied
Diltiazem HCl Immediate Release	90 – 420 mg	Divided tid or qid	Tablet 30mg, 60mg, 90mg, 120mg
Diltiazem HCl Sustained Release (Cardizem SR®)	120 – 420 mg	Divided bid	Sustained release capsule 60mg, 90mg, 120mg, 180mg
Diltiazem HCl Extended Release (Cardizem CD®, Dilacor XR®, Tiazac®, Cartia XT®)	180 – 420 mg	Once daily	Extended release capsule 120mg, 180mg, 240mg, 300mg, 360mg
Diltiazem HCl Extended Release Tablet (Cardizem LA)	120 – 540 mg	Once daily	Extended release tablet 120mg, 180mg, 240mg, 300mg, 360mg, 420mg
Verapamil HCl (Calan®, Isoptin®)	80 – 320 mg	Divided tid or qid	Tablet 40mg, 80mg, 120mg, 160mg
Verapamil HCl Long Acting (Isoptin SR®)	120 – 480 mg	Once daily or divided bid	Extended release tablet 120mg, 180mg, 240mg
Verapamil HCl Sustained Release Capsules (Verelan®)	120 – 360 mg	Once daily	Sustained release pellet filled capsule 120mg, 180mg, 240mg, 360mg
Verapamil HCl Extended Release Capsules (Verelan PM®)	100 – 400 mg	Once daily at bedtime	Extended release capsule 100mg, 200mg, 300mg
Verapamil HCl (Covera HS®)	120 – 360 mg	Once daily at bedtime	Extended release tablet 180mg, 240mg

Alpha-Blockers

Mechanism of action: Selectively inhibits alpha-1 adrenergic receptors causing a reduction in systemic vascular resistance

Precautions: High incidence first dose postural dizziness, use with caution in patients with hepatic dysfunction

Side Effects: Syncope, postural dizziness/orthostatic hypotension, vertigo, fatigue, peripheral edema, dyspnea, leukopenia

	Usual daily dose	Usual frequency	How supplied
Doxazosin mesylate (Cardura®, Cardura XL®)	1 – 16 mg	Once daily	Tablet 1mg, 2mg, 4mg, 8mg Extended release tablet 4mg, 8mg
Prazosin HCl (Minipress®)	2 – 20 mg	Divided bid or tid	Tablet 1mg, 2mg, 5mg
Terazosin HCl (Hytrin®)	1 – 20 mg	Once daily or divided bid	Tablet 1mg, 2mg, 5mg, 10mg Capsule 1mg, 2mg, 5mg, 10mg

Combined Alpha and Beta-Blockers

	Usual daily dose	Usual frequency	How supplied
Carvedilol (Coreg®)	6.25 – 100 mg	Divided bid	Tablet 3.125mg, 6.25mg, 12.5mg, 25mg
Carvedilol phosphate (Coreg CR®)	10 – 80 mg	Once daily	Extended release capsule 10mg, 20mg, 40mg, 80mg
Labetolol HCl (Normodyne®, Trandate®)	200 – 800 mg	Divided bid	Tablet 100mg, 200mg, 300mg

Mechanism of action: Adrenergic receptor blockers with both selective α-$_1$ and nonselective β blocking actions

Contraindications: Severe bradycardia, second or third degree heart block, cardiogenic shock, severe decompensated heart failure, sick sinus syndrome (in patients without a pacemaker)

Precautions: Bronchspastic disease, severe hepatic dysfunction, severe peripheral vascular disease, diabetes mellitus (may mask signs of hypoglycemia), hypotension, thyrotoxicosis (may mask sign of hyperthyroidism), avoid abrupt withdrawal

Side Effects: Bradycardia, hypotension, dizziness, nausea, elevated liver function tests

Central Agonists

	Usual daily dose	Usual frequency	How supplied
Methyldopa (Aldomet®)	250 – 1000 mg	Divided bid	Tablet 250mg, 500mg

Mechanism of action: Stimulates central inhibitory α adrenergic receptors by a false neurotransmitter which reduces sympathetic outflow from the central nervous system to the heart, kidneys, and peripheral vasculature

Contraindications: Active hepatic disease

Precautions: History of hepatic dysfunction

Adverse effects: Dry mouth, drowsiness, dizziness, constipation, sedation, headache, weakness, edema, bradycardia, bone marrow suppression, parkinsonism, positive coombs test, hemolytic anemia, hepatic dysfunction

	Usual daily dose	Usual frequency	How supplied
Clonidine HCl (Catapres®)	0.1 – 0.8 mg	Divided bid	Tablet 0.1mg, 0.2mg, 0.3mg
Clonidine Extended Release Oral Suspension	0.17 mg (2mL) – 0.52 mg (6mL) Note: 0.17mg (2mL) ER suspension daily is equivalent to 0.1mg BID of clonidine HCl immediate release tablets	Once daily	ER oral suspension 0.09mg/mL
Clonidine Extended Release Tablets	0.17 – 0.52 mg Note: 0.17mg ER tablet daily is equivalent to 0.1mg BID of clonidine HCl immediate release tablets	Once daily	ER Tablet 0.17mg, 0.26mg
Clonidine HCl transdermal (Catapres-TTS®)	0.1 – 0.3 mg	Once weekly	Transdermal patch 0.1mg/24hr, 0.2mg/24hr, 0.3mg/24hr
Guanfacine HCl (Tenex®)	0.5 – 2 mg	Once daily	Tablet 1mg, 2mg

Mechanism of action: Centrally acting α agonist which reduces sympathetic outflow from the central nervous system leading to decreased peripheral vascular resistance, renal vascular resistance, heart rate, and blood pressure

Precautions: Avoid abrupt withdrawal

Adverse effects: Bradycardia, dry mouth, drowsiness, dizziness, constipation, and sedation

	Usual daily dose	Usual frequency	How supplied
Reserpine (Serpasil®)	0.1 -0.25 mg	Once daily	Tablet 0.1mg, 0.25mg

Mechanism of action: Depletes stores of catecholamines and 5-hydroxytryptamine in many organs, including the brain and adrenal medulla causing decreased sympathetic nerve function resulting in decreased heart rate and a lowering of arterial blood pressure

Contraindications: Depression/suicidal tendencies

Precautions: Use with caution is patients with active peptic ulcer, ulcerative colitis, or gallstones

Side Effects: Bradycardia, hypotension, peripheral edema, dizziness, headache, drowsiness, fatigue, mental depression, parkinsonism, syncope, rash, increased gastric acid secretion, blurred vision, thrombocytonpenia

Direct Vasodilators

	Usual daily dose	Usual frequency	How supplied
Hydralazine HCl (Apresoline®)	25 – 100 mg	Divided bid or tid	Tablet 10mg, 25mg, 50mg, 100mg

Mechanism of action: Causes relaxation of arteriolar vascular smooth muscle, peripheral vasodilation and decreased systemic vascular resistance

Precautions: Coronary artery disease, mitral valve rheumatic heart disease

Adverse effects: Headache, nausea, vomiting, tachycardia, angina, antipyridoxine effect (peripheral paresthesia, numbness, tingling). Rare: reduction in hemoglobin and red blood cell count, leucopenia, agranulocytosis, rash, eosinophilia, hepatitis

	Usual daily dose	Usual frequency	How supplied
Minoxidil (Loniten®)	2.5 – 80 mg	Once daily or divided bid	Tablet 2.5mg, 10mg

Mechanism of action: Direct acting peripheral vasodilator which reduces systolic and diastolic blood pressure by decreasing systemic vascular resistance in all systemic vascular beds.

Contraindications: pheochromocytoma

Adverse effects: Edema. Rare adverse effects: rash, thrombocytopenia, pericarditis, pericardial effusion, and cardiac tamponade

Cholesterol Lowering Drugs

Statins	Usual daily dose	Usual frequency	How supplied
Atorvastatin (Lipitor®)	10 – 80 mg	Daily	Tablet 10mg, 20mg, 40mg, 80mg
Fluvastatin (Lescol®)	20 – 80 mg	Daily or divided bid	Capsule 20 mg, 40mg
Fluvastatin (Lescol XL®)	80 mg	Daily	XL tablet 80mg
Lovastatin (Mevacor®)	10 – 80 mg	Daily or divided bid	Tablet 10mg, 20mg, 40mg
Lovastatin XL (Altoprev®)	20 – 60 mg	Daily	XL tablet 20mg, 40mg, 60mg
Pravastatin (Pravachol®)	10 – 80 mg	Daily	Tablet 10mg, 20mg, 40mg, 80mg

Statins	Usual daily dose	Usual frequency	How supplied
Pitavastatin (Livalo®)	1 – 4 mg	Daily	Tablet 1mg, 2mg, 4mg
Rosuvastatin (Crestor®)	5 – 40 mg	Daily	Tablet 5mg, 10mg, 20mg. 40mg
Simvastatin (Zocor®)	5 – 80 mg	Daily	Tablet 5mg, 10mg, 20mg, 40mg, 80mg Orally disintegrating tablet 10mg, 20mg, 40mg, 80mg

Combination medications: Advicor® (lovastatin + niacin), Caduet® (atorvastatin + amlodipine), Simcor® (simvastatin + niacin) Vytorin® (simvastatin + ezetimibe)

Mechanism of action: Decreases cholesterol production by competitively inhibiting HMG-CoA reductase, the rate-limiting enzyme that converts 3-hydoxy-3-methylglutaryl-coenzyme A to mevalonate, a precursor of sterols, including cholesterol.

Precautions: Check for drug interactions, especially CYP3A4 inhibitors or other drugs that are metabolized by CYP3A4 (except for pravastatin)

Contraindications: Pregnant or nursing mothers, active hepatic disease, unexplained persistently elevated liver function tests

Adverse effects: Dyspepsia, abdominal pain, constipation, flatulence, elevated LFTs, myalgia, rhabdomyolsis, acute renal failure

Resins (bile acid sequestrants)	Usual daily dose	Usual frequency	How supplied
Cholestyramine (Questran®, Questran® Light, Prevalite®, Locholest®, Locholest® Light)	1 -4 packets or scoopfuls	Daily or divided bid preferably at mealtimes (may be divided up to 6 times daily if necessary)	Powder for oral suspension 4gm packets/scoopful
Colestipol (Colestid®)	2 – 16 grams	Daily or divided bid	Tablet 1gm Granules for oral suspension 5gm packets/scoopful
Colesevelam (WelChol®)	6 tablets (3.75 grams)	Daily or divided bid	Tablet 625mg Packet for oral suspension 1.875gram, 3.75gram

Mechanism of action: Absorb and combine with bile acids in the intestine to form an insoluble complex which is excreted in the feces. Loss of bile acid leads to an increased oxidation of cholesterol to bile acids, a decrease in LDL plasma levels and a decrease in serum cholesterol levels.

Contraindications: Complete biliary obstruction

Precautions: Check for drug interactions concomitant use may decrease absorption of other medications

Adverse effects: Constipation, abdominal discomfort, flatulence, nausea, vomiting, vitamin deficiencies (A, D, K), osteoporosis, rash, intestinal obstruction

Fibrates	Usual dose range	Usual frequency	How supplied
Gemfibrozil (Lopid®)	1200 mg	Divided bid (30 minutes before meals)	Tablet 600mg

Fibrates	Usual dose range	Usual frequency	How supplied
Fenofibrate	Tablets: 54 – 160mg Capsules: 67 – 200mg	Daily Daily	Tablc 54mg, 107mg, 160mg Capsule micronized 67mg, 134mg, 200mg
Fenofibrate (Antara®)	43 – 130 mg	Daily	Capsule micronized 43mg, 87mg, 130mg
Fenofibrate (Fenoglide®)	40 – 120 mg	Daily	Tablet 40mg, 120mg
Fenofibrate (Lipofen ®)	50 – 150 mg	Daily	Capsule 50mg, 100mg, 150mg
Fenofibrate (Tricor®)	48 – 145 mg	Daily	Tablet 48mg, 145mg
Fenofibrate (Triglide®)	50 – 160 mg	Daily	Tablet 50mg, 160mg
Fenofibrate (Trilipix®)	45 – 135 mg	Daily	Delayed-release capsule 45mg, 135mg

Mechanism of action: Inhibits peripheral lipolysis and decreases the hepatic extraction of free fatty acids thereby reducing hepatic triglyceride production. Inhibits the synthesis and increases the clearance of the VLDL carrier, apolipoprotein B, leading to decreased VLDL production.

Contraindications: Hepatic dysfunction, severe renal dysfunction, biliary cirrhosis, gallbladder disease

Precautions: Increased risk of rhabodomyolysis when given in combination with statins; check for drug interactions (especially with anticoagulants)

Adverse effects: Dyspepsia, abdominal pain, appendicitis, cholelithiasis, gallstones, myopathy, rhabdomyolysis, increased liver function tests.

Ezetimibe (Zetia®)

Mechanism of action: Inhibits sterol transport, which decreases the absorption of cholesterol from the small intestine, leading to a decrease in the delivery of intestinal cholesterol to the liver, thereby reducing hepatic cholesterol stores and increasing cholesterol clearance from blood

Usual dose: 10mg daily

Contraindications: Severe hepatic disease, unexplained elevated liver function tests, pregnant or nursing mothers

Precautions: Check for drug interactions (especially with anticoagulants)

Adverse effects: Arthralgia, dizziness, diarrhea, increased liver function tests, myalgia, rash, urticaria, anaphylaxis, angioedema

How supplied: Tablets 10mg.

ICU Opioid Analgesics and ICU Sedation - See Attached Charts

Vasopressors and Inotropes – See Chart

Niacin (Niaspan®)

Mechanism of action: Reduces total cholesterol, triglycerides, LDL and increases HDL. May cause partial inhibition of free fatty acid release from adipose tissue and increased lipoprotein lipase activating leading to increased rates of chylomicron triglyceride removal from plasma. Decreases the rate of hepatic synthesis of VLDL and LDL.

Usual dose: 500 – 200mg nightly (at bedtime), may pre-treat with aspirin 325mg 30 minutes prior to Niaspan dose to decrease flushing reaction

Contraindications: Acute hepatic dysfunction,

Precautions: History of liver disease

Adverse effects: Flushing, rash, diarrhea, nausea, vomiting; rare adverse effects: severe hepatic toxicity, rhabdomyolysis (risk increased with concomitant administration of HGM CoA reductase inhibitors)

How supplied: Tablet 500mg, Extended-release tablet 500mg, 750mg, 1000mg

	Usual Dose	Receptor Subtype					Select clinical effects
		α_1	β_1	β_2	DA	Other	
Dopamine	1-3 mcg/kg/min	+/-	++	+/-	++++		Possible renal, coronary, mesenteric, and cerebral arterial vasodilation and natriuetic response
	3-10 mcg/kg/min	++	+++	+	++		Can induce tachyarrhythmias, theoretical effets on renal blood flow may be lost at higher doses due to predominant α1 effects
	10-20 mcg/kg/min	+++	+++	0	+		
Norepinephrine (Levophed®)	0.5 – 30 mcg/min	++++	+++	0	0		Increases SVR, at high doses can decrease renal perfusion, and/or induce tachyarrhythmias
Phenylephrine (Neosynephrine®)	100 -200 mcg/min intitially, then titrate down to 40-60 mcg/min Max: 300 mcg/min	++++	0	0	0		Selective α1 agonist, increases SVR, can cause reflex bradycardia
Epinephrine	1 – 10 mcg/min	+++	+++	++	0		Positive inotropic and chronotropic effects can induce myocardial ischemia at higher doses.
Vasopressin (Pitressin®)	0.01 – 0.04 units/min	0	0	0	0	V_1 – vascular V_2 – renal V_3 – pituitary	Direct stimulation of V1 receptors causes increase in SVR, no adrenergic activity. Doses > 0.04 units/min can be associated with mesenteric and myocardial ischemia
Dobutamine	2 – 20 mcg/kg/min	+	+++	+	0		Positive inotrope, increases cardiac output, can cause tachyarrhythmias,
Milrinone (Primacor®)	50 mcg/kg bolus over 10 min, then 0.375 – 0.75 mcg/kg/min	0	0	0	0	Phosphodiesterase inhibitor	Positive inotrope, phosphodiesterase inhibition leads to increase in cAMP resulting in increased myocardial contractility along with venous and arterial dilation (decreases preload and SVR), renally eliminated – effects are prolonged in renal dysfunction.

0= no effect, ++++ = maximal effect, SVR = systemic vascular resistance, cAMP = cyclic adenosine monophosphate, DA = dopamine receptor.

ICU Opioid Analgesics (References [20, 21, 22])

Opioid Analgesic	Comparative IV Dose	Usual ICU dose	Onset of Action	Half-life	Duration	Metabolism/ Elimination	Notes:
Morphine	10mg	Intermittent: 1-4 mg IVP q1-2 h Continuous infusion: 1-30 mg/h	5-10 min	3-7 h	2-4 h	Glucuronidation, Morphine-6-glucuronide, active metabolite which accumulates in renal dysfunction.	- Associated with the most histamine release leading to hypotension, flushing, bronchoaspasm, urticaria, and puritus.
Fentanyl	100 – 200 mcg	Intermittent: 0.35-1.5 mcg/kg IVP q 0.5-1 h Continuous infusion: 0.7 – 10 mcg/kg/	Immediate	1.5-6 h	2-4 h (prolonged with liver failure)	Hepatic CYP3A4 substrate No active metabolites, parent compound can accumulate	- May accumulate in patients with renal dysfunction - May cause muscle rigidity at high doses - Can be safely used in patients with a suspected allergy to morphine
Hydromorphone	1.5mg	Intermittent: 10-30 mcg/kg IVP q1-2 h Continuous infusion: 7 – 15 mcg/kg/h	5-10 min	2-3 h	2-4 h	Glucuronidation	- Opioid of choice for patients with ESRD
Meperidine	75 - 100mg	Not recommend for analgesia For shivering or rigors: 12.5 – 50 mg IVP q4 -6 h	5 min	3-4 h	2-3 h	Demethylation and hydroxylation Active metabolite: normeperidine accumulates with renal dysfunction	- Normeperidine is neurotoxic - Avoid use with MAOIs and SSRIs
Remifentanil		Loading dose 1 mcg/kg IVP over 1 min Continuous infusion: 0.6 – 15 mcg/kg/h	1-3 min	3-10 min	10-20 min	Tissue esterases	- No accumulation in hepatic or renal dysfunction - May cause hypotension, bradycardia

ESRD = end stage renal disease, MAOI = monoamine oxidase inhibitor, SSRI = selective serotonin-reuptake inhibitor.

Shared adverse effects: respiratory depression, nausea, vomiting, agitation, hallucinations, constipation, illeus, urinary retention.

Reversal agent: Naloxone 0.4 mg IVP (For opioid dependent patients dilute 1:10 and give 40 – 80 mcg IVP repeated as necessary).

Withdrawal symptoms: agitation, hypertension, tachypnea, and sweating.

Benzodiazepine Sedatives	Usual ICU Dosing	Onset of Action (minutes)	Half-life (hours)	Duration	Metabolism/ Elimination	Notes	Shared Adverse Effects
Midazolam (Versed®)	Intermittent: 2-5 mg IVP q 1-2 h Continuous infusion: 1-20 mg/h Status epilepticus:	2 – 5	3 – 12	1-4 h (longer in CHF, liver failure, ESRD, or obesity)	- Hepatic hydroxylation to active 1-hypoxymidazolam glucuronide (CYP3A4/5) - Active metabolite excreted renally	- Water soluble in solution, becomes highly lipid soluble after injection (at blood pH) - Potential for many drug interactions (CYP3A4) - Duration of action can be significantly prolonged with continuous infusion, especially in obese patients	- respiratory depression, continuous infusion generally requires mechanical ventilation - Paradoxical agitation - delirium - Withdrawal symptoms and seizures with acute discontinuation Reversal agent: Flumazenil 0.2 mg IVP q1 min up to a total of 1mg.
Lorazepam (Ativan®)	Intermittent: 2-6 mg IVP q4-6 h Continuous infusion: 1-10 mg/h	5 – 20	10 – 20	6-8 h (longer in ESRD, liver dysfunction, or elderly)	Hepatic glucuronidation to inactive metabolites	- If using continuous infusion > 1 mg/kg/day monitor osmol gap for potential propylene glycol toxicty	

ICU Sedation (Continued)

Other Sedatives	Usual ICUDosing	Onset of Action (minutes)	Half-life (hours)	Duration	Metabolism/ Elimination	Notes
Propofol (Diprivan®)	5-150 mcg/kg/min	1 – 2	1.5 – 12	3-10 mins (dose dependent)	Hepatic hydroxylation and glucuronidation (CYP2B6)	- Short-acting hypnotic, $GABA_A$ agonist - Lipid emulsion, delivers 1.1 kcal/mL - Reduces ICP after TBI - Decreases CBF and metabolism Adverse effects: - Respiratory depression - Hypotension (peripheral vasodilation) - Hypertriglyceridemia - Pancreatitis - Monitor for propofol infusion syndrome, PRIS (metabolic acidosis, rhabdomyolysis, acute renal failure, bradyarrhythmias, hyperkalemia, hypotension, rapid progressive heart failure)
Dexmedetomidine (Precedex®)	Loading dose (optional): 0.5-1 mcg/kg over 10 mins Continuous infusion: 0.2-0.7 mcg/kg/hr (doses up to 1.5 mcg/kg/hr have been tolerated in recent trials)	< 1 min	2	6 mins (prolonged with liver dysfunction)	Hepatic CYP450 and glucuronidation	-Selective central α_2-adrenergic receptor agonist - Does not decrease respiratory drive - Has some analgesic activity - May cause hypotension, bradycardia

References

[1]   Cottrel JE, Patel K, Turndorf H, et al. *ICP changes induced by sodium nitroprusside in patients with intracranial mass lesions.* J Neurosurg 1978;48:329-31.

[2]   Varon J and Marik PE. *The diagnosis and management of hypertensive crises.* Chest 2000;118:214-227.

[3]   Sherman DG, Albers GW, Bladin C, Feischi C, Gabbai AA, KAse CS, O'Riordan W, Pineo GF; PREVAIL investigators. *The efficacy and safety of enoxaparin versus unfractionated heparin for the prevention of venous thromboembolism after acute ischaemic stroke (PREVAIL Study): an open-label randomized comparison.* Lancet 2007 Apr 21;369(9570):1347-55.

[4]   Raslan AM, Fields JD, and Bhardwaj A. *Prophylaxis for Venous Thrombo-embolism in Neurocritical Care: A Critical Appraisal.* Neurocrit Care 2010;12:297-309.

[5]   Geerts AH, Bergqvist D, Pineo GF, Heit JA, Samama CM, Lassen MR, and Colwell CW. *Prevention of Venous Thromboembolism: American College of Chest Physicians Evidence-Based Clinical Practice Guidelines (8th Edition).* Chest 2008;133:381-453.

[6]   Spinal Cord Injury Thromboprophylaxis Investigators. *Prevention of venous thromboembolism in the acute treatment phase after spinal cord injury: a randomized, multicenter trial comparing low-dose heparin plus intermittent pneumatic compression with enoxaparin.* J Trauma 2003;54:1116-26.

[7]   Morgenstern LB, Hemphill JC 3rd, Anderson C, Becker K, Broderick JP, et. al. *Guidelines for the Management of Spontaneous Intracerebral Hemorrhage. A Guideline for Healthcare Professionals from the American Heart Association/American Stroke Association.* Stroke 2010;41. (E-published ahead of print)

[8]   Ansell J, Hirsh J, Hylek E, Jacobson A, Crowther M, and Palareti G. *Pharmacology and Management of the Vitamin K Antagonists: American College of Chest Physicians Evidence-Based Clinical Practice Guidelines (8th Edition).* Chest 2008;133:160-198.

[9]   Starke RM, Kim GH, Fernandez A, Komotar RJ, Hickman ZL, et al. *Impact of a protocol for acute antifibrinolytic therapy on aneurysm rebleeding after subarachnoid hemorrhage.* Stroke. 2008;39:2617-21.

[10] Hirsh J, Bauer KA, Donati MB, Gould M, Samama MM, and Weitz JI. *Parental Anticoagulants: American College of Chest Physicians Evidence-Based Clinical Practice Guidelines (8th Edition)*. Chest 2008;133:141-59.

[11] *Guidelines for the Management of Severe Traumatic Brain Injury (3rd Edition)*. Journal of Neurotraum 2007;24(Suppl.1):S1-106.

[12] Forsyth LL, Liu-Deryke X, Parker D, and Rhoney DH. *Role of Hypertonic Saline for the Management of Intracranial Hypertension After Stroke and Traumatic Brain Injury*. Pharmacotherapy 2008;28(4):469-84.

[13] Hartl R, Medary MB, Ruge M, Arfors KE, Ghahremani F, Ghajar J. *Hypertonic/hyperoncotic saline attenuates microcirculatory disturbances after traumatic brain injury*. J Trauma 1997;42(suppl):S41-7.

[14] Osorio I, Reed RC. *Treatment of refractory generalized tonic-clonic status epilepticus with pentobarbital anesthesia after high-dose phenytoin*. Epilepsia 1989;30:464-71.

[15] Eisenberg HM, Frankowski RF, *Contant CF et al. High-dose barbiturate control of elevated intracranial pressure in patients with severe head injury*. J Neurosurg 1988;69:15-23.

[16] Lowenstein DH and Alldredge BK. *Status epilepticus*. NEJM 1998;338(4):970-6.

[17] Lee MW, Deppe SA, Sipperly ME, Barrette RR, and Thompson DR. *The efficacy of barbiturate coma in the management of uncontrolled intracranial hypertension following neurosurgical trauma*. J Neurotraum 1994;11(3):325-31.

[18] Towne AR, Garnett LK, Waterhouse EJ, Morton LD, and DeLorenzo RJ. *The use of topiramate in refractory status epilepticus*. Neurology 2003;60:332-334.

[19] Pickard JD, Murray GD, Illingworth R, Shaw MD, Teasdale GM, et al. *Effect of oral Nimodipine on cerebral infarction and outcome after subarachnoid haemorrhage: British aneurysm nimodipine trial*. Br Med J 1989;298:636-42.

[20] Devlin JW and Roberts RJ. *Pharmacology of commonly used analgesics and sedatives in the ICU: benzodiazepines, propofol, and opioids*. Crit Care Clin. 2009 Jul;25(3):431-49.

[21] Jacobi J, Fraser GL, Coursin DB, et al. *Clinical practice guidelines for the sustained use of sedatives and analgesics in the critically ill adult*. Crit Care Med 2002;30(1):119-41.

[22] Sessler CN, Varney K. *Patient-focused sedation and analgesia in the ICU.* Chest 2008;133(2):552-65.

[23] Riker RR, Shehabi Y, Bokesch PM, et al. *Dexmedetomidine vs. midazolam for sedation of critically ill patients: a randomized trial.* JAMA. 2009;301(5):489-499.

[24] Pratik P. Pandharipande; Brenda T. Pun; Daniel L. Herr; et. Al. *Effect of Sedation With Dexmedetomidine vs. Lorazepam on Acute Brain Dysfunction in Mechanically Ventilated Patients: The MENDS Randomized Controlled Trial.* JAMA. 2007;298(22):2644-2653.

Index

D

E

F

J

K

L

M

N

O

Q

R

S

T

X

W

Y

Z